New Choices in
NATURAL
HEALING
for Women

Drug-Free Remedies from
the World of Alternative Medicine

By Barbara Loecher, Sara Altshul O'Donnell

and the Editors of **PREVENTION** Magazine Health Books
Edited by Sharon Faelten

Adriane Fugh-Berman, M.D., Medical Adviser

D1473852

Rodale Press, Inc.
Emmaus, Pennsylvania

Library of Congress Cataloging-in-Publication Data

Loecher, Barbara.
New choices in natural healing for women : drug-free remedies from the world of alternative medicine / by Barbara Loecher, Sara Altshul O'Donnell and the editors of Prevention Health Books ; edited by Sharon Faelten.
    p.   cm.
Includes index.
ISBN 0–87596–387–0 hardcover
1. Women—Health and hygiene. 2. Alternative medicine. 3. Self-care, Health. I. O'Donnell, Sara Altshul. II. Faelten, Sharon. III. Prevention Health Books. IV. Title.
RA778.028   1997
615.5'082—DC21   97–2481
     ISBN 1–57954–129–1 paperback

Distributed to the book trade by St. Martin's Press

2 4 6 8 10 9 7 5 3   hardcover
2 4 6 8 10 9 7 5 3 1 paperback

Visit us on the Web at www.preventionbookshelf.com, or call us toll-free at (800) 848-4735.

───── OUR PURPOSE ─────

We inspire and enable people to improve their lives and the world around them.

Notice

This book is intended as a reference volume only, not as a medical manual. The information given here is designed to help you make informed decisions about your health. It is not intended as a substitute for any treatment that may have been prescribed by your doctor. If you suspect that you have a medical problem, we urge you to seek competent medical help.

Safety limits have been noted for potentially harmful nutrients. However, you should not go on any vitamin or nutritional therapy program without first consulting your doctor.

While the use of general descriptive names, trade names or trademarks in a publication, even if not specifically identified, does not imply that these names are not protected by the relevant laws and regulations, we wish to acknowledge the following trademarked names that appear within this book.

Jin Shin Do, Feldenkrais, Feldenkrais Method, The Feldenkrais Guild, Functional Integration, Awareness Through Movement, Trager, Rolfing, Mentastics, Therapeutic Touch, Reiki, Accommotrac

New Choices in Natural Healing for Women
Editorial Staff

Managing Editor: **Sharon Faelten**
Staff Writers: **Barbara Loecher, Sara Altshul O'Donnell**
Contributing Writer: **Caroline Saucer**
Assistant Research Manager: **Anita C. Small**
Book Project Researcher: **Sandra Salera-Lloyd**
Editorial Researchers: **Susan E. Burdick, Kelly Elizabeth Coffey, Raymond DiCecco, Carol J. Gilmore, Toby Hanlon, Sarah Wolfgang Heffner, Nicole A. Kelly, Terry Sutton Kravitz, Betsy Lyman, Paris Mihely-Muchanic, Jennifer Pierce, Staci Ann Sander, Jennifer Schaeffer, Therese Walsh, Shea Zukowski**
Cover Designer: **Debra Sfetsios**
Cover Photographer: **Masao Ota**
Book Designer: **Kristen Morgan Downey**
Layout Designer: **Kathleen J. Cole**
Illustrators: **Lydia Hess, Karen Kuchar**
Senior Copy Editor: **Kathy D. Everleth**
Copy Editor: **Linda Mooney**
Manufacturing Coordinator: **Melinda B. Rizzo**
Office Manager: **Roberta Mulliner**
Office Staff: **Julie Kehs, Mary Lou Stephen**

Rodale Health and Fitness Books

Vice-President and Editorial Director: **Debora T. Yost**
Executive Editor: **Neil Wertheimer**
Design and Production Director: **Michael Ward**
Research Manager: **Ann Gossy Yermish**
Copy Manager: **Lisa D. Andruscavage**
Studio Manager: **Stefano Carbini**
Book Manufacturing Director: **Helen Clogston**

Board of Advisers

Adriane Fugh-Berman, M.D.
Former head of field investigations for the Office of Alternative Medicine at the
National Institutes of Health in Bethesda, Maryland

Clarita E. Herrera, M.D.
Clinical instructor in primary care at the New York Medical College in Valhalla,
New York, and associate attending physician at Lenox Hill Hospital in New
York City

Debra Ruth Judelson, M.D.
Senior partner with the Cardiovascular Medical Group of Southern California
in Beverly Hills and Fellow of the American College of Cardiology and
president of the American Medical Women's Association

JoAnn E. Manson, M.D.
Associate professor of medicine at Harvard Medical School and co-director of
women's health at Brigham and Women's Hospital in Boston

Mary Lake Polan, M.D., Ph.D.
Professor and chairman of the Department of Gynecology and Obstetrics at
Stanford University School of Medicine in California

Lila A. Wallis, M.D.
Clinical professor of medicine at Cornell University Medical College in New
York City and director of "Update Your Medicine," a series of continuing
medical educational programs for physicians at Cornell University Medical College in New York City

Carla Wolper, R.D.
Registered dietician and clinical coordinator of the Obesity Research Center at
St. Luke's-Roosevelt Hospital Center in New York City

CONTENTS

PART 1
NATURAL HEALING AND YOU

PART 2
THE BEST NATURAL-HEALING THERAPIES

PART 3
PUT NATURAL HEALING TO WORK FOR YOU

ACKNOWLEDGMENTS

Special thanks to Adriane Fugh-Berman, M.D., chairperson of the National Women's Health Network in Washington, D.C., former head of field investigations for the Office of Alternative Medicine at the National Institutes of Health in Bethesda, Maryland, and author of *Alternative Medicine: What Works*, for serving as medical adviser to the writers, researchers and editor who worked on this book.

We'd also like to thank the numerous other physicians and health care practitioners who shared their expertise with us.

INTRODUCTION
A Source You Can Trust

I served as editorial director of *Prevention* Book Club for eight years. In selecting health and fitness books offered to our readers, I reviewed many books on alternative healing. With each passing year, I noticed more and more books on aromatherapy, acupuncture, herbal medicine, reflexology, yoga, meditation, massage and dozens of other natural-healing techniques.

Most of our book-club customers are women. Books on alternative therapies sold pretty well, suggesting that women were eager to learn all that they could about these "new" treatments. We met face-to-face with some of our best readers—women just like you—to find out why they were turning to alternative medicine. What they told us was fascinating. Some women had suffered from problems like allergies, headaches or menstrual problems for years. They said they were discouraged by medications that either didn't work, put them to sleep or triggered other unwanted side effects. So they looked to natural methods to relieve their pain without disrupting their lives.

Still other women turned to natural healing as a way to prevent health problems from occurring in the first place, supporting their bodies' innate ability to stay strong and ward off disease.

Hundreds of alternative therapies are now in use. And more and more conventional doctors are embracing the use of alternative therapies. Yet many women rely on books as their primary source of information on what works. Physicians freely admit that there's only so much information that they can offer their patients in a routine office visit, so books can fill in the gap.

While many alternative therapies are safe and effective—and more are being studied all the time—some alternative practitioners and books suggest the use of herbs that are strong enough to do harm, without providing proper warnings for use by pregnant women or people with underlying health problems. And sometimes the directions for use aren't very clear. Since the therapies sound mysterious and unfamiliar, there's too often room for error.

Like other women, you're probably looking for a single book that takes the guesswork and risk out of alternative therapies, that focuses on what natural healing offers women. An easy-to-use reference book that women can trust.

To research and write this book, we attended conferences and workshops sponsored by medical schools that are now training physicians to use alternative medicine. We consulted the most respected experts in widely used therapies such as acupuncture, massage, yoga, meditation and reflexology, among others. We talked to women like you and your friends who have used alternative medicine successfully. And we consulted Adriane Fugh-Berman, M.D., former head of field investigations for the Office of Alternative Medicine at the National Institutes of Health in Bethesda, Maryland, to help us determine what therapies are safe and effective.

We also tried many of the therapies firsthand, to take the mystery out of alternative medicine and explain it in practical everyday ways.

Part 1 of this book explains why natural healing makes sense, especially for women. In part 2 of this book, you'll find an in-depth discussion of 30 individual therapies, from acupuncture to yoga. Here, in easy-to-understand terms, you'll find out how each therapy evolved and how and why it works. You'll find out what it feels like to go to an alternative practitioner for the first time. And you'll learn how to locate a qualified practitioner in your area.

Physicians who advocate natural healing say that the key is providing a variety of options so that people can select what works best for them as individuals. This book offers those options. In part 3, you'll discover how to use alternative remedies for dozens of health problems, from aches and pains and menstrual cramps to insomnia, anxiety to vaginal infections, and more.

We've paid special attention to finding out what alternative treatments work best for the health conditions unique to women—breast problems, menstrual discomforts, menopausal changes, pregnancy and urinary tract infections, among others. You'll also find natural treatments for conditions that affect more women than men—such as varicose veins, irritable bowel syndrome and chronic fatigue syndrome. Plus, you'll read about hopeful treatments for conditions that stymie medical doctors, like fibromyalgia (a painful condition that leaves your whole body sore and tired) and chronic pain, among others.

Throughout this book, you'll also read first-person stories from women who've healed themselves naturally: Yoga for digestive problems. Acupressure for migraine headaches. A vegetarian diet for the pain of rheumatoid arthritis. Evening primrose oil for tender breasts. And many more. In these highly personal, authentic accounts, the women that we interviewed tell how natural healing works.

This is the first book to offer the best in alternative medicine, geared specifically toward women. We hope that you enjoy reading—and using—this exciting new book.

Sharon Faelten

Sharon Faelten
Managing Editor

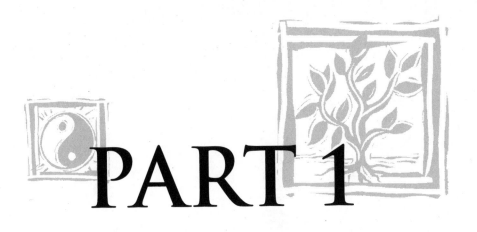

PART 1

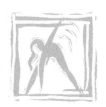

NATURAL
HEALING
AND
YOU

WHAT NATURAL HEALING OFFERS WOMEN
Made-to-Order Options for Total Health

Have you ever soaked in a hot, fragrant bath at the end of a stress-filled day? Or iced a bruise or used a hot-water bottle to ease menstrual cramps?

Have you ever had, or given, a back rub? Have you ever kissed away a child's pain?

If you answered yes to any of these questions, you've tried natural healing. Your therapeutic repertoire in those instances? Aromatherapy, hydrotherapy, massage and one form of therapeutic touch.

If you're like many women, you might think that natural healing therapies are mysterious and exotic. Paradoxically, natural healing is quite simple. In fact, you may already be using natural healing to help yourself and your family stay healthy, without even realizing it. Many of the therapies are as familiar as hot-water bottles and back rubs.

A RENAISSANCE OF NATURAL THERAPIES

A therapy is considered natural if it relies more on your body's innate power to heal itself than on invasive interventions such as drugs and surgery. Some natural therapies, like acupuncture, are considered conventional in non-Western countries such as China. Others, like herbal medicine, are practiced widely in one form or the other in nearly every culture of the globe. In this country, however, natural therapies are variously referred to as unconventional, alternative, complementary or unorthodox.

Unless doctors make a special effort to explore alternative medicine on their own, they don't generally learn about aromatherapy, massage, herbs or other forms of alternative medicine in medical school—yet. Nor are

3

these and other alternative therapies used in most hospitals. But you can expect alternative medicine to become even more familiar as we enter the twenty-first century, according to a landmark study by doctors at Harvard Medical School. The study reports that far more people than previously thought are utilizing unconventional therapies.

The Harvard study estimates that Americans make 37 million more visits to alternative practitioners than they do to conventional physicians, and that a third of all the people studied have used at least one unconventional therapy within the last year.

To further demonstrate that natural healing is becoming more mainstream, consider this.

- The National Institutes of Health established the Office of Alternative Medicine (OAM) in 1992 to research unconventional therapies. The OAM funds studies on health concerns as diverse as menopause and AIDS. In the first five years, the OAM budget more than quadrupled.
- In 1995, a National Institutes of Health panel found various alternative treatments to be effective for chronic pain and insomnia. Included were meditation, hypnosis, biofeedback, cognitive behavior therapy and relaxation techniques such as yoga and breathing exercises.
- The World Health Organization (WHO) says that more than 70 percent of the world's population relies on what Western physicians consider alternative healing methods.

Dozens of America's most respected university medical schools—including Harvard, Yale, Georgetown University in Washington, D.C., Tufts University in Boston, Columbia University in New York City and Stanford—have begun to add courses in various forms of alternative medicine to their curricula.

What's more, there are three schools of medicine devoted solely to naturopathy, a form of medicine that emphasizes the use of vitamin and mineral therapy, acupuncture and other alternative therapies over the use of drugs or surgery. They are Bastyr University of Naturopathic Medicine in Seattle, Southwest College of Naturopathic Medicine and Health Sciences in Tempe, Arizona, and the National College of Naturopathic Medicine in Portland, Oregon. So don't be surprised if one day soon, your family doctor recommends a natural treatment to you—if she hasn't done so already.

"I've been involved in alternative medicine for a long time," says Michael Carlston, M.D., assistant clinical professor at the University of California, San Francisco, School of Medicine. "We are in the midst of a huge transition in the way that we practice—and teach—medicine. Younger doctors feel comfortable with alternative medicine, and many are becoming certified in alternative treatments."

A NATURAL FOR WOMEN

You've probably noticed that interest in alternatives to Western medicine, like herbal remedies, is at an all-time high. Frequently featured in news magazines, major newspapers and broadcast media, natural healing has even figured into the story lines of television comedies and medical dramas. Suddenly, natural healing is everywhere. And that bodes well for women's health.

The preventive philosophy supports the "Dr. Mom" role that so many of us play.

"Women have traditionally been the gatekeepers for the health of their families," says Adriane Fugh-Berman, M.D., former head of field investigations for the Office of Alternative Medicine at the National Institutes of Health in Bethesda, Maryland. "Natural medicine stresses the importance of maintaining wellness, and it offers gentle, safe and effective remedies that women can use to care for themselves and for those they love.

"Many natural medicine systems, like Traditional Chinese Medicine, provide good models for self-care and wellness," says Dr. Fugh-Berman. These modalities emphasize good nutrition, stress reduction and other habits that help prevent health problems—not just fix what goes wrong.

Furthermore, health problems unique to women, such as menstrual problems, breast discomfort and hot flashes, can often be eased by natural therapies like herbal medicine, acupuncture, homeopathy and other therapies, says Dr. Fugh-Berman.

Take premenstrual syndrome (PMS), for example. "Over 200 symptoms are attributed to PMS," says Joyce Frye, D.O., an obstetrician/gynecologist and chairperson of the gynecology department at Presbyterian Medical Center and a clinical faculty member at Jefferson Medical College, both in Philadelphia.

"Some doctors say, 'Here's a women with PMS. She needs Prozac (a major antidepressant drug),'" explains Dr. Frye, who integrates natural-healing techniques with osteopathy. In contrast, she says, an alternative practitioner may evaluate the same woman and say, "Here's a woman who needs to improve her nutrition. She needs to exercise. Let's try vitamin supplements and other natural treatments that won't trigger uncomfortable—or even dangerous—side effects."

When it comes to relieving discomforts associated with menopause, alternative medicine offers gentle, safe choices for women who decide against taking hormone replacement therapy.

"For example, herbal medicine will ease hot flashes and other symptoms for some women," says Dr. Fugh-Berman. "Other women find that taking vitamin E helps. Still others report that simple deep-breathing exercises make hot flashes more bearable. It's natural medicine for a natural transition."

THE SPIRITUAL SIDE

Some natural traditions encourage women to consider the spiritual essence of being female.

"The Iroquois called menstruation a woman's vision time," says Kathleen Maier, a physician's assistant, herbalist and director of Dreamtime Center for Herbal Studies in Flint Hill, Virginia, and former adviser on botanical medicine for the National Institutes of Health. "They believed that during menstruation, women's energies are much more sensitive to external stimuli and their surrounding environments and that women should use the time to rest and reflect. Even though these teachings have not been part of our culture, the concept is important to consider," Maier says.

FOCUS ON PREVENTION

In these days of medical miracles like organ transplants, bypass surgery and drugs that end common killer diseases, what place does natural healing play? First strike? Last resort? An add-on to other, more conventional therapies?

The answer is all of the above, depending on your circumstances. No competent natural healer would ever suggest that you bypass the emergency room if you're seriously injured in an accident. Nor should you forgo medical help if you suddenly come down with a life-threatening illness. No one should stop taking prescription medicine for serious conditions like cancer or heart disease in favor of a highly questionable therapy with no track record or scientific basis, says Dr. Fugh-Berman.

But natural healing and conventional medicine can and should peacefully co-exist. "Natural medicine is great for preventing illness and treating minor and chronic conditions, and it's a great complement to conventional treatments for heart disease and cancer," says Dr. Fugh-Berman.

Herbal medicine, for example, has tonics that help support heart function while you take your regularly prescribed medication. Some herbs can ease the discomfort of cancer treatments. And mind-body therapies like visualization, yoga, meditation and breath work can help reduce stress—an essential aspect of treatment for a long list of conditions, says Dr. Fugh-Berman.

What's more, alternative therapies are often appropriate for a long list of everyday complaints that can be safely and effectively treated at home—from cuts and scrapes to insomnia, indigestion and headaches.

Finally, "natural medicine can be an excellent alternative choice for treating chronic problems, such as irritable bowel syndrome and fibromyalgia (painful 'trigger points' in the muscles), which have no good conventional treatments," says Dr. Fugh-Berman.

"Western medicine has big guns to solve life-threatening problems and medical emergencies: space-age diagnostic equipment, intricate surgical procedures, powerful drugs and the like," says Christina Stemmler, M.D., a Houston physician who uses acupuncture and Traditional Chinese Medicine in her practice and previously headed the American Academy of Medical Acupuncture. "But we don't have or use weapons that can handle the little problems before they become chronic conditions. Instead, we use tools like acupuncture, dietary therapy and massage, which can halt the progression or reverse an illness before it becomes unmanageable."

Indeed, treating health problems before they become chronic may be the common denominator for therapies as diverse as Traditional Chinese Medicine, osteopathy, chiropractic, naturopathy, yoga and herbal medicine. In fact, perhaps the most important advantage offered by many natural-healing disciplines is their ability to help you stay healthy.

NATURAL HEALING AND YOU

If you decide to try an alternative therapy, tell your family physician about your plans. She may need to monitor your progress or adjust your medication.

And be patient. Don't expect natural-healing methods to work in quite the same way that Western medicine does.

"We're used to quick-fix treatments that work almost immediately," says Dr. Fugh-Berman. "Natural medicine tends to be slower, gentler and often easier on your system." So listen to your body, find what works for you and give it time.

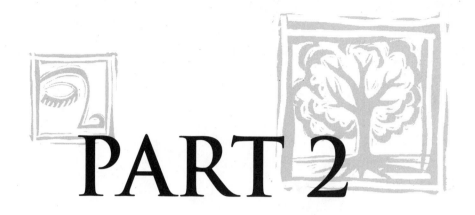

PART 2

THE BEST
NATURAL-HEALING
THERAPIES

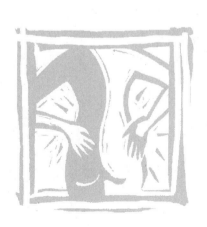

ACUPRESSURE
Health and Vitality, at Your Fingertips

It's the start of a new school day and in classrooms across China, school children are practicing preventive health.

Sitting at their desks, they press their index fingers between their eyes, pull their fingers down below their cheekbones, and press. With the middle three fingers of each hand, they press between their brows, pull out to their temples and press once more.

In China, no one is too young to learn the fundamentals of acupressure, an integral element of centuries-old Traditional Chinese Medicine.

More than 2,500 years ago, the Chinese concluded that they could relieve pain, lessen other symptoms of illness and promote health by pressing their fingers and hands on strategic points on the body. Pressing a point two inches above the wrist crease, on the inside of either wrist, between the tendons, it turned out, relieves and helps prevent nausea. Pressing the webbing between the thumb and index finger helps soothe and prevent headaches.

Today, millions of Chinese rely on acupressure to alleviate and prevent stress-related aches and pains, migraines, allergies, sinus problems, premenstrual syndrome (PMS), menstrual and breast pain, nausea and constipation as well as to help heal sports and other injuries and lessen fatigue, stress, eyestrain, wrinkles, anxiety, depression and insomnia.

"Anyone who has grown up in China in the last 30 years has learned simple self-acupressure techniques in school," explains Mark Nolting, licensed acupuncturist, naturopath and associate professor and chairman of the Department of Acupuncture and Oriental Medicine at Bastyr University of Naturopathic Medicine in Seattle.

Though it's less well-recognized in the United States than acupuncture, which uses needles rather than fingers and hands on strategic points, acupressure is gaining ground here. Thousands of practitioners, from massage therapists to acupuncturists and even some physicians, practice acupressure in the United States. Though the American Medical Association considers both acupressure and acupuncture to be unproven, research designed to test claims that acupressure relieves nausea has found that it works quite well. A growing number of medical doctors are using acupressure, acupuncture or a combination of the two in their practices.

"With acupressure and acupuncture, you assist the body in healing itself," says Glenn S. Rothfeld, M.D., clinical instructor in the Department of Community Health at Tufts University School of Medicine in Boston and a practitioner in Arlington, Massachusetts. Dr. Rothfeld uses both acupuncture and acupressure in his practice. "I like combining Western and Eastern techniques. With Western medicine, you treat a specific illness but don't address the body's ability to heal itself."

Like acupuncture, acupressure is virtually side-effect-free, Dr. Rothfeld and other practitioners point out. And though it isn't generally regarded as being as potent as acupuncture, it's something that patients can learn to use on their own.

For women in particular, that's a bonus, says Dr. Nolting. "Many practitioners find that a large percentage of their patients are women," he explains. "Acupressure can do a lot to assist women with problems associated with menstruation and childbirth."

Getting**Started**

Acupressure

Acupressure is widely practiced by acupuncturists, massage therapists and other health professionals, including physicians.

Number of practitioners in the United States: Unknown.

Qualifications to look for: Membership in the American Oriental Bodywork Therapy Association (AOBTA) is helpful but not required. Licensed acupuncturists may also be qualified to practice acupressure. Massage therapists and other alternative practitioners may be qualified as well.

Professional associations: American Oriental Bodywork Therapy Association, Glendale Executive Campus, Suite 510, 1000 Whitehorse Road, Voorhees, NJ 08043.

To find a practitioner: Contact the AOBTA at the address listed above.

Approximate cost: $40 to 100 per hour, depending on where you live.

WHY IT WORKS—THE EASTERN VIEW

Acupressure is an offshoot of acupuncture. According to legend, acupuncture originated with China's Yellow Emperor and his ministers in 2500 B.C. Historians, however, suspect that it evolved gradually. When the Chinese realized that they could achieve similar results simply by pressing on, rather than needling, specific points on the body, acupressure emerged as another way to stimulate healing.

According to traditional Chinese theory, both acupuncture and acupressure aid healing and promote health because they establish balance. Maintaining good health, the Chinese believe, is a matter of maintaining a harmonious balance of vital energy, or qi (also written as chi and pronounced "chee"), throughout the body. Qi is believed to flow through invisible, interconnected internal channels called meridians, which run from head to toe. (To see where meridians are on the body, see page 14.)

Normally, qi flows freely, but stress, poor nutrition, injuries, lack of exercise, poor attitude and exposure to the elements can cause blockages in the meridians and interfere with the flow of qi. Like a river that's been dammed, qi may flood some parts of the body and barely trickle into others. The resulting imbalance eventually leads to disease. Acupressure helps because pressure applied to appropriate "acupoints" along the meridians breaks up obstructions, allowing qi to flow freely and the body to begin healing itself, according to theory.

"When the energy is moving freely through the body, all of the body's systems are balanced," says Michael Reed Gach, Ph.D., acupressurist, director of the Acupressure Institute in Berkeley, California, and author of *Acupressure's Potent Points* and a series of acupressure audiotapes for women.

A TYPICAL VISIT, AND VARIATIONS

At the Jin Shin Do Foundation for Bodymind Acupressure in Felton, California, Judy lies on a table, cushions under her neck and knees.

Judy has been suffering from pelvic pain and constipation for several years, she tells Iona Marsaa Teeguarden, a certified acupressurist, the Foundation's director and author of *The Acupressure Way of Health*. Teeguarden listens, asks additional questions about Judy's medical history, then begins with pulse reading and point "palpation" (inquiring touch) to locate the main tension points and tender spots in Judy's neck, shoulders and torso.

Jin Shin Do, developed by Teeguarden, is one of several different schools of acupressure now practiced in the United States. Different

Full Body Acupressure Points

Acupressure points are found throughout the body and correspond to 12 main meridians (or energy channels), plus 2 extra meridians called the conception vessel and the governing vessel.

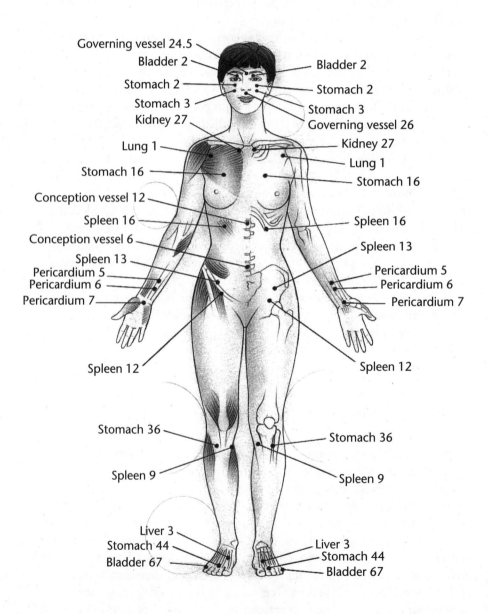

Governing vessel 24.5
Bladder 2
Stomach 2
Stomach 3
Kidney 27
Lung 1
Stomach 16
Conception vessel 12
Spleen 16
Conception vessel 6
Spleen 13
Pericardium 5
Pericardium 6
Pericardium 7
Spleen 12

Bladder 2
Stomach 2
Stomach 3
Governing vessel 26
Kidney 27
Lung 1
Stomach 16
Spleen 16
Spleen 13
Pericardium 5
Pericardium 6
Pericardium 7
Spleen 12

Stomach 36
Spleen 9
Liver 3
Stomach 44
Bladder 67

Stomach 36
Spleen 9
Liver 3
Stomach 44
Bladder 67

schools concentrate on different points on the body, some focusing primarily on acupoints along the meridians, others concentrating on tender points that turn up during palpation. According to these schools, tender points mark obstructions that interfere with the free flow of qi.

Depending on which school and which philosophy they train in, practitioners will use different therapeutic techniques as well—either holding, rubbing, kneading or vibrating points, or using a combination of those techniques—and will apply pressure to points for different periods of time.

Jin Shin Do practitioners use both meridian and tender points and hold pairs of points with a gentle but firm pressure. Also known as Bodymind Acupressure, Jin Shin Do emphasizes the interrelationship of mental, emotional and physical health, so treatment may include counseling.

While holding points in Judy's neck and shoulders, together with related "distal points," which help release the tension, Teeguarden asks Judy to pay attention to how her body feels. When Judy says that a point in her neck feels tender, Teeguarden suggests that she come up with an image or word to describe the feeling. "A tunnel," says Judy. "Stuck . . . frustration." Teeguarden uses body-focusing techniques to encourage Judy to describe the feeling more deeply. "Loneliness . . . sadness . . . a tight chest." While chest and arm points are held, Judy realizes a need for comfort and then grief for her father, who always supported and encouraged her. Though he died 20 years ago, Judy had only been able to cry a little once, 10 years ago. Working with acupoints in the abdomen, lower back and legs, Teeguarden reassures Judy that she can find the strength that she needs within herself.

Jin Shin Do practitioners sometimes lead you through visualization exercises during sessions. In other schools, including several schools of shiatsu, practitioners may also guide clients through deep-breathing exercises, meditation and stretching and offer dietary advice, explains Denise Shinn, certified practitioner of macrobiotic shiatsu and president of the American Oriental Bodywork Therapy Association in Voorhees, New Jersey.

After about an hour on the table, Judy says that her pelvic pain has disappeared. Alleviating the constipation problem, Teeguarden tells her, will probably require more sessions.

Long-standing health problems require more sessions, Dr. Gach explains. For chronic conditions, practitioners may begin with frequent sessions, once a week or more, then taper off once symptoms lessen, scheduling a "booster" session once a month. The typical session lasts about an hour, he says. "A session will leave you in a very deeply relaxed state. So it's beneficial to take a short nap afterward, if possible, to heighten the results," he adds.

Shiatsu: Press and Stretch to Release Blocked Energy

If it weren't for shiatsu, says Lise Ste-Marie, M.D., she might never have made it through natural childbirth. Fortunately, she was able to have a natural birth and shiatsu helped her to prepare for it.

A general practitioner in Quebec, Dr. Ste-Marie took a shiatsu therapist with her to the delivery room when her daughter was due. She was counting on shiatsu to help relieve labor pain, but it did more than that.

"My gynecologist said that the labor was taking so long that I might need a caesarean," recalls Dr. Ste-Marie, who started studying shiatsu shortly after finishing her medical degree. She recommends it to her patients who complain of pain, premenstrual syndrome, stress and breast tenderness. "But the shiatsu therapist kept working on the meridians and she helped the baby descend—and the birth was normal."

Shiatsu, the Japanese word for "finger pressure," is one of the best known forms of acupressure in North America. Though similar to other forms of acupressure in technique, shiatsu has a slightly different focus, says Robbee Fian, a licensed acupuncturist who practices acupuncture and teaches shiatsu in New York City.

While acupressurists focus on specific "acupoints" along the body's meridians—the invisible energy channels that run from head to toe— shiatsu therapists cover entire meridians, Fian says. "You tend to work the *whole* meridian—movement along the whole meridian is important."

There are several types of shiatsu. Some incorporate visualization, deep breathing, stretching, meditation and dietary advice. Others, like Five Element shiatsu, come with their own special diagnostic techniques as well. Another form, called Ohashiatsu, is designed to benefit both the person giving the shiatsu and the person to whom it's given.

"We teach how to move your body and how to let your body work so that you don't strain it" while you do shiatsu, says Wataru Ohashi, creator of Ohashiatsu; founder of The Ohashi Institute in 1974, a nonprofit educational institute in New York City; and author of *The Ohashi Bodywork Book* and *Do-It-Yourself Shiatsu.* "The giver is very much exercising in a very natural way. You limber your body. You are stretching places that Americans tend not to stretch, and you become more flexible." Though some massage therapists offer "shiatsu massage," that's a misnomer, according to Fian. What they're offering is really massage with a little shiatsu technique on the side—not true shiatsu, she says.

If you want to see what shiatsu can do, you're best off visiting a trained practitioner since it takes time and training to master the therapy, says Fian. You can, however, do some simple shiatsu on your own. One way that shiatsu opens meridians and stimulates the flow of energy is to stretch.

Specific shiatsu stretches use the body's own weight, applying pressure to the meridians as you lean this way and that way. By stimulating meridians, shiatsu stretches may assist in freeing up blocked energy and drawing it toward areas of weakness, thus releasing tensions and limbering you up for yoga or aerobic exercise— even if no practitioner is available to apply pressure to the shiatsu acupoints.

Interested? Fian, creator of Five Element shiatsu, recommends Makko-Ho, a daily five-step routine that takes five to ten minutes. "When people do this on a regular basis, everything seems to function much better," she says. "It helps relieve stress, and people say that they have more energy."

It is important to remember, when practicing the Makko-Ho exercises, that what matters is the action of beginning the stretch, not how far you can stretch. If in this exercise you can only lean back onto your palms, simply hold that position and stretch, breathe and relax. The more you practice, the easier the positions will become, adds Fian.

Shiatsu stretches are shown on the following five pages. Do these stretches each morning, before breakfast.

Shiatsu Stretch 1:
Bend Forward, Arms behind Back

Begin in a standing position. Inhale and place your hands behind your back and interlock your thumbs. Exhale as you gently allow your body to hang forward from your waist, allowing your arms and thumbs to raise up behind you, toward the ceiling. (You'll feel as though you're hanging from the ceiling by your thumbs.) Exhale as you hold this position. Inhale and straighten up. Repeat this stretch three to five times.

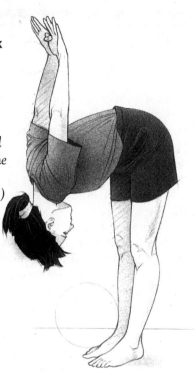

Shiatsu Stretch 2:
Sitting, Legs Tucked Under

Sit on your heels with your feet crossed, toes over toes, and with your back straight. Relax and breathe.

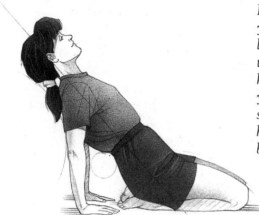

Put your arms behind you and your palms flat on the floor, then lean back, keeping your buttocks touching your feet and your knees together. Avoid arching your back. You should feel a stretch along your thighs as you hold this position. Relax and breathe.

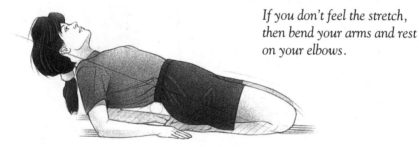

If you don't feel the stretch, then bend your arms and rest on your elbows.

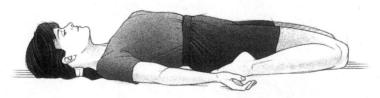

If leaning back on your arms is easy to sustain, try to sit between your legs with your buttocks touching the floor and then lean all the way back until your back is resting on the floor. Relax and breathe. Then sit up in stages: First prop yourself up on your elbows, then up to your palms and then back to a full sitting position. (If you suffer from any weakness or pain in the knees, skip this exercise.)

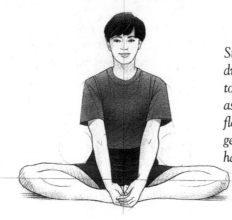

**Shiatsu Stretch 3:
Sitting Position**

*Sit on the floor, with your legs
drawn in and the soles of your feet
touching. Inhale deeply and relax
as you press your knees to the
floor. If this seems difficult at first,
gently push your knees with your
hands or elbows.*

*Next, exhale and bend forward
until your head comes as close to
the floor as possible. (Skip this step
if you are pregnant, since bending
forward will compress the area
around your uterus.) Relax and
hold this position for 15 to 30
seconds, then sit up and inhale. Repeat this stretch three to five times.*

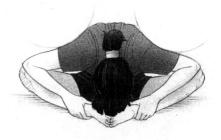

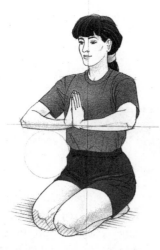

*Next, sit on your heels, bring your
palms together in front of your heart,
with your elbows out and fingers
touching. Breathe in.*

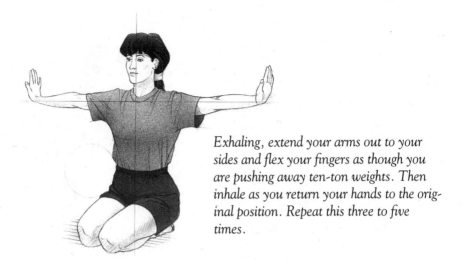

Exhaling, extend your arms out to your sides and flex your fingers as though you are pushing away ten-ton weights. Then inhale as you return your hands to the original position. Repeat this three to five times.

Shiatsu Stretch 4: Bend Forward, Legs Out

Sit on the floor with your back straight and stretch your legs out in front of you, keeping your feet flexed toward your body at a 90-degree angle. Inhale when settled in this position.

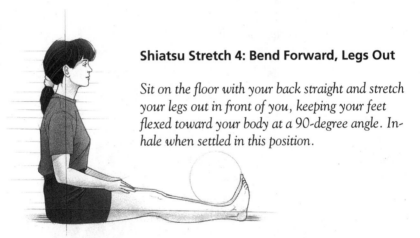

Exhale as you allow your body weight to pull you forward, and gently reach out to grab the soles of your feet—or your calves or knees, if that's as far as you can comfortably reach— so that you feel the stretch in your upper thighs. (If you are pregnant, stretch forward from your buttocks, without letting your torso collapse, bend or sag over your legs, so that you feel the stretch in your upper thighs.) Inhale and straighten up. Repeat this stretch three to five times, each time holding the stretch for 15 to 30 seconds, while continuously relaxing and breathing slowly and deeply.

Shiatsu Stretch 5:
Legs to Sides, Bend Forward

Sit on the floor with your legs as far apart as possible. Inhale and extend your arms toward the floor. (If you're pregnant, stretch forward without letting your torso collapse, bend or sag over your legs and without rounding your back.) Exhale and bend forward so that your head touches the floor (or in that general direction). Hold and relax for 15 to 30 seconds. Inhale and return to an upright position.

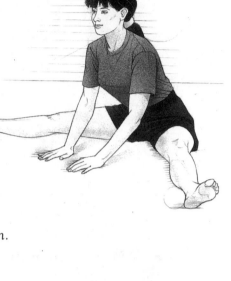

Exhale and stretch to the side, over your left leg, and stretch your right arm over your head, to your left. Breathe deeply as you relax for 15 to 30 seconds. Then inhale and return to the center position. Repeat on the opposite side.

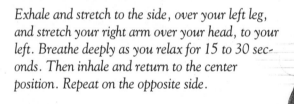

With your legs in the same position, exhale and turn your torso to the left. Leaning across your left leg, stretch and exhale. Hold this position and breathe, for 15 to 30 seconds. Inhale and return to an upright position. Repeat on the opposite side. Then repeat these step 5 stretches three more times.

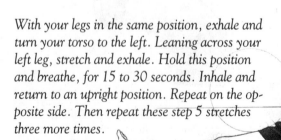

WHY IT WORKS—THE WESTERN VIEW

Western science has yet to uncover hard evidence that qi exists. Oriental theory is that qi is the flow through two opposing forces, yin and yang. An imbalance signifies disease. Acupressure attempts to re-establish this balance by pressure along specific points and meridians.

Some of the most intriguing research suggests that acupressure relieves symptoms of illness by triggering production of neurochemicals, chemical messengers that ferry information between your brain and the rest of your body. Several studies have shown that *acupuncture* prompts the body to produce neurochemicals responsible for relieving pain, producing feelings of well-being, reducing the inflammation that contributes to asthma and arthritis and regulating appetite.

Acupressure may do the same, says Bruce Pomeranz, M.D., Ph.D., neurophysiologist, professor at the University of Toronto School of Medicine and one of the world's foremost acupuncture researchers.

Acupressure's tension-relieving potential may also explain its effect on pain and other symptoms, suggests Dr. Gach. Numerous studies find that the body's physiological response to stress—increased blood pressure and an outpouring of adrenaline—can contribute to heart disease, depression, irritability, insomnia, headaches, difficulty concentrating, dampened immunity and other problems. "And it's often stress and anxiety that make us want to overeat, and worsen PMS as well," adds Dr. Gach.

Finally, acupressure improves circulation, says Dr. Rothfeld. And that may explain why it helps alleviate related problems, like muscle aches and pains, in people with poor circulation.

THE SCIENTIFIC EVIDENCE

The best documented benefit of acupressure is relief from nausea and dizziness. Studies show that it relieves queasiness and vomiting both during pregnancy and after anesthesia. In a North Carolina study, pregnant women who wore wristbands fitted with buttons that pressed against the antinausea acupoint reported a 50 percent reduction in queasiness and vomiting. And in a British study, men and women reported less severe postoperative nausea when wearing the wristbands.

Early research into acupressure's effect on pain has also been promising. Michael I. Weintraub, M.D., advocate of shiatsu, clinical professor of neurology at New York Medical College in Valhalla and head of neurology at Phelps Memorial Hospital in Tarrytown, New York, says a small study that he directed found that 86 percent of patients with herniated disks experienced pain relief with a combination of shiatsu and Swedish massage.

"And these were people who failed to respond to other treatments, such as drugs, physical therapy and chiropractic," says Dr. Weintraub, who teaches his patients simple shiatsu techniques for alleviating headaches, nausea, dizziness and spine pain.

Though there have been few controlled scientific studies examining acupressure's efficacy in alleviating symptoms other than nausea and pain, practitioners say that they get good results with a wide range of symptoms like headaches, menstrual cramps and stress.

"In general, anything that's caused by or exacerbated by stress and tension responds well," says Dr. Gach. The illustrations that follow demonstrate some of the most common uses for acupressure.

Lower Back Pain

Pressing two points located two inches from each side of your spine, on your lower back, can help relieve lower-back pain caused from sitting for too long or from menstrual cramps. If you have a weak back, these points may be tender, so see your doctor before trying acupressure on your lower back.

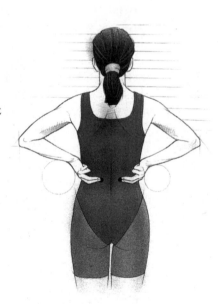

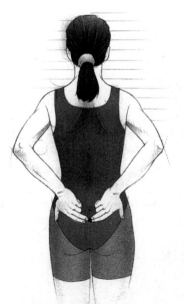

Disk and Hip Pain

Using your index and middle fingers of each hand, press on either side of your tailbone, about where the crease in your buttocks begins. These points can relieve sciatica, resulting from inflammation of the sciatic nerve that runs from the buttocks through the leg, or from a slipped or herniated disk. These points also ease hip pain.

Headache—Between the Eyes

Pressing a point called the Third Eye, located at the bridge of your nose between
the eyebrows, balances the pituitary gland
and relieves hay fever, headaches, indigestion, ulcer pain and eyestrain.

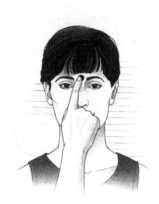

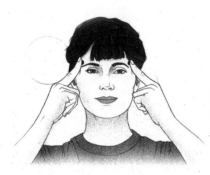

Headache—Sides of Forehead

Pressing the index finger of your left hand
to your left temple and the index finger of
your right hand to your right temple can
treat headaches.

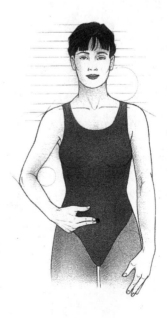

Menstrual Discomforts

Pressing a point called the Sea of Energy,
located two finger-widths below your
belly button, aids premenstrual
syndrome, menstrual cramps, irregular
vaginal discharge, irregular periods and
constipation. Use your index and middle
fingers.

Menstrual Pain

To help combat menstrual cramps, press your index and middle fingertips to the point outside your knee, about three finger-widths below your kneecap.

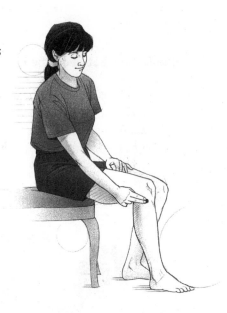

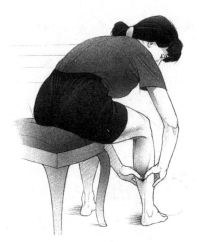

Leg and Back Pain

Pressing both thumbs at a point called the Supporting Mountain, located in the center of the base of your calf, eases leg cramps in your calf and can help fight knee pain, lower-back pain and swelling in the feet.

Insomnia and Anxiety

Applying acupressure to the Spirit Gate point, located on the outside of your wrist, below the first crease and in line with your pinkie finger, relieves anxiety, cold sweats and insomnia brought on by being overexcited.

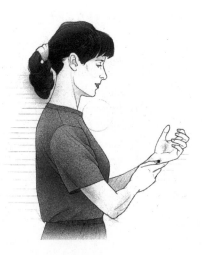

Insomnia and Pain

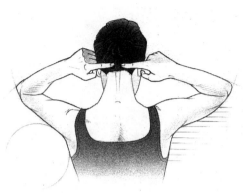

To ease arthritis, headaches and neck pain that can cause insomnia, press your left index finger against your hairline about one-half inch to the left of your spine and your right index finger against your hairline about one-half inch to the right of your spine.

Coughing and Congestion

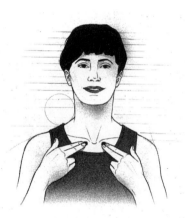

Pressing the acupoints located below your collarbone and alongside your breastbone relieves coughing, chest congestion and breathing difficulties.

Out-of-Control Coughing

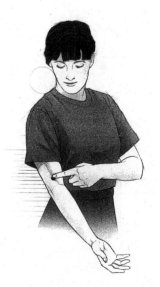

To control coughs, press the point located at the bottom of your biceps and slightly to the outside of your arm.

Hiccups

Pressing the point called Heaven Rushing Out, in the hollow at the base of your throat, eases hiccups, bronchitis, throat spasms, sore throats, chest congestion and heartburn.

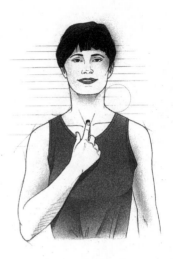

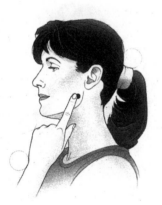

Toothache and TMJ Pain

To relieve jaw pain and spasms, toothaches or temporomandibular disorders, press this point, called the Jaw Chariot, located above the end of your jaw, on the side of your face that hurts.

Tennis Elbow

To relieve the pain of tennis elbow, press the outside of your knuckle on the pinkie finger of your opposite hand.

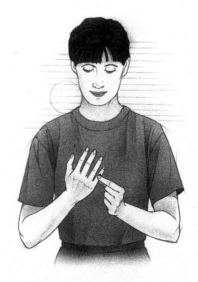

An alternate way to relieve tennis elbow is to locate the point of greatest pain near your elbow, then press the same point but on the opposite elbow.

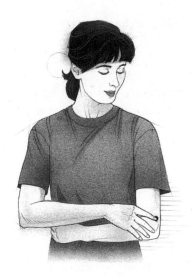

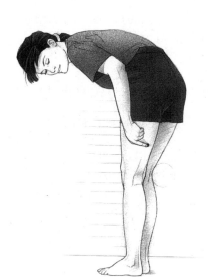

Hamstring Pain

Some people find that they can relieve hamstring pain by pressing the point midway between the back of the knee and the bottom of the buttocks, on the leg opposite the one that hurts.

WHEN TO GO

If you're not feeling well, Dr. Pomeranz suggests that you see your physician for a diagnosis. If you're diagnosed with a health problem that conventional medicine really can't help, or a problem that acupressure has a good track record with, or you want to add acupressure to conventional medical therapy, see a practitioner trained in acupuncture or acupressure, suggests Adriane Fugh-Berman, M.D., former head of field investigations for the Office of Alternative Medicine at the National Institutes of Health in Bethesda, Maryland. "Once you learn what points work for you, you can use the technique at home."

Acupuncture (not a do-at-home technique) is a more potent way to stimulate healing. If your symptoms are severe—you're in extreme pain, for instance—you'll need acupuncture, Dr. Pomeranz says. If they're mild, acupressure should do the trick.

One of the advantages of acupressure is that you can do it on your own on a daily basis, Dr. Pomeranz points out.

"We've shown that daily treatment is much more effective than less frequent treatment," says Dr. Pomeranz. "The good thing about acupressure is that you can do it without making an appointment." You can also do it immediately—as soon as your head starts to hurt or your stomach begins to pitch, he adds.

SELF-ACUPRESSURE FOR GOOD HEALTH

You can learn simple self-acupressure techniques from a trained acupressurist or licensed or certified acupuncturist, or from tapes or books.

Before you give it a try, here are a few pointers on proper technique and some caveats to keep in mind.

Get trim. Trim your nails before you start so that you don't dig into the skin surface.

Stick to the middle. Your middle finger is the longest and strongest and the best suited for self-acupressure. If it's not strong enough, try using your knuckles, your fist or a pencil eraser, suggests Dr. Gach.

Keep doc in mind. If you have a serious or chronic illness, such as heart disease, cancer or high blood pressure, or if you're pregnant, talk to your physician and a professional acupressurist before using self-acupressure. Pressing on some points is forbidden in pregnancy because doing so may encourage abortion, and using acupoints for this purpose is also dangerous, as it may invite hemorrhaging, adds Teeguarden.

Tread carefully. Avoid applying acupressure to areas with scars, infections, ulcers or recent burns. Don't apply pressure directly over an artery or over the genitals. And go easy on the abdominal area. Touch, don't press, sensitive areas on the throat, below the ear or on the outer breast near the armpit, according to Dr. Gach.

Don't eat and press. If you've just eaten a heavy meal, wait an hour before beginning an all-body regimen, says Dr. Gach. "Many of the meridians cross the stomach, and if there's a lot of food in the stomach, the energy can get blocked, causing nausea."

Zero in. Search for acupoints by carefully probing with your thumb. Acupoints are usually much more sensitive than the surrounding area, so be on alert for sensitivity.

Make it "hurt good." One of the most common mistakes that novices make is to press too lightly. "You have to press hard enough," says Dr. Pomeranz. "Press until you get an aching sensation. A lot of people don't do that. They're too timid."

Press your fingertips in firmly—at a 90-degree angle to the skin—exploring until you find the sensitive spot. Push hard but not to the point that you puncture the skin. Often, you'll feel the same sensation that you get when you hit your funny bone—part pain, part numbness, part tingle. If you have well-developed muscles, you'll need to use deeper pressure. Women often need less pressure than men. Don't press any point that's excruciatingly painful. Acupressure should "hurt good," according to Dr. Gach.

Make it last. Maintain pressure for 15 to 30 seconds per spot. Use a stopwatch or count "one thousand one, one thousand two" to pace yourself. If you're working a spot that has been injured or is painful or tense, hold it until the hurt lessens, but no more than five minutes, Dr. Gach says. If you're just starting to use self-acupressure, don't work the same spot more than two or three times a day. "If you do more than that, you could release too much energy in that area, and this could create blockages in other places," he says.

Do it daily. Make sure that you apply acupressure often enough to get results. Dr. Pomeranz recommends doing your regimen every day.

A Daily Self-Acupressure Regimen

Chinese school children learn and follow a simple finger acupressure regimen daily.

"It's good for all sorts of things—for maintaining skin tone in the face, for vision, for preventing sinus problems and headaches," says Mark Nolting, licensed acupuncturist, naturopath and associate professor and chairman of the Department of Acupuncture and Oriental Medicine at Bastyr University of Naturopathic Medicine in Seattle.

For your own daily self-acupressure routine, follow these simple steps.

1. Place each of your index fingers beside the tear ducts of your eyes, press in against your face at the bridge of your nose and hold to a count of five or ten. Now pull your index fingers down, along the sides of your nose, until they touch your nostrils. Press for five to ten seconds.
2. Press two or three fingers of each hand between your eyebrows, hold for five to ten seconds, then pull out toward your temples. Press again for five to ten seconds.
3. Repeat the routine several times.

ACUPUNCTURE
New Evidence for an Ancient Therapy

Basking in the warm glow of a heat lamp, Sara MacKay stretches out on the table like a sunbather on a beach.

"This is so-o-o-o relaxing," she murmurs.

About to doze off, she shifts, sending a shiver down a row of sharp stainless-steel needles protruding from her neck, back and shoulders.

This is MacKay's second visit to David Molony, Ph.D., licensed acupuncturist and executive director of the American Association of Acupuncture and Oriental Medicine, who practices in the northern suburbs of Philadelphia. A 40-year-old writer from New York City, MacKay has come looking for relief from a constant dull pain in her hands.

After prodding her with his index finger, Dr. Molony has found two dozen tender spots on her shins, back, shoulders, neck and fingers and has inserted a two-inch-long needle in each area.

The needles stung when they went in, MacKay says, but they don't hurt anymore. And now, after two sessions, her hands don't hurt anymore either. That's the important part.

"My hands used to hurt so much that I couldn't write a letter longhand, and I was taking ibuprofen several times a day," she explains. "Now, I've stopped taking Advil, and I can write again."

ANCIENT PRACTICE, NEWLY DISCOVERED

The Chinese have been practicing acupuncture—inserting needles at strategic points in the body to relieve pain, treat illness and promote health—for centuries. Acupuncture is just one facet of Traditional Chinese Medicine, which dates back some 5,000 years. Despite that long history, acupuncture was largely unknown in the United States until 1972, when former President Richard Nixon reestablished ties with China. *New York Times* correspondent James Reston, covering the event, suffered an attack of appendicitis. After an emergency appendectomy and a post-op recovery eased by acupuncture, Reston wrote a column testifying to its pain-relieving potential.

Today, millions of Americans get acupuncture yearly, most often for relief from chronic pain, back problems, addiction, headaches, menstrual discomfort and arthritis. Acupuncturists use the therapy to treat a wide array of other health concerns, from weight problems to insomnia to morning sickness.

Though the American Medical Association considers acupuncture unproven, scientific research is building a convincing case for the age-old practice, finding it effective in treating a variety of ills. Some medical schools offer acupuncture courses to medical students. Impressed by its track record and the fact that side effects are minimal, an estimated 5,000 M.D.'s and more than 7,000 Oriental medicine practitioners practice acupuncture in the United States. Increasingly, insurance companies are covering the treatment.

Getting**Started**

Acupuncture

Alternative practitioners and medical physicians alike use acupuncture for a wide variety of ailments, from pain relief to nausea. If you're considering acupuncture, these guidelines can help you to pursue this option.

Number of practitioners in the United States: Approximately 8,000.

Qualifications to look for: Certification by the National Certification Commission for Acupuncture and Oriental Medicine (NCCA) in Washington, D.C. To become certified, practitioners must finish a training program and pass a national certifying exam or licensing exam in the state in which they practice. To protect against blood-borne infection, make sure the acupuncturist uses disposable acupuncture needles.

Professional associations: The American Association of Oriental Medicine, 433 Front Street, Catasauqua, PA 18032; American Academy of Medical Acupuncture (AAMA), 5820 Wilshire Boulevard, Suite 500, Los Angeles, CA 90036.

To find a practitioner: Contact the NCCA, P.O. Box 97075, Washington, D.C. 20090-7075. The NCCA will send you a list of certified practitioners in your state or the complete national list, for a fee. Or contact the American Association of Oriental Medicine or the AAMA (both listed above).

Approximate cost: $35 to $125 per session.

MAINTAINING HARMONIOUS BALANCE

How can needles inserted in the back, shoulders, neck and shins relieve pain in the hands or, for that matter, treat arthritis?

In the traditional Chinese view—a perspective less mechanistic than our own—it's simple. According to ancient Chinese precepts, maintaining

Acupuncture Meridians: Front View

Chinese healers classify the hundreds of acupuncture points into 12 main groups joined by lines called meridians, shown here. Each meridian is named for an organ or area of the body and runs along both the right and the left sides of the body. (The kidney meridian is shown on one side only.)

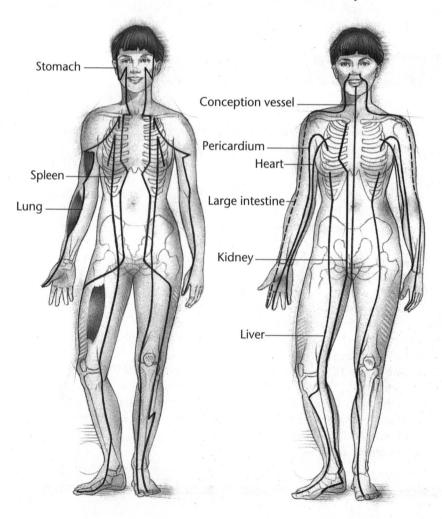

Stomach

Conception vessel

Pericardium

Heart

Spleen

Lung

Large intestine

Kidney

Liver

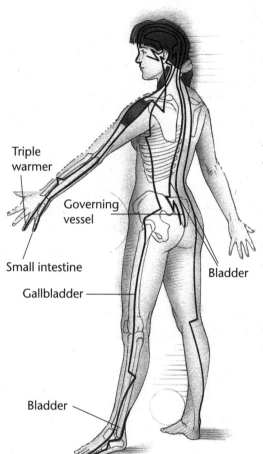

Acupuncture Meridians: Rear and Side View

The Chinese believe that qi, the energy of life, flows along the meridians the way that water flows along a river or impulses flow through a nerve. The triple warmer refers to the three sections of the body's trunk. It ensures proper movement of qi and fluids throughout the body. Another meridian known as the governing vessel passes through the rear center of the body. Stimulating points along its path can relieve headaches, stiff necks and backs and pain of hemorrhoids.

Triple warmer

Governing vessel

Small intestine

Gallbladder

Bladder

Bladder

good health is a matter of maintaining a harmonious balance of *qi*, or *chi*, (pronounced *chee*), or vital energy, in the body.

Normally, qi flows freely along invisible internal channels, or "meridians," that traverse the body. Stress, poor nutrition, injuries or lack of exercise, however, can create obstructions in the meridians that keep qi from flowing freely. Like a stream that's been dammed, qi overflows in certain parts of the body but barely trickles into others.

"This imbalance leads to weakness, and weakness can lead to disorder," explains Dr. Molony. As a result, the body may be more susceptible to disease.

Acupuncture needles, inserted at certain "acupoints" along the meridians, trigger healing because they break up obstructions, stimulate energy or drain energy in a meridian, bringing the body back into balance and allowing qi to flow freely again, Dr. Molony explains. Of course, the needles need to be in the right spots in the correct meridians to do the trick. The right acupoint can be a distance from the ailing area.

Dr. Molony has decided in MacKay's case that an obstruction in her gallbladder meridian is leading to the pain in her hands. In the traditional Chinese view, the gallbladder and liver meridians are the organs responsible for muscles and tendons.

Since the gallbladder meridian runs through the shoulder and also runs through the hip and the leg, Dr. Molony inserts acupuncture needles in these areas. Before he inserts the needles, though, he palpates for sensitive spots. According to theory, the spots that need to be "stimulated" with needles will most likely be tender.

"The needles are so small, there usually isn't any bleeding, except in some areas with a lot of blood vessels, like the hands," he says. There's a small drop of blood where each needle has pierced MacKay's little finger—but nowhere else. (If you see an acupuncturist, make sure disposable needles are used to prevent transmission of blood-borne illnesses. Most acupuncturists use them.)

VARIATIONS ON THE ART OF ACUPUNCTURE

Acupuncturists sometimes twirl needles after inserting them or connect the needles to a low-voltage electrical source to increase stimulation of acupoints (a technique called electroacupuncture). They may also train heat lamps on the needles to increase stimulation. Some use lasers rather than needles to stimulate acupoints.

They may also use "moxibustion," placing small cones of an herb called mugwort on acupoints and burning it to produce penetrating heat. Moxibustion cones can be applied directly to the skin in such a way that prevents burns, or indirectly, on salt or a slice of ginger or other barrier or wrapped around the needle.

The protocol—how many needles are used, how deeply they're inserted, how long they're left in and whether they're used with electricity or heat—depends on the diagnosis and the preferences of the acupuncturist. So do the frequency and duration of treatments. The more advanced and entrenched the health problem, the longer the therapy.

Traditionally trained practitioners like Dr. Molony may treat patients with a combination of acupuncture, massage, acupressure (which uses finger pressure, rather than needles, on acupoints), Chinese herbs and dietary advice.

Some M.D.'s combine acupuncture and other traditional Chinese therapies, too. Others use it as an adjunct to conventional drug therapy and surgery. Acupuncture, says Christina Stemmler, M.D., a Houston physician who uses acupuncture in her practice and previously headed the

American Academy of Medical Acupuncture, enables some patients to get the same results with less medication.

Dr. Stemmler says the combination of acupuncture and Western medicine can work better than either one alone. Dr. Molony, however, finds that conventional medicines sometimes interfere with acupuncture treatments. So treatment plans must be individualized.

For MacKay, Dr. Molony prescribes a few dietary changes, an herbal remedy and acupuncture. If she sticks to the regimen, MacKay should be symptom-free after a few more sessions, he says, since the treatment should clear the obstruction in her meridians and reestablish a harmonious balance of qi. If she doesn't make some necessary lifestyle changes, though, the balance of qi may shift again, especially during changes of season. Her symptoms may recur, and she may need to come back for further treatments, says Dr. Molony.

WHY IT WORKS: THE WESTERN VIEW

After devoting 20 years to the scientific study of acupuncture, Bruce Pomeranz, M.D., Ph.D., neurophysiologist, professor at the University of Toronto School of Medicine and one of the world's foremost acupuncture researchers, has yet to find compelling evidence that meridians and qi exist. But he has found compelling evidence that acupuncture works and has formulated a convincing Western-style theory to explain *why* it works—at least in some cases.

In a major breakthrough in 1976, Dr. Pomeranz discovered that acupuncture affects the nervous system, triggering the release of endorphins—neurochemicals that naturally alleviate pain. These findings appear to explain why acupuncture both relieves pain and alleviates addicts' withdrawal symptoms: Endorphins "may replace the missing morphinelike substances produced by the brain and ease withdrawal that way," he explains.

In subsequent research, Dr. Pomeranz and others have discovered that inserting needles at acupoints or stimulating the points with low-voltage electricity can trigger the release of the neurochemicals serotonin and cortisol. Since serotonin promotes feelings of well-being and cortisol reduces inflammation, these results may account for acupuncture's success in the treatment of depression, arthritis and asthma. He believes that more research is needed in these areas.

Although researchers have yet to document exactly how acupuncture influences hormones and metabolism, Dr. Stemmler says that, in her experience, people who undergo acupuncture seem to be able to lose excess weight effortlessly while being treated for other health conditions. Dr. Stemmler often calls weight loss a fringe benefit of acupuncture.

Some researchers speculate that acupuncture may actually retrain the nervous system so it releases appropriate amounts of neurochemicals, thereby correcting certain chronic conditions.

The neurochemical theory, however, doesn't explain everything, Dr. Pomeranz acknowledges. At this point, it doesn't explain why acupuncture relieves nausea, for instance.

"Acupuncture probably has many different mechanisms," says Dr. Stemmler, who credits acupuncture with alleviating osteoarthritis and asthma in many of her patients. She speculates that the therapy may also correct bioelectrical abnormalities in the body that contribute to illness.

THE SCIENTIFIC EVIDENCE

Hands down, the most accepted benefit of acupuncture is pain relief. Controlled clinical studies find it considerably more effective than placebo, or dummy, treatment in relieving pain. Many studies have divided patients into two groups: those who have had actual treatment (needles inserted at appropriate acupoints) and those who have had "sham" acupuncture (needles inserted at the wrong places). According to Dr. Pomeranz, who has reviewed more than a dozen such studies, 55 to 85 percent of patients who got the real thing reported relief from chronic pain, compared with just 35 percent of those who got the placebo treatment.

Several controlled clinical trials suggest that acupuncture can play a role in treating addiction as well. Research at Florida's Metro-Dade County Outpatient Substance Abuse Treatment Facility concluded that it can help drug addicts and alcoholics kick their addictions. "Whether it's effective with smoking is still up in the air," Dr. Pomeranz says.

Studies show that acupuncture can also help relieve nausea, whether it's the result of a turbulent car ride, chemotherapy or pregnancy. And other research suggests that acupuncture may help treat arthritis, asthma, bronchitis, cold symptoms, migraines, premenstrual syndrome (PMS) and tennis elbow. It may also speed recovery from stroke, partially reverse nerve damage caused by diabetes, ease bladder problems, lessen depression, lower blood pressure, speed labor and relieve hot flashes during menopause.

"But these areas are less well studied than pain relief at this point and are not as well nailed-down scientifically," Dr. Pomeranz says.

Nonetheless, practitioners and some physicians are using acupuncture in many of these less well-studied areas. The treatment seems to help, they note, and it doesn't cause the side effects that accompany drug therapy and surgery, according to Dr. Stemmler. Inserting needles at certain acupoints appears to induce labor, however, and can harm the fetus in early pregnancy. If you're pregnant and want to have acupuncture, get approval from your obstetrician first, and before treatment begins, tell the acupuncturist that you're pregnant, she adds.

"I treat most of the pain conditions that wouldn't respond to surgery," says Dr. Stemmler, who also uses acupuncture to treat sinusitis, asthma, chronic bladder inflammation, certain types of urinary incontinence, insomnia and poststroke paralysis.

Another physician, Abegael Lorico, M.D., assistant professor of obstetrics and gynecology at Allegheny University of the Health Sciences MCP–Hahnemann School of Medicine and a licensed acupuncturist, says that she offers the women she treats the option of prescription drugs or acupuncture treatment for PMS and other gynecological problems, following a complete evaluation.

"For treatment of allergies, acupuncture is beyond belief," says Haig Ignatius, M.D., a Maryland otolaryngologist who uses the ancient technique in his practice. "In effect, acupuncture gets the body's immune system to make a better decision, to stop overreacting (or being hypersensitive), and so allergy symptoms will likely improve or clear up."

WHEN TO SEE AN ACUPUNCTURIST

Even the most enthusiastic advocates of acupuncture acknowledge that Western medicine has advantages of its own. "Conventional treatment is famous for diagnosis, so I'd say go to a Western doctor for a diagnosis," Dr. Pomeranz says.

"It's always a good idea to get a diagnosis from an M.D. or a D.O.," agrees Adriane Fugh-Berman, M.D., former head of field investigations for the Office of Alternative Medicine at the National Institutes of Health in Bethesda, Maryland. "Infections should be treated with antibiotics, but many chronic conditions respond better to acupuncture than conventional treatment. And sometimes, a combination of Western and Eastern medicine works best."

ALEXANDER TECHNIQUE

Finding the Perfect Posture

When your mother nagged you about "sitting up like a lady," you probably squared your shoulders for a second and then resumed slouching.

Who'd have thought Mom actually knew what she was talking about? As it turns out, good posture actually *can* affect your life—and your health.

Just ask Judith S., a 48-year-old who suffered severe, unexplained neck pain and headaches for months. "I was going crazy," says the New York City magazine editor. "It was just extremely uncomfortable."

When doctors couldn't figure out the root of her problem, Judith went to a teacher of the Alexander Technique—a movement-training program in which an instructor studies how you sit, stand, walk and bend in order to correct postural and tension-related mistakes and help you increase your awareness of how you might move more naturally.

The results were dramatic. "What the Alexander Technique did was teach me how to use my body more efficiently. I'd been holding my head, neck, back and legs wrong and was using more muscle tension than I needed," she notes. "I seldom have any pain or headaches now."

The technique was developed by F. M. Alexander, a Shakespearean actor from Australia who lost his voice due to overuse during the late 1800s. Studying himself in three-way mirrors, he discovered his tendency to tighten his neck, jut his jaw forward and hold his rib cage as he spoke, thereby cutting off breath support to his voice.

Alexander, who became known as the Breathing Man, began teaching his technique by the mid-1890s, a pursuit that took him to England.

Rather than concentrating on the old good-posture axiom of "chin up, shoulders pushed back and stomach in," the Alexander Technique helps you restore the effortless way of carrying yourself without compressing your spine, says Vivien Schapera, director of the training course at the Alexander Technique of Cincinnati.

"The hallmark of the Alexander Technique is if a movement takes effort, it's wrong. What's causing you to slouch is the excessive unconscious contraction of muscles—in the stomach, the back, the shoulders—throughout your body," she says. "The Alexander Technique shows you how to free up your body so that you stop pulling on your skeleton with your habitually tense muscles."

When your body parts are compressed and pulled in, you don't function at your utmost efficiency, says Judith Stern, physical therapist on the faculty at the American Center for the Alexander Technique in New York City. Whether it's the joints, blood vessels, digestive tract, stomach or heart, when you press down on an organ or body part, there isn't enough space for them to work as well, she says.

HEADING OFF TROUBLE

By taking stress off the body, the technique can help ease backaches, neck pains, joint problems, headaches, temporomandibular disorder, repetitive strain injury syndrome and voice strain. It can even be used to help with the swayback posture that pregnancy causes, to aid with childbirth and to lessen breathing woes caused by asthma.

Environmental factors, including fashion, can induce poor posture. For example, two-inch heels and three-pound purses make women especially vulnerable to fashion-induced bad posture, says Don Krim, chairman of the North American Society of Teachers of the Alexander Technique and an instructor in Beverly Hills, California.

Many women often feel compelled to conform to certain body images. If you're a woman that is "too tall," especially as a teen, slouching can become the perfect camouflage. Similarly, younger large-breasted women may hunch their shoulders to hide their chests.

IT'S ALL ABOUT TECHNIQUE

An Alexander Technique instructor can teach you to be more fully aware of yourself when you're walking, standing, sitting and working. Your teacher will combine manual guidance and verbal instruction, and you will be able to apply what you learn in your lesson to your daily life. "The technique is virtually impossible to learn to do on your own," says Schapera.

The learning takes place in two ways, says Deborah Caplan, physical therapist and teacher of the Alexander Technique in New York City. "You learn as the principles are taught to you verbally by a teacher, and you learn on a kinesthetic level by the teacher gently guiding you with her hands into applying the correct use."

Usually, the teacher puts her hand near your head and spine while you sit, stand or move. This helps remind you to keep your head easefully balanced on your spine and helps you maintain a noncompressing posture, says Stern.

Practioners use mirrors to show you the difference between what you feel you're doing with your body and what you're really doing. It can be an eye-opening experience. For example, when your shoulder muscles relax, you might feel like you're slouching, but the mirror shows you standing effortlessly upright, says Schapera.

"The teacher guides you through everyday activities, such as sitting, bending, breathing and talking," Schapera says. "If you were a musician, for example, I would ask you to bring in your instrument so I could see what you do while you play."

Poised for Success

When you think of grace, you picture Fred Astaire and Ginger Rogers flowing across the dance floor in a fluid, athletic whirl.

Well, effortless poise might have come naturally to both of them, but many dancers and actors need a little help. That's why they're among the most common students of the Alexander Technique, says Don Krim, chairman of the North American Society of Teachers of the Alexander Technique and an instructor in Beverly Hills, California.

Today, it's still a vital part of education for any classically trained actor, with Kevin Kline and Kenneth Branagh as just a few of the stars who've had Alexander training, says Krim.

What are the payoffs of studying the Alexander Technique? "It means good posture and coordination," says Judith Stern, physical therapist on the faculty at the American Center for the Alexander Technique in New York City. "The person moves gracefully and easefully, has natural balance and is poised."

And who exemplifies natural grace and ease of movement? Krim mentions Marilyn Monroe, Audrey Hepburn, Whitney Houston, Steffi Graf, Cary Grant, Denzel Washington and, of course, Fred Astaire. Stern puts Mikhail Baryshnikov, Arthur Ashe, Bjorn Borg and diver Greg Louganis on the list as well.

"When you look at them it's so beautiful, and they make it look so easy," says Stern. "Michael Jordan is a perfect example. You watch him and you'd love to be able to move like that. It's a combination of reaching a goal yet staying perfectly free physically."

You'll also learn what Alexander Technique teachers call constructive rest, says Stern. You lie down on your back on the floor or a table, knees bent and feet flat on the surface, and learn to release excess muscle tension in your body.

"Allow your neck to release so that your head balances delicately on top of your spine, then allow your torso to release in length and width," she says. "Then you allow your legs to release from your torso and allow your arms to release from your torso."

How many lessons will you need? While this varies from person to person, it usually takes at least 30 visits to make a lasting difference on your postural habits, says Krim, who recommends scheduling at least one lesson a week.

FREE YOUR BODY

As toddlers, most of us start out with picture-perfect posture, with our heads up and our limbs loose. But around age three we start looking up to our parents—both literally and figuratively, says Krim.

"We model our posture and movement from our parents," Krim says. "For example, a lot of people say lower-back pain runs in their family, and they just assume it's hereditary. But it could actually be from modeling their parents' movements and postural patterns."

People commonly walk with the head pulled back and down on the neck. This compresses the joints and disks of the neck and back disks and can lead to physical woes such as headaches, says Caplan. "The head weighs about 12 pounds, and the vertebrae at the top of the spine are very delicate," she says. "People should ask themselves, 'Could I have less tension in my neck and shoulders?' "

Bad posture also affects breathing, notes Stern. The diaphragm, the muscle separating the chest from the abdomen—has to move down in the torso to draw breath in. "If it's all compressed and crunched, there's no place for the diaphragm to go," Stern says. "When there's more room for the diaphragm to descend, breathing automatically gets fuller."

That's how the Alexander Technique can aid people with asthma, a condition of recurrent attacks of breathlessness and wheezing, by teaching them to take in a full amount of air with each breath, says Stern. "One thing that happens with asthma is that you panic and can't get breath. This helps to quiet the system rather than getting it all worked up," she says. "It doesn't take away asthma—it's a coping mechanism."

Like Lamaze, the Alexander Technique teaches you to work with pain during childbirth and stay calm. You learn not to pull in and contract all your muscles against the pain but to stay relaxed, Stern says. "Your habitual response to pain is to close down and to hold until the pain passes, but this technique is a way of counteracting that."

Pregnant women learn how to counteract their shift in balance, she says. They're taught how to stop the standard pregnancy swayback as well as how to lie down and stand differently, with the head leading and the spine following.

BALANCING YOUR BODY

Here are a few hints from top Alexander Technique instructors about how to put your posture into tip-top form.

Kick off your heels. High-heeled shoes are an enemy to good posture because of the way they slant the foot and throw the body out of alignment, notes Caplan. Flats with cushioned soles give the best support. "Walking in high heels jars the whole body," she says. "The foot is designed

Getting**Started**

Alexander Technique

The Alexander Technique teaches you new posture and movement patterns, to reduce wear and tear on your body as you go about your everyday activities.

Number of practitioners in the United States: Between 700 and 800.

Qualifications to look for: Certification from a professional association or a teacher-training course. Certified teachers of the Alexander Technique typically undergo a minimum of 1,600 hours of specialized training over a period of approximately three years.

Professional associations: Alexander Technique International, 1692 Massachusetts Avenue, Cambridge, MA 02138; American Center for the Alexander Technique, 129 East 67th Street, New York, NY 10023; North American Society of Teachers of the Alexander Technique, 1-800-473-0620.

To find a practitioner: Contact one of the professional associations listed above.

Approximate cost: $45 to $60 for a 30- to 45-minute one-on-one session with an instructor.

to absorb the shock of walking, but with heels the result is a tremendous amount of stress on the back."

Unlock those legs. Perhaps more than men, women commonly cross their legs and hold the inner thighs together, which can lead to back problems because of a twist it creates in the lower spine and pelvis, notes Krim. "They're often told to keep their legs together. But keeping your legs together as you move can distort the balance between the hip, knee and ankle joints, causing strain."

Rather than pulling your knees together after you sit down, keep each knee lined up with your feet. If you wear miniskirts and want to maintain decorum in dress, you may have to trade in your miniskirts for long dresses and slacks in order to sit correctly.

Sit up tall. Many working women spend their days slouched behind a computer, says Caplan. For good sitting posture, it's most important to have a chair that supports the lower back—one that's not so deep or high that your feet can't rest comfortably on the floor. "Slouching undermines support of the spine and weakens the muscles, stretches the ligaments and strains the facet joints in the back of the spine and the disks," she says. "Plus, the shoulders slip forward and put strain on the neck."

Try to avoid sitting in peculiar positions. Tucking one leg under the other might give you a sense of support, for instance, but it actually causes the body to twist and contort, notes Schapera. It is ideal to sit with your feet apart and have them resting on an adjustable footrest or flat on the floor, which gives more support to the back.

Bend with care. When you reach down to pick something up, make sure that you're not just bending at the waist, says Stern. "You should be bending over so that the hips, knees and ankles are doing the work," she says. "When you bend at your waist, the spine has no hinge joints at that point. It's a real strain because the back muscles aren't designed for that kind of work."

Hold 'em high. Sitting at your computer typing all day won't be as big of a strain on your neck and back if you adjust your body, says Stern. "Your hands shouldn't be down too low. They should be up near chest level so that you don't have to keep dropping your head to see the screen or keyboard," she says. Your work area should be more like an architect's drawing board, which is nearer to chest level, Stern explains.

Stand up for yourself. Long hours of sitting without a break are sure to aggravate posture problems, notes Schapera. "All you need to do is stand up every 20 minutes or so and then sit back down again. Otherwise, your muscles get fatigued and have no choice but to tighten and collapse into themselves."

The Wrong Way to Sit

Sitting with the body heavily slumped and the head pulled back into the neck puts tension on the ligaments and joints supporting the spine. Slouching also strains the neck and undermines breathing.

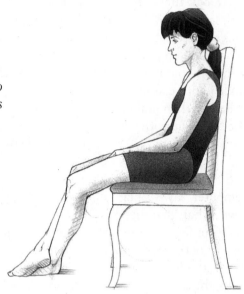

The Right Way to Sit

To lengthen your spine and release tension in your neck, sit back in your chair with your feet flat on the ground. To breathe more fully, hold your head up.

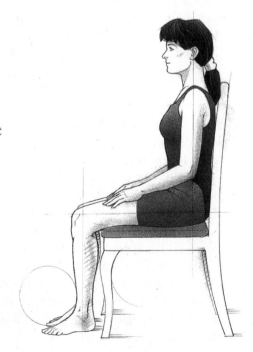

The Wrong Way to Sit at a Computer

Sitting with your hands too low on the keyboard and your computer screen at chest level forces you to continually look from your screen to your keyboard. When that happens, your shoulders tend to slouch, causing neck and back tension.

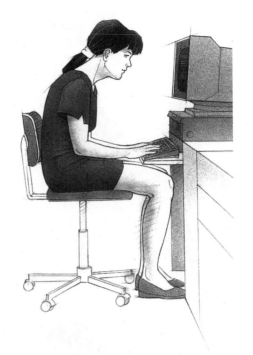

The Right Way to Sit at a Computer

To keep your spine aligned, your torso lengthened and your neck and shoulders pain-free, raise your keyboard to chest level and keep your screen at eye level.

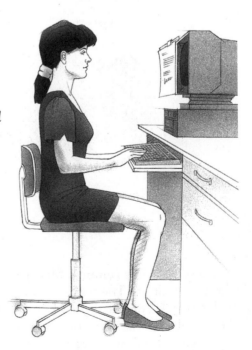

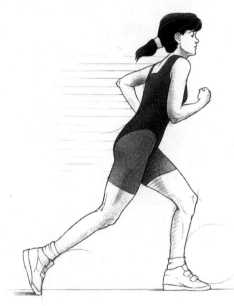

The Wrong Way to Run

Pulling your head back and down while running throws it out of alignment with your torso and legs, putting pressure on your back.

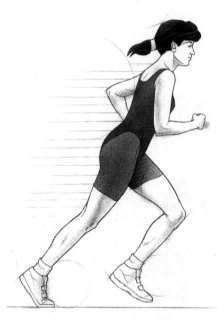

The Right Way to Run

To run with ease, hold your head upward, keep it balanced above your neck and lengthen your spine.

Do some heady running. Most people jog with their heads back and down, says Stern. The result is that you end up pulling your head back rather than keeping it aligned with your torso and legs. "Don't move your head in the opposite direction of your legs," says Stern. "Keep your head balanced and your spine lengthened."

Don't hold the phone. If you're on the phone all day—especially if you're typing while talking—you harm your body by pressing the receiver to your shoulder, says Stern. Use a headset to avoid spine compression and body contortion, she says.

The Right Way to Read

To support your back and arms and prevent discomfort as you read, rest your book on a sloped surface with your feet flat on the ground and lean forward at the hips.

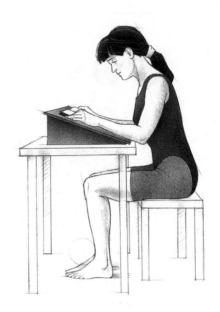

Read at an angle. Want plenty of support while you're reading? Reclining chairs are best, says Schapera. If you're sitting at a table, rest your book at a slope in front of you rather than flat on the table. If you're sitting in a chair, put a pillow in your lap and place the book on that. Your arms won't tire, and you'll avoid the temptation to slump.

Cue yourself to remember. Post notes reminding yourself to be aware of your posture, Stern suggests. "You could stick a note on your computer that says, 'Think.' You'll start paying attention to how you're holding yourself: Are your legs relaxed? How are you breathing? Things like that," she says.

Ditch the bag-lady look. Hauling an enormous purse can throw your body out of alignment, so it's important to find a good balance, says Krim. Although backpack-style purses have straps going over both shoulders, they tend to make women contort their bodies differently. "I see people with backpacks who completely collapse forward or collapse backward until the backpack is digging into the lower back," he notes.

"Don't contort yourself to fit the bag. The key is to find a good balanced state—to carry the bag and not let the bag carry you," says Krim.

AROMATHERAPY
Healing with Nature's Scents

Close your eyes and picture yourself strolling through a formal rose garden on a warm June day. The air is still, and the intensely lush, sensuous perfume from hundreds of full-blown blooms utterly envelopes you.

Scene change.

Now you're deep within the bosom of an aromatic pine forest. Each step you take crushes pine needles under your feet, releasing even more crisp, invigorating fragrance as you walk.

How did those two mind-strolls make you feel?

According to those who practice the art of aromatherapy, the answer, quite likely, is "quite different."

The scent of roses, for example, is thought by aromatherapists to be soothing and spiritually uplifting. In contrast, pine is known for its stimulating, revitalizing qualities.

NATURE IN A BOTTLE

Aromatherapy takes the soothing or energizing powers of scent one step further. Pure essential oils are distilled from plants, which are then inhaled or applied to the skin in various ways. Aromatherapists believe that each essential oil possesses unique healing qualities, and they recommend the oils for everything from arthritis and high blood pressure to fluid retention and cellulite, among numerous other health concerns. Essential oils are utilized in various forms—diffused into the air and inhaled, added to the bath, applied (during massage) or incorporated into compresses, creams and lotions.

And though the roots of aromatherapy are ancient, it took a twentieth-century French chemist named René-Maurice Gattefossé to coin the term *aromatherapie* and spark the development of aromatherapy as a healing art.

While working for his family's perfume company, Gattefossé learned the hard way that essential oils had healing powers when he plunged his badly burned hand into a vat of pure lavender oil. His hand healed within hours, unscarred and uninfected, prompting Gattefossé to begin exploring the use of essential oils in dermatology and cosmetics.

FOR WOMEN, AN EMOTIONAL LINK

Almost everyone can benefit from using essential oils, according to Michael Scholes, president of Michael Scholes School of Aromatic Studies in Los Angeles and author of *Aromatherapy Pocket Guide*, who holds a degree in advanced aromatherapy from the Bretland School in London.

But, Scholes notes, "Ninety-five percent of the people I train to practice aromatherapy are women, possibly because aromatherapy makes such sense to them and because it's so familiar. Historically, there's a connection between women and plants and between women and aromatherapy."

According to aromatherapist Joan Clark, Scholes' partner and vice-president of Michael Scholes School of Aromatic Studies, aromatherapy can help women stimulate the process of emotional healing.

"Lots of women aren't taking the time for themselves that they should," says Clark. "Especially business women who may feel the need to put forth lots of male energy and sublimate their essential feminine natures. When a woman like this comes in for an aromatherapy session, she gets the undivided time and attention of a therapist who anoints her body with essential oils that make her feel wonderful. That alone is a very powerful healing tool."

What is it about the essential oils that stimulate a woman's emotional healing?

"True essential oils, as opposed to the lifeless synthetic compounds that comprise most commercial fragrances, are distilled from plants and flowers—living creations that have energy," says Clark. "When you use essential oils with aromas that please you, their energy can stimulate and uplift you, or relax and calm you, based on your needs."

"Most of the women who see me want a natural antidote for stress and insomnia, and some ask me for aromatherapy to help boost their energy," says Francois Michel, founder of the American Society of Aromatherapy and aromatherapy instructor at Temple University in Philadelphia. "When a client consults me, I interview her carefully to determine her needs and lifestyle. Then I can create a personalized blend of essential oils that helps her feel better."

SCIENCE OR FOLKLORE?

If you're wondering exactly how various aromas can alleviate disease, so are plenty of other people. Does it work? Is there any proof to the health claims?

Getting science to back the benefits of aromatherapy is tricky. To show that a drug (or treatment) works, scientists rely on carefully controlled double-blind studies—that is, they test two identical drugs (or treatments): a fake one and the real thing. The fake (placebo) drug must be undistinguishable from the real drug; neither the researcher nor the individuals tested can know who gets which, to minimize the power of suggestion.

For attempts to test aromatherapy oils, that presents a real problem. The oils by nature are readily distinguishable by their aromas, according to J. R. King, associate fellow in the Department of Psychology at the University of Warwick in Coventry, England. So, according to scientists, good research on aromatherapy is hard to find.

"Most of the information you read about aromatherapy's benefits is based on folklore," says Susan Knasko, Ph.D., an environmental psychologist at the Monell Chemical Senses Center in Philadelphia. "There just isn't a lot of scientific research to back it up."

"But that's not to say that if aromatherapy were studied, it wouldn't show some benefits," adds Dr. Knasko. "For example, there's a handful of studies on the effect of odor on mood. And although there are a lot of conflicting results, it seems that in general, pleasant odors tend to put people in a good mood while unpleasant odors tend to put people in a bad mood."

One way aromatherapy may be beneficial is by making your everyday experience more pleasant, says Dr. Knasko. "Anything that makes your environment more pleasant seems to be good for you emotionally," she continues. "Therefore, aromatherapy has the potential to be an effective stress-buster. Scenting a room with a pleasing fragrance, taking a warm bath with a scent you especially like, choosing music that relaxes you and lighting that soothes you—these are techniques that can help you gain control over a stressful environment." And, she adds, exercising control over a stressor or even just thinking that you have control over it can be an excellent way to combat the negative effects of stress.

OILS AGAINST STRESS

For general relaxation, renewed energy or stress relief, aromatherapy is easily learned at home. Essential oils can be added to your bath, diluted in a carrier oil (a neutral, nonaromatic oil) and used in massage, applied to hankies or compresses, placed on lightbulb fragrance rings or used in special aromatherapy diffusers. You can also put a few drops of oil in a bucket of hot water and place the bucket in the tub when you shower.

"The best way to familiarize yourself with aromatherapy is to read up on the subject, learn about the healing properties of the major essential oils and learn how to put its stress-balancing benefits to work for you," says Jane Buckle, R.N., a certified aromatherapist and aromatherapy teacher in England and author of *Clinical Aromatherapy in Nursing.*

Though scores of different essential oils are used for therapeutic effect,

The Divinely Relaxing Aromatherapy Massage

Many massage therapists, spas and beauty salons offer aromatherapy massages—with good reason. Experiencing an aromatherapy massage has been described as heavenly bliss.

As those hands work rhythmically up and down your back, neck and shoulders, kinks and knots will melt away. Then, ever so gently, those hands will smooth away worry, tension and stress as they play over the frown lines on your face. And by the time those hands apply themselves to each and every one of your toes and fingers, you may hear yourself sighing audibly in pure pleasure.

If you decide to make an appointment, count on spending an hour or more, and plan on bringing sweats to wear après massage so you don't get oil residue on your good clothes.

You'll be draped in soft sheets, and you'll lie on a padded massage table while warm, strong hands apply oil chosen especially for you to your body.

"Before I give you an aromatherapy massage, I'll question you thoroughly about your medical history and about what you'd like me to work on," says Margot Latimer, a certified massage therapist who practices in Doylestown, Pennsylvania.

Latimer calls stress, muscle aches and other concerns not problems but projects that the proper combination of essential oils and hands-on healing can help relieve. After a 20- to 30-minute interview, Latimer will look through the oils in her special purple box and select no more than four that she determines will be the most effective. Before she adds them to the pure grapeseed oil that she'll use to massage you, she may give you some choices. She says, "It's critical that the woman really likes the blend that is created."

here are the ones aromatherapists say that they most frequently use as stress-busters.

Basil: nature's nerve tonic. Aromatherapists call basil a natural nerve tonic. Try mixing one to five drops of pure essential oil in a thimbleful of alcohol such as vodka before mixing with four ounces of distilled water in a clean spray bottle (usually in housewares departments or drugstores). Store in the refrigerator. Shake well and, avoiding your eyes, spritz it on your skin as a refreshing pick-me-up. Or mix pure essential oil with a thimbleful of milk and add it to your bath.

Clary sage: the mood elevator. Clarysage oil is "an absolutely brilliant confidence restorer and mood elevator," says Buckle. Don't mix it with alcohol, however.

Geranium: the hormonal balancer. One to five drops of geranium makes a delightful accompaniment when added to your bath or mixed into your lotion. Aromatherapists say it can help balance mood swings and ease depression, premenstrual syndrome and irregular or painful periods.

Lavender: the insomniac's friend. Considered one of the most important of the essential oils, aromatherapists believe lavender has relaxing effects that can calm anxiety and help you sleep. They believe lavender has painkilling properties. Use it for massage, inhalation or in the bath.

Roman chamomile: for bad dreams or bad moods. Aromatherapists praise the scent of chamomile for its effects as a mild sedative and antidepressant. Used during a massage or a bath, on compresses or diffused, you might even try it to relieve nightmares or stall your toddler's tantrum. If you're allergic to ragweed, avoid chamomile—they're closely related.

Sweet orange: an emotional pick-me-up. "To lift your spirits, try a few drops of oil of sweet orange in a bath, or blend it with lavender for an emotional boost," says Michel.

GROUND RULES

For best results, Buckle advises following these simple rules when using aromatherapy at home.

Dilute your oils. Always dilute essential oils before applying them to the skin, says Buckle. She suggests blending essential oils with a cold-pressed carrier oil such as grapeseed oil, available in some health food stores.

Beware the sun. Some oils, like bergamot, angelica root and all essential oils obtained from citrus peels, can cause phototoxicity. That means that using them on skin exposed to sunlight might cause a rash or burning sensation. Never apply essential oils to exposed skin when you're going to be out in the sun.

Please don't drink the oil. Never take essential oils internally except under the guidance of a qualified health care professional. Many are toxic.

Talk to your doctor. If you are receiving chemotherapy or radiation treatment or you are taking any medication, check with your doctor before using essential oils—they could interact with your treatment.

Store your oils in a safe place. Essential oils are concentrated substances and should be treated like medicines. So store them as you would any medicine—out of the reach of children. And keep in mind that vials are not childproof. "Even one teaspoon of eucalyptus oil, for example, could be fatal to a child," notes Buckle.

Getting**Started** ●

Aromatherapy

Aromatherapists are commonly trained in other forms of therapy. If you want to experience the rejuvenating effects of aromatherapy, ask reflexologists, massage therapists and chiropractors in your area if they incorporate essential oils in their practice. And be wary of practitioners who make claims that certain aromas can cure serious health conditions.

Number of practitioners in the United States: Approximately 3,000.

Qualifications to look for: Completion of courses in aromatherapy offered by schools or professional associations. Aromatherapists are certified in Europe but not the United States.

Professional associations: American Society of Aromatherapy, P.O. Box 95, Wallingford, PA 19086; National Association for Holistic Aromatherapy, P.O. Box 17622, Boulder, CO 80308.

To find a practitioner: Contact the professional associations of aromatherapists listed above.

Approximate cost: $50 to $100 per session.

Purchasing information: Always buy pure essential oils, labeled with the correct botanical name, from a reputable supplier (ideally, someone recommended by an aromatherapist) who guarantees that the essential oil is steam-distilled and medicinal strength.

Due to variations in the amount of plant material needed to produce essential oils, the cost varies greatly—$3 to $25, depending on the oil you select.

ART THERAPY
Let the Pictures Do the Talking

Women being treated at the University of Washington Medical Center in Seattle sometimes get modeling clay with their chemotherapy, paint pots with their postsurgical painkillers or pastels with their kidney dialysis treatment.

That's because in addition to the usual complement of surgeons, cardiologists, oncologists, orthopedists and assorted other medical specialists, the Seattle hospital employs its own artist-in-residence, Dianne Erickson. On any given day, you might find Erickson sketching a young girl in pediatrics, giving a woman in dialysis tips on using pastels or helping someone being treated for cancer piece together a collage.

The hospital's artist-in-residence program, one of several nationwide, is colorful testimony to the potential benefits of recreational art.

"We've found that recreational art relieves patients' boredom, distracts them from pain, provides a pleasurable respite from treatment and gives them something to do when they return home after treatment," says Lynn Basa, the program's director. "They discover they actually like making art once someone's shown them how."

While the Seattle program is completely recreational, other programs incorporate art as outright therapy. At Shands Hospital, an affiliate of the University of Florida at Gainesville, nurses who introduced an art program found that it helped alleviate anxiety and loneliness among those they cared for.

The benefits aren't limited to hospital settings, either. Using biofeedback equipment to measure stress in children, a researcher at the College of Notre Dame in Belmont, California, found that drawing helped ease anxiety. In a similar experiment, another researcher found that adolescents' anxiety levels dropped significantly when they worked on collages using reproductions of great masterpieces.

"Just looking at the works of the old masters greatly reduces stress levels," says Doris Arrington, Ed.D., an art therapist, licensed psychologist, and professor and director of the art therapy and marital and family therapy program at the College of Notre Dame. Dr. Arrington often uses the technique in stress-reduction workshops with adults, asking them to make collages from copies of old-master paintings.

"When you look at art, it moves you out of the ordinary," she explains. "If you're worrying or obsessing over something, looking at art can take you out of that cycle and all of a sudden enable you to move forward."

ART, HEALING AND THE MIND

Though effective in helping patients deal with chronic physical pain, art finds a wider application in the treatment of emotional pain.

Most art therapists are psychotherapists trained in both art and psychotherapy. In institutional settings and private practices, they help men and women being treated for disabilities, trauma or stroke express themselves through art. They work with individuals struggling with chronic mental illness, addictions, depression, anxiety, stress, grief, troubled relationships and legacies of abuse.

Men and women seem to do equally well in art therapy. "But women are likely to be a little more interested in art therapy for self-exploration," notes Harriet Wadeson, Ph.D., a registered art therapist, professor and coordinator of the art therapy graduate program at the University of Illinois at Chicago and author of *Art Psychotherapy* and *The Dynamics of Art Psychotherapy*. "I think women are more interested in self-exploration, period."

IN THE STUDIO

What happens in art therapy depends on the therapist's style and your goals. A therapist might recommend couples or family therapy for relationship problems. For clients who have trouble relating to nonfamily members or who would benefit from peer support, she might suggest group sessions. Groups usually bring together people with similar histories or goals—breast cancer survivors, for instance, or women who want to strengthen their self-esteem.

To get things rolling during a session, a therapist might suggest a specific exercise—asking you to draw what you would find if you wandered through a cave, for example. Participants choose their media, anything from paint to clay to papier-mâché. To get a woman to talk about the work she's creating, Virginia Minar, a registered art therapist and past president of the American Art Therapy Association in Mundelein, Illinois, asks questions like, "What does that image mean to you?" or, "Who does this figure represent?"

Though art therapists may cover the same turf talk therapists do, art therapy offers several advantages, according to Dr. Arrington and others.

For starters, it's easier to express troubled feelings through art than through talk because art allows distance, explains Bruce Moon, a registered art therapist and director of the Marywood College art therapy program in Scranton, Pennsylvania. We might not be able to talk about how we feel, but we can talk about how the woman that we drew feels.

"You don't even have to be an art therapist to see the connection," Moon says. "It helps them, though, to create that distance."

While working with images, we're also less likely to censor ourselves, Dr. Wadeson adds. Since we're accustomed to using words to communicate, we're more adept at screening out comments that might be frightening or threatening. Communicating through art, however, we're more likely to have the occasional revealing "slip of the brush."

Artistic ability isn't required in art therapy. "Anyone can make marks on paper. The results can be surprising, and the discoveries that the art provides can be illuminating," says Dr. Wadeson.

WHEN WORDS FAIL

Sometimes, simply expressing feelings through art is enough. "One of the hardest things for many breast cancer survivors is that their families don't want them to talk about the cancer after they've been in remission awhile," explains Minar. "But they're really afraid of a recurrence and they need to express this. Expressing it in art helps ease the fear."

Simply by offering an opportunity to create, art therapy can be empowering, Moon adds. "Making an image or sculpture is putting yourself in a position of being a creator, rather than a victim," he explains. "There's a sense of mastery that enhances one's self-regard."

Art also offers a way to work through difficult experiences, make sense of them and find meaning, Dr. Wadeson notes.

"After my father died, I made art and wrote poetry about it," she says. "Doing that brought about a transformation of the pain I felt. It helped me integrate the pain. Doing something creative helped with the grieving."

Finally, art offers women the chance to explore options, Dr. Wadeson says. One of her clients, she recalls, explored the possibility of divorce. The woman joined therapy after a suicide attempt. "She tried traditional therapy with a psychiatrist, but her feelings were very locked up inside her."

Not so in art therapy. To her surprise, the woman began to draw vivid pictures of herself—violently attacking her husband. Most of her life, it turned out, she'd sacrificed her own wishes for those of her children and her demanding spouse. In art therapy, she realized that she was furious with him. She also drew pictures that spoke of her own sadness—in one she showed her brain, brimming with trapped tears. After she'd spent time exploring and expressing her feelings, the woman began to get more perspective on her situation.

"Eventually, she said that she realized the problems weren't all her husband's fault, and she was able to take some responsibility, too," Dr. Wadeson says. She explored various options in her art, including divorce, depicting herself and her life as it would be if she ended her marriage. Ultimately, she decided against that but began doing more for herself. She started working on art outside therapy, and selling her work, Dr. Wadeson notes.

TRY IT YOURSELF

If you're seriously depressed or struggling in the aftermath of a traumatic experience, it's a good idea to seek professional counseling, say experts. But

Getting**Started**

Art Therapy

Most art therapists are psychotherapists trained in both art and psychotherapy. They may work privately or as a member of a team of caregivers and can be found in hospitals, clinics and schools.

Number of practitioners in the United States: Approximately 4,000.

Qualifications to look for: Registered Art Therapist (A.T.R.) or Board-Certified Registered Art Therapist (A.T.R.–BC). Registration requires a master's degree in art therapy or a master's degree with an emphasis in art therapy.

Professional associations: American Art Therapy Association, 1202 Allanson Road, Mundelein, IL 60060; Art Therapy Credentials Board, 401 North Michigan Avenue, Chicago, IL 60611.

To find a practitioner: Contact one of the organizations listed above.

Approximate cost: $25 per hour or more at a hospital or in a group setting or $50 to $90 per hour for private sessions.

if you're simply bored, under stress or looking for a way to improve communication with loved ones, you can use art on your own.

Here's how to get started.

Set up a "mini-gallery." Simply looking at art can help relieve stress, Dr. Arrington says. Buy a calendar of artwork you like and put it on your wall, or pick up a glossy art book and keep it near your desk.

Dabble. If you want to create your own art and have little or no experience, choose media that are easy to use and require little preparation or clean up. Dr. Wadeson and others recommend colored pencils, pastels, felt-tipped markers and modeling clay. You can find basic art supplies in the toy, craft or office supply sections of discount stores, drugstores and even grocery stores.

Pound away tension. "Clay is a wonderful medium because it's totally forgiving and allows you to vent a lot of feeling. You can pound it, poke it, rip it, whatever you like," Dr. Wadeson says.

Doodle as you dawdle. Doodling is a reliable stress reducer, Minar says. Keep colored pencils, felt-tipped pens, chalks or pastels in your desk drawer for stressful days at work. Toss your colored pencils into your purse with some paper so you can doodle on the go.

Write your own captions. "I encourage people to keep a journal that includes both writing and drawings," Dr. Arrington says. That way, you can jot down what you were thinking and feeling as you sketched.

BIOFEEDBACK
Listen to Your Body

The weather. Aging. Traffic. Income taxes. Rude people. Unfortunately, a list of all the things you can't control in life is practically endless.

But there's also some good news. You can learn to control most of the vital functions that affect your health—from blood pressure to pulse rate to body temperature, among others. Imagine learning how to divert blood away from your head to alleviate your migraine. Or relaxing specific muscles to relieve neck pain or fibromyalgia. Or even controlling incontinence by learning to contract certain muscles.

Women are great at reading other people's emotions, but the ability to read your body's reactions is something that comes with practice—and a little biofeedback training.

That's right—biofeedback. It might sound complicated, but it's actually just the monitoring of blood pressure, temperature, muscle tension, heartbeat or brain waves, which is turned into easy-to-interpret sounds, temperature or video images for the person being monitored.

Medical science first tuned in to biofeedback in the 1960s. Now it's used by mainstream medical doctors, psychologists and psychiatrists to help women relieve stubborn migraine headaches and other stress-related complaints, among other health conditions.

You begin with about ten one-hour sessions of supervised biofeedback training on a specially designed apparatus, then you practice—and apply biofeedback—on your own, says Angele McGrady, Ph.D., professor of psychiatry and physiology at the Medical College of Ohio in Toledo and past president of the Association for Applied Psychophysiology and Biofeedback based in Wheatridge, Colorado.

HOOK UP, TUNE IN

Typically, you sit in a chair with three wired metal sensors attached to a band on your head. From a pair of headphones, you hear something resembling static. Each click of the static means your brain is emitting an alpha wave, associated with relaxation. The more you relax, the faster the clicks keep coming. By listening to the clicks, you can gauge how well your body responds and learn how to modify your response.

"Paying attention is crucial in biofeedback," notes Susana A. Galle, Ph.D., director of the Body-Mind Center and clinical assistant professor of pediatrics at Georgetown University Medical School, both in Washington, D.C. "By monitoring audiovisual signals such as pictures or musical tones from a computer connected to the biofeedback equipment, you establish a bridge between stress and its physiological effects. Then you can start to control it."

The specifics of biofeedback will vary from session to session and practitioner to practitioner. Generally, during the first session, the practitioner will try to get a sense of how you react to stress.

First, the practitioner takes a baseline reading of your relaxation level. While hooked up to a monitor, you relax as the practitioner measures your muscle tension, temperature and heart rate for four minutes. During the next four minutes, you perform a challenging mental task such as counting backward by sevens, which usually raises blood pressure and lowers the temperature of the hands. Then it's back to relaxation mode. Next is a period where you talk about an emotional problem, with the last four minutes spent achieving relaxation again.

"It's important for the practitioner to first observe a woman's level of stress and then how quickly she recovers," says Dr. Galle. "If a woman doesn't recover quickly, it means her stress baseline is high. Biofeedback helps a woman see how she reacts to stress and how she can control it by regulating how her body and mind work."

LEARN TO EASE UP

Having sensors and wires hooked to your body while monitors flash and tones beep might resemble a scene from a science fiction movie, but biofeedback's premise is downright simple, notes Dr. McGrady. "The idea is to take a body function that previously was thought to be uncontrollable, then show it to a person and teach them how to change that function."

Perhaps the simplest biofeedback exercise involves learning to warm up your hands (considered a sure sign of being relaxed). By pinching a sensor at the end of a wire attached to a handheld digital monitor, you measure your peripheral body temperature (which is slightly lower than your core temperature of 98.6°F). With the help of meditation or yoga or whatever relaxation method works best, you concentrate on raising that tempera-

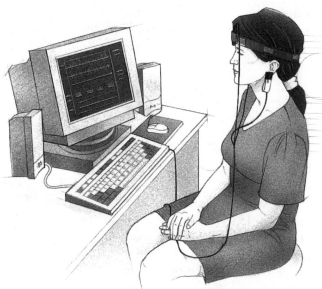

A Typical Biofeedback Set-Up

Biofeedback machines vary in design. Fairly high-tech but easy to use, they monitor physiological responses such as heartbeat, blood pressure or muscle tension. Sensors translate those responses in various ways—through a computer monitor (shown here), a meter, a light or a tone. Reading and understanding these signals can allow you to control your body's reaction to pain or stress.

ture, with the ultimate goal being 95°F, explains George Fritz, Ed.D., a psychologist with the Pain Management and Biofeedback Institute in Bethlehem, Pennsylvania.

"Relaxation is a skill like any other—it can be taught," notes Dr. Mc-Grady. "I have women tighten the muscles in their arms or in their foreheads and let them hear the beeps, then tell them to relax and compare."

REAPING THE BENEFITS

Because stress causes neurochemical changes in your body, many ailments that women suffer are brought on or aggravated by it. These are the conditions for which biofeedback works best—decreased appetite and diminished sex drive if related to anxiety, high blood pressure triggered by stress, and certain types of depression and pain.

Studies show that biofeedback works. It's been effectively used to treat many stress-related disorders that commonly plague women—certain forms of urinary incontinence, migraine and tension headaches, fibromyalgia (painful "trigger points" in muscles) and temporomandibular disorder.

Biofeedback is especially useful for women because they're more likely to get vasoconstrictive disorders—that is, blood vessels that misbehave—causing migraine headaches, Raynaud's disease and cold hands and feet. For similar reasons, practitioners also find that biofeedback training helps relieve hot flashes and premenstrual syndrome.

With the use of biofeedback, men and women with diabetes can be taught to increase the skin temperature in their feet and legs, according to a study conducted at the University of Wisconsin in La Crosse.

Biofeedback has even been shown to boost women's immune systems. The results of a study of 13 women who had undergone modified radical mastectomies suggest that a daily routine of relaxation, imagery and biofeedback training help boost the immune system by increasing the number of killer T-cells. Since these T-cells are champion disease-fighters in your body, when you increase their number, you're elevating your body's immune power.

SOLO FEEDBACK

The whole goal of biofeedback is to be able to do it on your own, notes Dr. McGrady.

"Women who are taught biofeedback learn to react not with tension and anxiety but with relaxation," she notes. "Eventually, women should start being able to read their own body's stress responses with no external monitors and remember how to counteract them."

"You want to maintain a baseline relaxation response so you're not revving your engines," explains Joseph P. Primavera III, Ph.D., psychologist and co-director of the Comprehensive Headache Center at Germantown Hospital and Medical Center in Philadelphia. "If your boss is a tremendous pain, you can't smack him in the head or quit, so you start revving your engine. And that's not a healthy thing to do. Biofeedback is a way to measure how well you control your fight-or-flight response. It just gives you feedback about whether your relaxation technique is causing physiological change," he explains.

"Women say, 'I know how to relax. After I get the kids fed and help them with their homework, I take a bath and light a candle at around 10:00 P.M.,'" says Dr. Primavera. "But learning to ease up and let go isn't that easy, especially in a world where women are expected to do it all. Biofeedback is a technique that's pretty easy to build into any lifestyle. Women can do it sitting in their cars or standing—whenever they need it."

PRACTICE, PRACTICE, PRACTICE

The whole key to biofeedback is to eventually be able to do it sans apparatus. So practice is the key, notes Dr. McGrady.

Here are a few ways to help you get the most out of biofeedback training.

Pick a technique, any technique. For biofeedback to work, you need to employ some kind of relaxation technique, such as visualization or meditation. (For more on visualization and meditation, see pages 204 and 233.) Or try passive relaxation, which means that you simply concentrate on the words or phrases that help you relax. Dr. McGrady suggests phrases such

Getting**Started**

Biofeedback

A variety of health practitioners—from psychologists to dentists and from physicians and nurses to physical therapists—use biofeedback. Here's how to locate a practitioner trained in the use of this technique.

Number of practitioners in the United States: Between 5,400 and 7,200.

Qualifications to look for: Certification by the Biofeedback Certification Institute of America (BCIA). If certified, BCIA-C will be added to their credentials. This certification, however, is not mandatory in order to practice biofeedback.

Professional associations: Association for Applied Psychophysiology and Biofeedback (AAPB), 10200 West 44th Avenue, Suite 304, Wheatridge, CO 80033.

To find a practitioner: Contact your state chapter of the AAPB through the address listed above, or send a self-addressed, stamped envelope to the Biofeedback Certification Institute of America (also at the AAPB address above) and ask for a list of certified biofeedback specialists in your area.

Approximate cost: Varies according to the area in which you live.

as, "I feel calm; I feel relaxed; my arms and legs are heavy," or phrases related to warmth.

Do it daily. You should find a quiet place and get into a comfortable position, but not one so comfortable that you'll fall asleep, notes Dr. McGrady. "Then take 10 to 15 minutes two times a day to practice your relaxation technique," she says.

Monitor your progress. To get an idea of how well you're relaxing, Dr. Fritz suggests that you use an inexpensive handheld digital thermometer, similar to those used in office sessions. Available from many practitioners or in stores that sell alternative healing products, a handheld thermometer can provide a quick affirmation of your relaxation level by showing if your peripheral temperature is dropping or rising.

BREATH WORK

Deep Breathing for Better Health

A holistic psychiatrist, C. Shaffia Laue, M.D., sees women with a wide range of problems—everything from anxiety and depression to chronic fatigue. Even so, she says that the same treatment may be helpful to all of them as part of their therapy.

"I tell them to breathe," says Dr. Laue, who practices in Lawrence, Kansas. The treatment that she offers always involves psychotherapy, but it often includes breathing lessons as well.

Truth be told, most of us have forgotten how to breathe correctly. Proper breathing not only helps alleviate psychological problems but it also helps soothe physical ones like premenstrual syndrome (PMS), asthma and insomnia, says Dr. Laue and other advocates of the therapy known as breath work.

We're born breathing the right way, says Dr. Laue. The right way to breathe is deep down in our abdomens. Watch a newborn's tummy slowly rise and fall with each inhalation and exhalation and you'll see how it's done. Unfortunately, most of us unwittingly switch from deep abdominal breathing to shallow "chest breathing" over time. We hold our stomachs tight and start breathing shallowly.

Shallow breathing spells trouble because it delivers less air per breath to our lungs, says Robert Fried, Ph.D., professor of psychology at Hunter College, City University of New York, director of the Stress and Biofeedback Clinic at the Institute for Rational Emotive Therapy in Manhattan and author of *The Breath Connection*. Less air per breath means that we take more frequent breaths, but this only makes matters worse, triggering a series of physiological changes that constrict our blood vessels.

"The end result of the whole process is that less oxygen reaches the brain, the heart and the rest of the body," says Dr. Fried.

This undersupply of oxygen can leave us feeling dizzy and shaky, groggy and ill-equipped to make decisions. A chronic undersupply of oxygen can contribute to fatigue, depression, stress, anxiety and even panic attacks and phobias, explains Dr. Laue.

Shallow chest breathing can also contribute to stress-related disorders such as PMS, menstrual cramps, headaches, migraines, insomnia, high blood pressure, asthma, back pain and allergies, says Jeff Migdow, M.D., a holistic medical doctor and director of yoga teacher–training at the Kripalu Center for Yoga and Health in Lenox, Massachusetts, and co-author of *Take a Deep Breath.*

Since rapid shallow breathing leads to the constriction of blood vessels, it can boost blood pressure and even trigger arterial spasms, says Dr. Fried.

THE GENESIS OF BREATHING DISORDERS

What makes us switch from deep, satisfying abdominal breathing to shallow chest breathing in the first place? Stress, among other things, Dr. Laue says.

When you're under stress, your diaphragm—the internal muscle between your chest and abdomen—contracts partway. This shrinks the space in your chest into which your lungs can expand, Dr. Fried explains. Your breathing becomes shallow and rapid, your blood vessels contract and you start selling yourself short on oxygen. Since rapid shallow breathing also contributes to stress, it creates a vicious cycle. Stress leads to shallow breathing, which leads to stress, and so on.

Throwing your shoulders back, sucking your stomach in and puffing your chest out—the way your mother told you to—can also keep your lungs from expanding fully and lead to shallow chest breathing, adds Dr. Laue.

Respiratory problems such as asthma can also trigger rapid shallow

Check Your Breathing

Most of us breathe shallowly, from our chests, says C. Shaffia Laue, M.D., a holistic psychiatrist who uses breath work in her Lawrence, Kansas, practice. To determine if you're a chest breather, try this simple self-test.

Sit comfortably in a chair and put one hand on your chest and one on your abdomen. Inhale. If the hand on your chest rises more than the hand on your abdomen, you're chest breathing, says Dr. Laue. Follow the exercises in this chapter to correct your breathing. If the hand on your abdomen rises more than the hand on your chest, congratulations! You're breathing the right way—from your abdomen.

breathing, says Dr. Fried. Since shallow breathing also exacerbates asthma, this, too, can start a vicious cycle of asthma attacks, shallow breathing and more asthma attacks.

BREATHING LESSONS

Fortunately, most of us can relearn deep abdominal breathing by practicing simple relaxation and breathing techniques.

"When people start abdominal breathing, they're less anxious, less depressed and less stressed, and they sleep better and have more energy," says Dr. Laue. Women with asthma and PMS have told her that they suffer less severe symptoms on those fronts, too, once they start breathing abdominally.

Dr. Migdow says that a combination of relaxation exercises and abdominal breathing has helped ease headaches, menstrual cramps and back pain and helped lower the blood pressure of those he treats.

The best way to learn how to breathe properly is to find a physical therapist or psychotherapist who does breath work or a doctor who can teach you breathing exercises, watch you do them and correct any mistakes, says Dr. Laue. Unfortunately, physicians and psychotherapists who use therapeutic breath work are still few and far between. If you can't find one, a yoga, qi gong (chi gung) or martial arts teacher may be able to help you, since abdominal breathing is an important part of those disciplines. Failing that, look for a good video, Dr. Laue suggests.

If you have diabetes, low blood sugar or kidney disease, says Dr. Fried, you should not practice breath work without your physician's approval.

First, relax. Relax before practicing abdominal breathing and you'll find the job easier, Dr. Laue says. She suggests the following progressive relaxation exercise. Though some therapists teach a progressive relaxation exercise that actually has you tense your muscles first, Dr. Laue says that some people have a hard time relaxing their muscles after doing that. She prefers this version in which you *imagine* tensing your muscles.

- Wearing comfortable clothes, lie down.
- Starting at your feet and working up to your head, imagine tensing and then relaxing each part of your body.
- Imagine tensing your feet for four or five seconds; then imagine releasing the tension for four or five seconds.
- Moving up to your calf muscles, imagine tensing and relaxing those muscles. Imagine the wind blowing leaves along the gutter on a windy day. In your mind's eye, feel your breath moving the tension down your body and out the bottoms of your feet.

- Continue moving upward through your hips, abdomen, arms and chest. While you are focusing on your heart, imagine the sun melting the snow on an early spring day. Feel the energy of the sun melting the tension in your body and then the tension running off your body like the spring melt. Continue with your shoulder, neck and head muscles, ending with your forehead. Finish by imagining yourself tensing and relaxing in a quiet place in nature where you feel very safe and peaceful.

Breathe by the book. Once you're relaxed, remain lying down and place a book on your abdomen. When you inhale, push the book upward, using your stomach muscles. When you exhale, pull the book downward with your stomach muscles. Make sure that your inhalations and exhalations are of equal duration, Dr. Laue says. "If you breathe out to a slow

Getting**Started**

Breath Work

Practitioners of breath work vary and may include psychotherapists, physical therapists, yoga instructors and physicians. Shallow chest breathing may be a sign of an oxygen-depleting condition like kidney disease, says Robert Fried, Ph.D., professor of psychology at Hunter College, City University of New York, director of the Stress and Biofeedback Clinic at the Institute for Rational Emotive Therapy in Manhattan and author of *The Breath Connection.* So Dr. Fried recommends that most people have their breathing capacity evaluated as part of routine medical examinations.

Number of practitioners in the United States: Unknown.

Qualifications to look for: Interview practitioners about their background and experience before deciding with whom you would like to work. Your instructor should have training in human physiology and proper breathing techniques. If you choose a yoga instructor, she should have studied yoga extensively, be committed to daily yoga practice and regularly attend yoga teacher training.

Professional associations: None.

To find a practitioner: Ask your doctor, a physical therapist or a yoga instructor to teach you breath work or recommend a breath-work teacher.

Approximate cost: $10 to $12 per session for a yoga class. Costs for individual yoga instruction, including breath work, range from $40 to $50 per session.

count of three, breathe in to a slow count of three." Practice for 10 to 20 minutes twice a day, and eventually you'll be breathing from your abdomen automatically—even when you sleep, Dr. Laue says.

Imagine. Imagery can also help you breathe correctly, says Nancy Zi, a classical opera singer, voice teacher, practitioner of qi gong and innovator of chi yi, a system of breathing exercises. Chi yi, Zi explains, is a cross between traditional Chinese qi gong breathing exercises and the breath training that professional singers get. Author and executive producer of the book and videotape *The Art of Breathing,* Zi suggests this simple exercise as a starter: Imagine that your body is a giant upside-down eyedropper. Your mouth and nose are the dropper's opening, and your stomach is its bulb. With your hands on your stomach, breathe in deeply, imagining the air filling the bulb. Your stomach should expand when you do this. Then exhale, tightening your abdominal muscles as if squeezing the eyedropper bulb.

Branch out. Once you master basic abdominal breathing, you can learn variations on the technique that'll help you breathe most efficiently in different situations. For details on other breathing exercises that can help you deal with stress, ease pain, counter asthma attacks and pacify insomnia, see pages 491 (for asthma), 545 (for insomnia), 539 (for pain) and 402 (for stress).

CHIROPRACTIC
Getting It All into Alignment

Crossing a street in Jersey City one wintry afternoon, Mary Lou Zubel was hit by a van and wound up with serious back, neck and leg injuries and severe pain that wouldn't quit.

"My orthopedist recommended surgery on my neck and knee," says Zubel, a former purchasing director in her mid-forties. "But I'm trying to avoid that."

So, twice a week for a couple of months, she lets chiropractor Frank Zolli, D.C., adjust her spine.

Dr. Zolli, dean of the University of Bridgeport College of Chiropractic in Connecticut, starts each session with a series of orthopedic and neurologic tests to evaluate Zubel's coordination, flexibility and pain: Does the pain worsen when he bends her legs this way? How about when he moves her neck that way? This morning, Zubel says that her lower back *really* hurts when he bends her legs at the knee.

So Dr. Zolli asks Zubel to lie on a padded examination table and begins massaging her back. Once she's relaxed, he palpates or feels the bones and muscles along her spine, looking for subluxations—chiropractic jargon for skeletal misalignments.

Having located the problem spots on Zubel's back, Dr. Zolli adjusts her spine by delivering a few quick thrusts along the length of her back. He then asks her to lie on her side, with her top leg bent at a right angle. Pushing her hip in one direction while gently pulling her shoulder the opposite way, he adjusts her pelvic bones.

Though a few of the procedures look like they might *cause* some pain, Zubel says otherwise. (Some chiropractic manipulations are accompanied by unsettling popping sounds, but the noises, caused by gas escaping from spaces surrounding the newly manipulated joints, aren't cause for concern, practitioners say.)

"Chiropractic is the route that's helped me the most with the pain," Zubel says. "Before, the pain was so bad that I couldn't walk or sit."

In addition to Zubel's twice weekly adjustments, Dr. Zolli recommends sessions with a physical therapist three times a week. Like most chiropractors, he also prescribes at-home exercises and recommends dietary changes. To enhance the effect of adjustments, chiropractors sometimes use gentle techniques like massage, ultrasound and heat. Chiropractic, he says, requires full patient participation. "That's why women tend to do particularly well with chiropractic—because they take better care of themselves than men do."

ONE IN THREE AMERICANS HAS TRIED IT

According to chiropractic theory, skeletal and joint misalignments—caused by accidents, strains, poor posture and stress—are responsible for many types of pain and disease. The aim of chiropractic manipulation is to correct subluxations.

These days, only the most traditional chiropractors believe that all illness is the result of subluxations and rely on manipulation alone to treat all health problems. Less traditional practitioners treat mostly muscular and skeletal problems such as head, neck and back pain and menstrual cramps and refer patients with other types of health problems to physicians

Getting**Started**

Chiropractic

According to the *Harvard Women's Health Watch*, chiropractors are the third largest group of health practitioners, behind medical doctors and dentists. If you're considering chiropractic for a health problem like lower-back pain, here's how to locate qualified practioners in your area.

Number of practitioners in the United States: Approximately 50,000.

Qualifications to look for: Doctor of Chiropractic (D.C.) degree. Doctors of Osteopathy (D.O.) are also trained to perform spinal manipulation.

Professional associations: The American Chiropractic Association, 1701 Clarendon Boulevard, Arlington, Virginia 22209; the National Association of Chiropractic Medicine, 15427 Baybrook Drive, Houston, Texas 77062.

To find a practitioner: Contact one of the organizations above.

Approximate cost: $25 to $65 per session.

for treatment. Research suggests that this is the better way to go. While studies confirm that chiropractic gets results with lower-back problems, its track record with other ailments is spotty.

Despite opposition from mainstream medical organizations such as the American Medical Association, chiropractic is thriving a century after its founding. According to one poll, 30 percent of American adults have seen a chiropractor. An estimated 15 to 20 million of us visit chiropractors yearly—primarily for back pain, neck pain and headaches.

Once chilly toward chiropractors, many physicians are now referring patients with muscular and skeletal problems to D.C.'s and are even setting up joint practices with them.

"I don't see how a physician can work without a chiropractor," says David Edelberg, M.D., director of the Chicago-based American Holistic Centers. "A number of my patients have managed to avoid major surgery by taking this combined approach—seeing a physician and a chiropractor," says Dr. Edelberg, who sends patients to chiropractors for head, neck and back pain.

Most insurance plans, including Medicare and many state Medicaid programs, cover chiropractic care. A significant body of research, in fact, confirms that spinal manipulation can help alleviate lower-back pain.

Other benefits, however, aren't as well documented. Research is needed to determine if spinal manipulation helps relieve menstrual pain and treat borderline high blood pressure, at least temporarily. Chiropractors claim success with treating other health problems, like ulcers, carpal tunnel syndrome and asthma, but evidence of those benefits is mostly word-of-mouth.

Why chiropractic seems to relieve symptoms—particularly symptoms of problems other than back pain—is a matter of debate.

"There are a lot of chiropractors who believe the traditional theory—that subluxations cause most diseases and disorders. Many others don't believe that, but they do believe that the correction of these misalignments increases the potential of the body to heal itself," says Patricia Brennan, Ph.D., dean of research at National College of Chiropractic in Lombard, Illinois. "I believe spinal-manipulative therapeutic intervention can affect organ systems, but I'm not sure what the mechanism is. No one is."

THE SCIENTIFIC EVIDENCE

Controlled scientific studies have found spinal manipulation to be at least as good as, if not better than, conventional care for treating back pain. When researchers analyzed data from nine published trials, they found that men and women suffering uncomplicated, acute lower-back pain were 17 percent more likely to recover after three weeks if they had spinal manipulation. A British study that tracked more than 700 men and women with lower-back pain over the course of three years concluded that those who had spinal manipulation fared better than those who got traditional hospital care.

"Chiropractic is ideal for lower-back pain," says Willard Dean, M.D., medical director of the Center for Self Healing in Santa Fe, New Mexico, who refers patients to D.C.'s for neck pain and backaches.

A small pilot study has found that women who get manipulation on the first day of their menstrual periods report relief from severe menstrual cramps. And a number of preliminary studies suggest that spinal adjustments may reduce blood pressure temporarily, says Christine Goertz, D.C., vice-president of research and policy at the American Chiropractic Association in Arlington, Virginia.

Though chiropractors report success with treating ear infections, fibromyalgia (painful "trigger points" in the muscles), asthma, carpal tunnel syndrome, ulcers and colic, so far, there is no scientific evidence beyond case reports to back up those claims, says Scott Haldeman, D.C., M.D., Ph.D., associate clinical professor in the Department of Neurology at the University of California at Irvine and editor of *Principles and Practice of Chiropractic*.

WHY IT WORKS—THE THEORIES

Chiropractic traces its unlikely origins to a summer day in 1895 when a deaf janitor stopped at the Davenport, Iowa, offices of a self-taught healer named Daniel David Palmer. The janitor had lost his hearing 17 years earlier. It happened suddenly, he told Palmer, after he felt something "give" in his back. Palmer examined the man, examined what he thought to be a misplaced vertebra in his spine, concluded that this was the problem and then pushed the bone back into place. "And soon the man could hear as before," Palmer wrote in his autobiography, published in 1910.

Palmer's experience with the janitor and a subsequent success treating a patient with heart trouble, convinced him that 95 percent of all diseases stemmed from spinal misalignments. Knocked out of place, vertebrae pinched surrounding nerves, interfering with the proper function of the nervous system, Palmer reasoned. Since the nervous system influenced all other bodily systems, these misalignments gave rise to diseases—everything from diabetes to strep throat. The way to cure virtually all disease was to press, push and pull the spine, pelvis and other bones back into their proper places, Palmer concluded.

Though traditionalists still share Palmer's view—and his opposition to drug treatment, surgery and immunization—many do not. "The concept that somehow misalignments cause the pinching of nerves and that *that* causes organs not to work properly has virtually been thrown out of academic circles because no one has been able to establish that this, in fact, occurs," says Dr. Haldeman.

Abnormal spinal mechanics *can* cause back, neck and head pain, he continues, but the mechanism doesn't appear to be as simple as Palmer believed. Misaligned bones may pinch surrounding nerves. But they also appear to lead to abnormal muscle contractions that hamper mobility and circulation and contribute to pain, Dr. Haldeman says. Manipulation probably helps relieve pain by relaxing the muscles, increasing mobility and improving circulation.

At least one study suggests that manipulation may also ease pain by prompting the body to release endorphins—the feel-good nerve chemicals responsible for "runner's high," he notes. Neurochemical activity may also explain why manipulation seems to offer at least temporary relief from

A Chiropractic Guide to the Spine

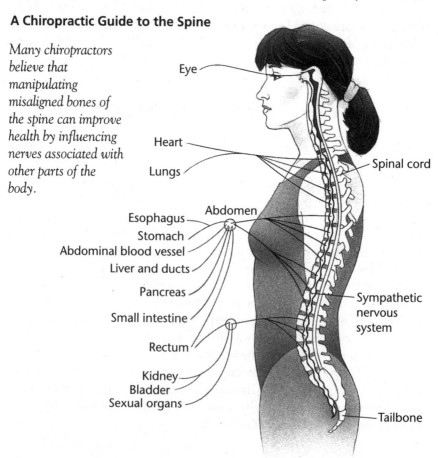

Many chiropractors believe that manipulating misaligned bones of the spine can improve health by influencing nerves associated with other parts of the body.

Eye

Heart

Lungs

Spinal cord

Abdomen

Esophagus
Stomach
Abdominal blood vessel
Liver and ducts
Pancreas
Small intestine
Rectum

Sympathetic nervous system

Kidney
Bladder
Sexual organs

Tailbone

menstrual cramps and other disorders that are neither muscular nor skeletal, Dr. Brennan says. In a preliminary study with women suffering menstrual pain, manipulation altered the blood levels of neurochemicals that can cause pain at high concentrations. Manipulation also appeared to trigger a drop in the levels of prostaglandin, a hormonelike chemical that contributes to pain. In women with dysmenorrhea (painful menstrual periods), Dr. Brennan notes, levels of prostaglandin are very high on the first day of menstruation. So it's possible that manipulation releases a compound that blocks prostaglandin synthesis, she adds.

Spinal manipulation—a tool used by both chiropractors and osteo-pathic physicians—may also help reprogram the nervous system, correcting glitches that cause pain and other symptoms, says Philip Greenman, D.O., associate dean and professor in the Department of Osteopathic Manipulative Medicine at Michigan State University College of Osteopathic Medicine in East Lansing.

Nerves that govern involuntary actions, such as breathing and digestion, run in the spinal cord and are linked to the function of the spine. So it's possible, for instance, that you could help ease stomach problems by manipulating the back in related segments of the spine to influence the nerves that run to the stomach, Dr. Greenman says.

In the end, research is likely to find that manipulation affects the body in a variety of ways, and all of these effects contribute to symptom relief under certain circumstances and to varying degrees, Dr. Brennan predicts. "I don't think that there's going to be any simple explanation."

WHEN TO SEE A PHYSICIAN FIRST

In light of the available evidence, when should you consider seeing a chiropractor?

For serious health problems—like cancer, diabetes, heart trouble or severe trauma—you should see a physician immediately. "I don't think chiropractors are equipped to deal with those problems," says Dr. Haldeman. If you're suffering simple back, neck or head pain, on the other hand, a visit to a D.C. makes a lot of sense, he says.

Dr. Edelberg suggests seeing a physician for a diagnosis first if you have unexplained, chronic back pain. However, "if you know you injured your back by lifting something, a visit to a physician isn't necessary," he says.

While orthopedists have better success rates treating progressive curvature of the spine than chiropractors do, a D.C. can help relieve the discomfort associated with mild spinal curvature. So seeing one for help with mild curvature also makes sense, Dr. Edelberg adds.

For carpal tunnel syndrome, Dr. Haldeman suggests that you see your chiropractor *before* surgery. "I always think that surgery is a last resort, and I like to try virtually everything else before surgery—taking anti-inflammatory drugs such as aspirin or ibuprofen, maybe going to a chiropractor or physical therapist or wearing wrist splints for awhile."

If you do go, be sure to give your chiropractor a complete medical history. You shouldn't undergo manipulation if you've had symptoms of a stroke or blood clot or have a condition that causes bone softening—such as cancers or infections that have spread to the bone, severe osteoporosis or severe rheumatoid arthritis, Dr. Haldeman says. But you can still see a chiropractor for physical therapy, nutritional and lifestyle advice and massage, ultrasound, heat or low-voltage electric current treatments to ease muscle tension.

Try five to ten treatments before making up your mind about chiropractic, advises Dr. Haldeman. If there's no change at all after ten treatments, discuss other treatment options with your physician. (As with other therapies, the frequency and duration of treatment varies with each condition.) "Patients who have problems as a result of a bad fall or a car crash have more damage and require more intensive care than the person who was reaching for something and felt a pop in her neck," explains Dr. Zolli.

You may want to ask your chiropractor at the outset how long therapy will take. One criticism of chiropractic care, Dr. Edelberg notes, is that D.C.'s drag it out.

A University of North Carolina study suggests that they might, indeed. According to the study, patients who saw chiropractors for acute back pain spent more for care than those who saw primary care physicians. Though the chiropractors charged less per visit, they scheduled many more sessions.

Some chiropractors will tell you to keep coming in for regular "preventive health" adjustments after you're back on your feet and feeling fine again. But you shouldn't, says Dr. Edelberg.

"Certain chiropractors earnestly believe that you should come in regularly for adjustments—until your next incarnation," he says. "But there's no reason to go for regular adjustments if you feel fine. Regular adjustments won't do anything except loosen up your ligaments, which isn't good."

COGNITIVE THERAPY

Healing with Positive Self-Talk

You're about to have your first job interview in years. You're as nervous as you can be. As you enter the office of your prospective employer, you're thinking:

(A) I'll never get this job. I'm so rattled that I'll blow the interview, and besides, they probably won't like me anyway.

(B) Plenty of people are this nervous when they're interviewed. And they called me right after they got my resumé—something about me must interest them.

If your answer is B, you already know a little something about cognitive therapy, a technique designed to chase away negative thoughts.

On the other hand, if you answered A, chances are you could benefit greatly from learning how to change your thinking habits.

UNCLOG YOUR "THINKING JAMS"

Cognitive therapy is an effective nondrug treatment for depression, anxiety and other common emotional problems. In contrast with long-term psychoanalysis, cognitive therapy is short-term and works by getting you to change your behavior and your general outlook and focus on the present, not the distant past. Experts say cognitive therapy can help you help yourself out of the "thinking jams" that can short-circuit success and happiness.

"Consider cognitive therapy instead of lengthy psychotherapy when you're beset with emotional problems such as depression, anxiety or eating disorders," says Judith S. Beck, Ph.D., director of the Beck Institute for Cognitive Therapy and Research, clinical assistant professor of psychology in psychiatry at the University of Pennsylvania in Philadelphia and author of a textbook on cognitive therapy.

The idea behind cognitive therapy is that emotional problems arise or get worse when your outlook and perceptions about yourself are distorted.

"Cognitive therapy looks at problems that women have in the here and now," says Dr. Beck, whose well-known father, Aaron T. Beck, M.D., developed the therapy in the 1960s. "It's a commonsense way of problem-solving that helps women handle the kind of negative thinking that affects them emotionally when they are distressed or depressed."

BEST OUT OF FIVE

Psychiatrists, psychologists and other mental-health practitioners have an arsenal of therapeutic treatments at their disposal to deal with the vast array of emotional problems that sometimes concern women.

So-called biomedical therapies use drugs, surgery or electric shock to alter behavior; only a psychiatrist or other medical doctor can administer these treatments.

Traditional psychoanalysis, originated by Sigmund Freud, is the mother of all talk therapies and relies primarily on free association and dream interpretation to resolve unconscious conflicts that cause emotional disorder. Treatment can last for years—or, in the case of Woody Allen's characters, a lifetime.

Group therapy brings together several people (six to ten, usually) under the supervision of a group therapist. Based on the principle of transference (that is, the assumption that you will react to group members as you do to your family), group therapy aims to reveal the distortions that people experience in relating to others.

In behavioral therapy, the focus is on your behavior rather than on the subconscious thinking that causes your behavior.

Proponents say that for many women, cognitive therapy may be a better choice than these four classic approaches.

"Research simply doesn't support the fact that long-term, traditional psychotherapy is effective," says Dr. Beck. "Cognitive therapy, on the other hand, has been shown to work in over 100 rigorously controlled studies," she says.

According to various researchers, including Dr. Beck, cognitive therapy has been shown to be effective for a long list of emotional and emotionally related problems, including anorexia, anxiety, back pain, bulimia, chronic fatigue syndrome, depression, fibromyalgia (painful "trigger points" in muscles), high blood pressure, marital difficulties, overeating and weight problems, panic and unexplained physical symptoms.

What's more, a small study at the University of California at Los Angeles indicates that cognitive therapy may actually affect the chemistry of the brain and may be an effective therapy for obsessive-compulsive disorder (the uncontrollable urge to repeat a certain ritual, like hand washing).

YOU'RE IN COMMAND

"Cognitive therapy alleviates distress and suffering in a short period of time—commonly, 8 to 12 weeks—by helping people look closely at the problems that disturb them," says Dr. Beck.

Generally speaking, certain aspects of cognitive therapy are radically different than traditional psychotherapy. The most striking differences are the active involvement of the therapist and the kind of work that you're expected to do. For example, Dr. Beck says that if you opt for cognitive therapy, you'll be encouraged to participate in the following areas.

Getting**Started**

Cognitive Therapy

You don't necessarily need to see a psychiatrist to learn cognitive therapy. Many counselors, psychologists, social workers and other mental-health professionals are trained in cognitive therapy. Here's how to find a mental-health professional trained in this technique.

Number of practitioners in the United States: 1,500 to 3,000.

Qualifications to look for: A mental-health professional with a background in cognitive therapy. Women with more severe disorders (obsessive-compulsive disorder, for example) should consult a licensed doctoral-level psychologist (Ph.D.) or psychiatrist (M.D.).

Professional associations: Beck Institute for Cognitive Therapy and Research and International Association for Cognitive Psychotherapy, 1 Belmont Avenue, Suite 700, Bala Cynwyd, PA 19004-1610.

To find a practitioner: Send a self-addressed, stamped envelope to the Beck Institute at the above address with your request for a referral.

Approximate cost: $10 to $65 per hour for group sessions or $65 to $125 per hour for private sessions.

Team up with your therapist. "The therapist and the client work to-gether actively, as a team," says Dr. Beck. You and your therapist will make decisions together, such as how often to meet, what to work on in each ses-sion and what kind of therapeutic homework you'll be assigned.

Focus on goals. In your very first session with a cognitive therapist, she will probably ask you to verbalize your problems and set specific goals for solving them. As you do, your therapist will begin to identify the mental roadblocks that make problem-solving difficult for you.

Structure your sessions. In traditional psychoanalysis, patients spend the whole session free-associating—just talking about whatever comes to their minds when the therapist throws out a series of words. In cognitive therapy, you'll have input into the structure of the sessions. Most likely, you and your therapist will:

- Briefly review your week
- Set a session agenda
- Give feedback on your last session
- Review your therapeutic homework
- Discuss agenda items
- Set new homework
- Summarize the session
- Provide feedback on this session

Work in the here and now. In most cases, your therapist will help you focus on solving whatever problems currently trouble you. Discussions of childhood events are explored to identify mind-sets you learned as a child, as in: "If I don't get good marks, then I'm a failure."

Apply new thinking to your daily life. As you learn about how your thoughts influence your emotions and behaviors, you'll also learn how to apply what you learn to prevent relapses from occurring.

Get results in months, not years. Dr. Beck says that most people with simple anxiety or depression require 4 to 14 sessions, although she notes that some patients who have personality disorders may need a year or two, or possibly longer, to change long-standing, rigid, dysfunctional beliefs and behavior patterns.

Identify dysfunctional thoughts and beliefs. By using a process that Dr. Beck refers to as guided discovery, your therapist will frequently ask you what your thoughts mean and will help you to see whether in fact they are valid. (Remember: "If I don't get good marks, then I'm a failure.") This will help you uncover underlying beliefs about yourself, your world and other people.

QUICK FIXES FOR COMMON DISTORTIONS

According to Dr. Beck, cognitive therapy empowers women by enabling them to help themselves out of depression and other emotional problems.

"There are certain classic distortions that people make in their thinking," says Dr. Beck. "Labeling these distortions is one way that therapists help you avoid some of the traps that can get you into emotional hot water."

Recognizing—and avoiding—these common distortions can go a long way toward easing emotional turmoil.

Black-and-white thinking. Viewing situations as being all black (bad) or all white (good) with no grays establishes unrealistic expectations and doesn't allow for partial satisfaction. Example: "If I don't do an outstanding job, then I'm a total failure." Instead, tell yourself: "So I made one little mistake. I'm human. It didn't ruin the entire project."

Catastrophizing. Don't assume the worst about a situation. Instead, consider positive outcomes. Example: "I'm so nervous; I know I'll blow the interview." Instead, tell yourself: "Everyone is nervous during interviews. She interviews hundreds of nervous applicants, so she's used to it and most likely won't count it against me."

Mind reading. Don't assume that you know what others are thinking—and don't assume that it's always negative. Example: "The man I met recently hasn't called because he thinks that I'm unattractive." Instead, tell yourself: "There could be hundreds of reasons for why he hasn't called. I'm not him. I can't know how he thinks."

Tunnel vision. Avoid the tendency to see only the negative aspects of a situation. Example: "The holidays will be a total disaster because I'll be at my in-laws' house." Instead, think: "So it's not my favorite place to be. At least the food is always good."

Personalization. Don't assume that you are the cause of others' actions. Example: "The repairman was gruff because I did something wrong." Instead, think: "That repairman needs an attitude adjustment. There's no excuse for being nasty to a customer."

Mental filtering. Avoid the temptation to focus on one negative detail instead of seeing the big picture. Example: "I got one low rating on my performance evaluation. I must be doing a lousy job." Instead, tell yourself: "Even though I need to improve my punctuality, my boss really likes the way I handle clients."

Overgeneralizing. Resist the habit of making sweeping negative statements that overlook the reality of a situation. Example: "I'm uncomfortable at parties. I don't have what it takes to make friends." Instead, think: "I always feel more comfortable when I socialize with people I have something in common with."

Writing off positive outcomes as dumb luck. Don't dismiss your achievements by telling yourself, "I'm not good—just lucky." In other words, don't fall into the trap of telling yourself that your positive qualities, deeds and experiences don't count. Example: "I didn't get that job because I earned it. I was just in the right place at the right time." Instead, say: "It takes more than being in the right place at the right time. It takes having the right stuff. If I didn't have what they wanted, they wouldn't have hired me."

EXERCISE

Prescriptions for Tranquillity, Flexibility and Energy

Carol Doepfner was losing hope: Climbing just one flight of stairs left her gasping for air. The slightest exertion made her sweat. Her doctor told her that her cholesterol was dangerously high. And after many years of being out of shape and overweight, the Dallas housewife wondered if she'd ever be fit and trim.

Then Doepfner started spending just 30 minutes a day on a treadmill. Instead of losing hope, Doepfner lost weight: 60 pounds, to be exact. And she lowered her cholesterol, reducing her risk of heart disease, stroke, diabetes and other life-threatening conditions. As a bonus, she also resolved a chronic back pain problem.

And what did Doepfner, who's in her early fifties, gain? A better, healthier body—and a new attitude. "I just feel so much better about myself," she says. "I have so much more energy. Like this morning, I got off the treadmill and started cleaning everything in the kitchen. Before, I was lucky if I could make a cup of coffee."

Of course, daily exercise wasn't the only answer. Doepfner now watches what she eats and simply moves whenever possible. "Instead of making one trip to pick things up around the house, I make two. When I do errands, I park farther away from the store so that I have to walk a bit," says Doepfner, who also has fewer colds and flus these days.

BETTER THAN DRUGS

Results like Doepfner's come as no surprise to Nicholas A. DiNubile, M.D., clinical assistant professor of orthopedics at the University of Pennsylvania in Philadelphia and author of *The Exercise Prescription*. Dr. DiNubile is convinced that exercise is as useful and as powerful as any drug.

"Doctors don't use exercise as a treatment for problems nearly enough," he says. "It's a medicine in itself; they could be using it as a first-line defense. I can hardly think of any woman—no matter what her age or condition—who wouldn't benefit from exercise. In fact, the Surgeon General's report demonstrates that inactivity is hazardous to your health. Being inactive is as bad for you, from a health standpoint, as smoking."

For many women like Doepfner—plagued by nagging health complaints and at risk for even bigger problems such as heart disease and high blood pressure—exercise can be the ticket to good health. Solid evidence shows that, performed regularly, even moderate exercise, such as treadmill walking, can:

- Reduce risk of heart disease
- Trim unwanted pounds
- Maintain weight loss
- Prevent excessive weight gain during pregnancy
- Shorten labor during childbirth
- Lower high blood pressure
- Strengthen bone
- Help diabetes
- Relieve lower-back pain
- Ease arthritis
- Ease menstrual discomfort
- Reduce risk of certain cancers, such as colon and breast
- Ease depression and boost self-esteem
- Sharpen memory
- Lessen the incidence of colds and flus

Research at the University of California, San Francisco, shows that exercise benefits both body and mind. In a two-year study of 1,758 adults with chronic conditions such as diabetes, high blood pressure, congestive heart failure or depression, people who exercised more tended to have more energy, less pain and fewer sleep problems and handled stress better than those who didn't.

BORN-AGAIN THERAPY

Like medicinal herbs, exercise has been valued for its therapeutic powers for hundreds—even thousands—of years. Ancient Greek philosophers and physicians extolled the benefits of exercise—at least for men. By the 1880s, a small segment of Americans was using weight machines, following the lead of Dr. Dudley Allen Sargent at Harvard University. In 1902, some 270 colleges had adopted physical education, 300 city schools required students to exercise and the YMCA had set up 500 gymnasiums—for men.

Until recent history, it seems, breaking a sweat was considered man's work. That changed in the 1970s, when Kenneth Cooper, M.D., discovered the benefits of aerobic exercise in his Dallas laboratory.

Joggers hit the road in droves—men and women both, says Dr. DiNubile. Several years later, weight lifting changed from something that only 250-pound he-men attempted into a craze that even grandmothers could (and should) do, he notes.

"It took someone like Arnold Schwarzenegger to bring weight lifting into the mainstream in the 1970s and 1980s," says Dr. DiNubile. "Before that, only an isolated group of so-called fanatics did it—definitely no women. Now we're seeing that it's even more important for women than men because of its benefits to bone health."

GOOD NEWS FOR WOMEN

If women were more active and also ate right and didn't smoke or drink, major health problems that often accompany menopause, such as breast cancer, heart disease and osteoporosis, might not occur as frequently, says William Wilkinson, M.D., medical director of the Cooper Institute for Aerobics Research in Dallas, founded by Dr. Cooper.

Evidence strongly shows that exercise can reduce your risk of breast cancer, for example. Researchers at Arizona State University in Tempe, in analyzing numerous studies, reported that women who pursued very active jobs, such as teaching physical education, could have up to a 50 percent less chance of getting breast cancer than those with sedentary jobs, such as office work.

Researchers suggest that moderate physical activity is a deterrent to certain cancers because exercise helps lower weight and body fat, which means that the body is exposed to lower levels of estrogen, a female hormone. Exposure to high levels of estrogen has been linked with breast, ovarian and endometrial cancers. Also, physical activity during adolescence delays the onset of your menstrual cycle, which means over the years your cumulative exposure to estrogen will also be reduced. Further, exercise boosts immunity—the body's natural way of fighting disease.

Among women in the United States, coronary heart disease outpaces everything else, including breast cancer, as the leading cause of death. Heart-smart workouts help make costly, risky medical procedures such as coronary bypass operations unnecessary, says Jerome Brandon, Ph.D., associate professor of kinesiology and health at Georgia State University in Atlanta.

In a study of 478 premenopausal and 44 postmenopausal women, those who exercised the most had 25 percent more high-density lipoprotein (HDL), or good cholesterol, and 20 percent less low-density lipoprotein (LDL), or bad cholesterol, than those in the low-fitness category. The HDL is desirable because it transports the bad LDL away from the artery walls, where it tends to accumulate and slow or block the flow of blood to the heart.

Exercise can also make pregnancy more manageable. "Pregnancy is like a marathon, and you're better off if you've been training for it," notes Dr. DiNubile. "It helps prevent excessive weight, it reduces prolonged labor and helps you feel better overall. Pregnancy is hard work!"

Being fit could help make for an easier childbirth, notes Dr. Wilkinson. "During delivery, you rely on lower abdominal muscles, so having these muscles in good shape is a tremendous help. If you've been exercising, the body is able to use and deliver oxygen to the muscles much more efficiently."

TRANQUILIZER, ENERGIZER

Every day, countless women call their doctors to renew their prescriptions for alprazolam (Xanax), a sedative that has long surpassed diazepam (Valium) as the anti-anxiety drug of choice among physicians and the women they treat. Millions of other women rely on regular jolts of coffee to get through their days. Performed regularly, exercise can serve as both a nondrug remedy for nervous tension and a natural energizer.

The benefits of exercise aren't just physical, says Dr. DiNubile. Exercise triggers biochemical changes, such as the release of natural painkilling compounds called endorphins. So a good workout can lift your spirits. Exercise has also been shown to ease anxiety and depression. It's a great stress-buster. And, he adds, breaking a sweat can even make you sharper mentally.

THE EXERCISE PRESCRIPTION

One of the best things about exercise is that it's never too late to start, says Dr. DiNubile. And you don't have to run marathons to adopt exercise as therapy. One study found that men and women who went from a sedentary lifestyle to doing just moderate activity, such as walking or gardening, saw relatively bigger gains in overall health status than those going from moderate to vigorous exercise, he notes.

In other words, just getting out and moving—doing anything that requires you to move your arms and legs and raises your heart rate for more than a minute or two—adds up to huge benefits later on, says Dr. DiNubile. Avoiding inactivity is the key.

You need to get your "exercise prescription" in three important ways, he adds.

- Aerobic activity, which gets your heart pumping and lowers your risk of heart disease and weight gain
- Strength training, also called resistance training or weight lifting, which strengthens muscle, increases bone growth and helps with weight control
- Stretching, which builds flexibility and prevents injuries

AEROBICS: PUMP UP YOUR HEART

Activities such as jogging, cycling and walking—movement that allows your muscles to work steadily with a constant supply of oxygenated blood—are known as aerobic exercise. This steady and sustained level of activity requires the heart to supply the muscles with oxygen, which is combined with fats and glucose to produce energy.

Are You Exercising Hard Enough?

Once you've decided to walk, run, bike or skate your way to better health, you need some way to see if you're working hard enough to reap the aerobic benefits. Your goal is to increase your heart rate to a range between 60 and 80 percent of the maximum number of beats that your heart can produce, says Jerome Brandon, Ph.D., associate professor of kinesiology and health at Georgia State University in Atlanta.

Figuring out your target heart rate is a lot faster and easier than doing your income taxes. You'll need a pocket calculator, a pencil and paper. Then follow these instructions.

1. Start out with your maximum heart rate—220 beats per minute.
2. From this, subtract your age. If you're 40, your maximum heart rate is 180 beats per minute.
3. Take 60 percent of that (.60 x 180 = 108), and then 80 percent (.80 x 180 = 144). So, your target range at age 40 would be between 108 and 144 beats per minute.

To best understand what aerobic exercise does, take a look at its effect on your most important muscle—the heart. If you get what doctors consider a good cardiovascular workout—30 minutes of exercise between 65 and 80 percent of your maximum effort—three times a week or more, your heart will become a more efficient pump that doesn't have to work as hard, says Dr. DiNubile.

"As you get into better shape, the heart doesn't have to work as hard to do its usual job," adds Dr. Brandon.

The result, says Dr. DiNubile, is a lower heart rate, lower blood pressure and lower incidence of heart disease.

For women, one of the biggest benefits of breaking a sweat is an increase in metabolic rate; that is, the rate at which your body burns calories. "If you consume more calories than you burn, you gain weight," says Jeffrey Rupp, Ph.D., associate professor of kinesiology and health at Georgia State University in Atlanta. "Conversely, to lose excess weight, you need to spend more calories than you take in. And there's no question that when you exercise, your metabolic rate increases." Taking in fewer calories isn't effective unless you exercise, though, says Dr. Rupp. The body reacts to food deprivation by lowering its resting metabolic rate to try to spare calories.

TAILOR YOUR WORKOUT

To incorporate aerobic exercise into your life, follow these guidelines.

Walk your dog (even if you don't have a dog). Dr. DiNubile says that he recommends walking most often for people who are just starting out. "It's easy, it's weight-bearing and anyone can do it. It's a good starting exercise."

Buy the right shoes. When you took your first steps as a toddler, your parents probably fitted you with supportive shoes to replace your crocheted booties. Now that you've gotten serious about walking (or other activities) as a form of aerobic exercise, supportive footwear is once again a high priority, says Dr. DiNubile. To prevent foot and leg injuries, he recommends a supportive walking or running shoe with good arch support and cushioning and plenty of room in the toe box at the front of the shoe.

"Every day in my office I see problems related to women's shoes and sneakers being too small," Dr. DiNubile says. "I recommend shopping at a store staffed by knowledgeable runners or athletes who can help you choose the best shoe for your particular foot type and activity."

Bring socks with you. Try on shoes with the socks that you're going to wear when you work out, says Dr. DiNubile. Also, feet tend to swell toward the end of the day, so this is the best time to shop for shoes.

Consider some variety. You could stick with walking as your primary exercise, says Dr. DiNubile. Or you could graduate to jogging or aerobic dance.

Other options include working out on a cross-country ski machine, biking, in-line skating or stair climbing, he says. Or you could cross-train, where you vary your activities to keep things interesting, says Dr. DiNubile. "That's a mixed-bag training program. One day you could be on the stationary bike, working your quads (thigh muscles), and the next day you could be swimming, working your back and upper body. They both effectively work your heart."

Most important, though, is that the workout you choose has to be something that you enjoy so that you'll stick with it. To determine which combination of exercise best meets your needs, see "A Mix and Match Guide to Exercise" on page 92.

Try before you buy. Before investing in a piece of aerobic equipment like a cross-country ski machine, a stair-climber or a stationary bicycle, it's a good idea to try it out for 20 minutes or so at the store or at a local health club, says Dr. DiNubile. "Make sure that you're comfortable using the equipment. And see how you feel the next day, to be sure that the machine isn't hard on some part of your body, like your knees." Most stores encourage such tryouts but, if not, shop somewhere else, he notes.

Slide into fitness. A great workout for the buttocks and tops and sides of your thighs is the slide board—a long, rectangular sheet of plastic on which you slide back and forth in nylon booties to simulate skating, notes Dr. DiNubile. You can also move your legs forward and backward to simulate cross-country ski movements. "It's not the same resistance as on a cross-country ski machine, but you can simulate the leg and arm movements. And it's a good aerobic program for balance and agility," he adds. It's also cheaper and easier to store than a machine.

Easy does it. You'll want to work up to 30 minutes of exercise a day, says Dr. DiNubile. But whatever form of exercise you choose, start off slowly, he warns. If you haven't had a walking workout before, start out doing it five minutes a day and don't increase your distance or time by more than 10 percent each week. "The 10 percent rule goes for anything," he says. "Don't increase weights by more than 10 percent or increase your time on the stair-climber by more than 10 percent a week."

Sweat with a buddy. It really helps you stay with a workout plan if you can use the buddy system, says Dr. Brandon. "Having someone with you who can motivate you on the days that you don't feel like exercising makes a big difference," he says. "Plus, it's more fun."

Make the time. Set aside 30 minutes a day, at least three times a week, designated for exercise, says Dr. DiNubile. "The biggest excuse is not having enough time. I tell people that when you exercise, you create time because it makes you more efficient the rest of the time: First, because

(continued on page 94)

A Mix and Match Guide to Exercise

To help you customize your exercise program, consult this chart—developed by Nicholas A. DiNubile, M.D., clinical assistant professor of orthopedics at the University of Pennsylvania in Philadelphia and author of *The Exercise Prescription*—as a general guideline.

Common activities shown here are rated for seven kinds of benefits: cardiovascular, flexibility, strength, fat burning, toning, bone strength and balance/agility. The exercises are ranked from 1 to 5, from least beneficial to most beneficial. Where a range is given, benefits depend on the intensity or range of motion used.

	POTENTIAL BENEFITS		
ACTIVITIES	Cardiovascular	Flexibility	Strength
Aerobic dance (low-impact)	5	4	3
Cross-country skiing	5	3	3
Cycling	5	1	2
In-line skating	4–5	2	3
Jogging	5	1	2
Martial arts	4–5	5	4
Rowing	5	2	3
Stair climbing	4–5	1	2
Stretching	1	5	1
Swimming	4	2	2
Tennis	3	2	2
Walking or hiking	4	1	2
Weight lifting	2–3	2	5

But Dr. DiNubile cautions that what you get out of each exercise depends on the effort that you put into it. For example, 30 minutes of brisk, intense walking could burn more fat than 30 minutes of a half-hearted workout on the cross-country ski machine, even though cross-country skiing rates higher in that category than walking does. Also, ratings in the strength category pertain to the muscle used in that exercise—for example, in-line skating rates a 3 for strength, but that applies to the legs and not to the arms, which don't get the same workout.

Fat Burning	Toning	Bone Strength	Balance/Agility
5	4	4	4
5	3	3	4
5	2	3	3
4	3	2–3	5
5	2	4	3
4	4	4	5
5	3	3	2
5	2	2	2
1	2	1	2
4	2	1	2
4	2	3	4–5
4	2	4	3
3–4	5	5	3–4

you're in better shape and, second, because you're more alert since blood is pumping to the brain," he says. "Also you add years to your life, so it's a great investment of time. All the busy, successful people that I know find time for that investment. The payback is great."

Dr. DiNubile points out that when he worked with Schwarzenegger on the President's Council for Physical Fitness and Sports, Schwarzenegger said that every hour you spend working out is one less that you have to spend in a doctor's office.

Pick a time, any time. Whether you work out in the morning, afternoon or evening isn't as important as sticking to a regular time, notes Dr. Brandon. "The vital thing is making it part of your routine and making it a priority—just like your job—so that you'll stick with it," he says.

Log in. For some people, recording the time or distance they walk, run or work out helps them make exercise part of their routine, like brushing their teeth, notes Dr. DiNubile. "Some people need that kind of feedback to stay motivated—to measure their progress and improve."

STRENGTH TRAINING: TONE UP FOR INNER HEALTH

Working your muscles against some form of resistance is, like aerobic exercise, important in the prescription for good health, says Alan Mikesky, Ph.D., exercise physiologist and director of the Human Performance and Biomechanics Laboratory at Indiana University Purdue University in Indianapolis. "That includes calisthenics, such as push-ups and leg lifts as well as weight lifting.

"Strength training improves strength, and it improves muscular endurance, which means you can work or play longer before you fatigue," he says. "It decreases the risk of injury, no matter what you're doing, and helps to maintain and improve flexibility."

As an added bonus, says Dr. Mikesky, building muscle increases your metabolism, helping to burn more calories, even while you're resting, which aids in maintaining weight. Strength training gives you added ammunition in the battle against excess weight.

And when it comes to bone health for women, nothing beats weight training, notes Susan Bloomfield, Ph.D., assistant professor in the Department of Health and Kinesiology at Texas A&M University in College Station. That's because the mechanical stress on the bones helps to improve bone density, which increases bone strength, in much the same way that muscle strength is influenced by repeated use of muscle, says Dr. Bloomfield. And the higher your bone mass, the better your odds of avoiding osteoporosis—a condition responsible for weak, easily broken bones in women past menopause.

By the way, don't worry that you'll look like the Incredible Hulk in heels after a few months of lifting weights, says Dr. Mikesky. "Women secrete very little testosterone, the hormone that contributes to the growth of muscle mass in men. So no matter how hard they work out, there's a natural limit to how large their muscles grow, he says.

GET PUMPED ON A BUDGET

So you've decided to put down that candy bar and pick up a barbell. Here's how to get started without spending hundreds of dollars on weight-training equipment and a membership at the gym.

Shop for free weights. "Strength training doesn't have to cost an arm and a leg," says Dr. DiNubile. If you don't belong to a gym, and a Nautilus-type machine may be out of your price range, you can purchase a pair of dumbbells, a barbell, a weight bench and free weights for far less money, he notes. "There's no magic equipment. For the most part, your muscles can't tell the difference between a $2,000 machine and a simple free weight."

Buy secondhand. To find good dumbbells and barbells, check sporting goods stores that sell used equipment, suggests Dr. DiNubile. Or check out ads in newspapers or cruise yard sales. Gyms often get rid of their weights or machines when they upgrade their equipment, so keep your eyes open for sales, he adds.

Try elastic bands. If you don't want to use weights, elastic bands can do the trick as well, notes Dr. DiNubile. These large rubber band–like loops that resemble bike inner tubes can be looped around your ankles for leg workouts or pulled up by your hands while looped under one foot to work your shoulders and arms. "They're inexpensive, easy to store and allow you to work all areas. They are also great for travel workouts," he says.

Do it right. It's a good idea to have a trainer at a gym or health club show you how to properly perform the resistance exercises that you will be using—especially your first time out, says Dr. Mikesky.

Warm up first. It's important to loosen up for three to five minutes before you start pumping iron, notes Dr. Mikesky. Jogging in place, treadmill running or riding a stationary bike for a few minutes will increase breathing and heart rate and promote blood flow to your muscles, getting them ready for resistance work.

Work your way down. First work the larger muscle groups—the thighs, chest and back, says Dr. Mikesky. Then work the smaller muscle groups—

the arms, calves and abdominals. Follow the step-by-step illustrations for strength training, shown below.

Know your limits. Knowing how much weight to use is trial and error, says Dr. Mikesky. If you can only do 10 lifts properly without overstraining, only do 10. Don't sacrifice exercise technique to lift a heavier weight or perform more repetitions. Most beginners should use a resistance that allows them to do between 10 and 15 lifts.

"If you can't get to 10 repetitions, then you're trying too much weight. If you can easily do more than 15, it's too light," he says. If you are a beginner to strength training, you'll do one set of repetitions for each muscle group in the course of a workout. As your training progresses over the next six to eight weeks, repeat the process until you can do three sets of repetitions for each exercise.

Bent-Over Dumbbell Row

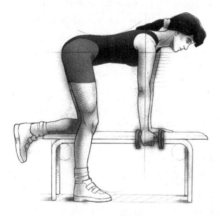 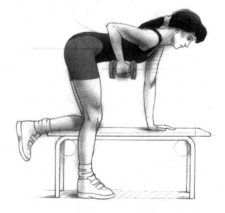

With your left leg, kneel against one end of a padded weight bench while keeping your right leg on the floor, slightly bent. Support yourself with your left arm and hold a dumbbell in your right hand. Your back should be slightly arched.

Inhale and lift the dumbbell until your right elbow is a few inches higher than your back. Exhale and bring the dumbbell back to the starting position. Repeat, then switch sides.

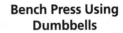

Bench Press Using Dumbbells

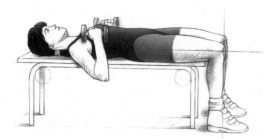

Lie on a padded weight bench with your feet flat on the floor and shoulder-width apart. Hold a dumbbell in each hand at chest level with an inward grip.

Inhale and begin to raise the dumbbells. Exhale after passing the most difficult part of the lift, which may be slightly beyond the midway point. Pause when your weights have reached the top position and your arms are fully extended. Inhale as you lower the weights back to your chest. Pause for a second and then repeat.

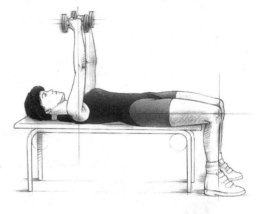

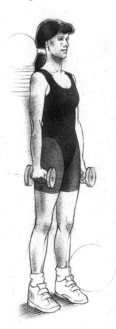

Dumbbell Front Lunge

Hold dumbbells at arm's length with your palms facing in. Hold your head and your back straight, with your feet about six inches apart.

(continued)

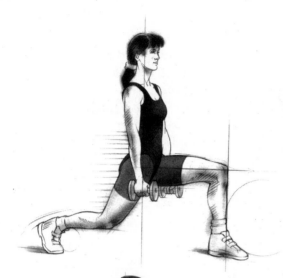

Step forward with your left leg until your left thigh is almost parallel to the floor. Inhale as you step out. Keep your right leg as straight as possible. Step back to the starting position. Exhale as you step back. Repeat with the right leg.

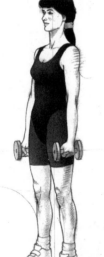

Standing Dumbbell Curl

Hold dumbbells at arm's length with your palms facing in. Your head should be up, your back straight and your feet shoulder-width apart.

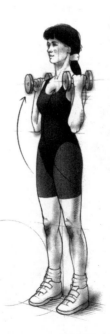

Keeping your upper arms close to your sides, bring the dumbbells up to shoulder height. Inhale as you are lifting. Bring the dumbbells back down. Exhale as you are bringing dumbbells back down. Repeat.

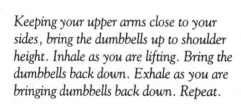

Triceps Kickback Using Dumbbells

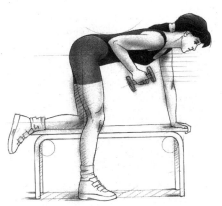

With your left leg, kneel against one end of a padded weight bench while keeping your right leg on the floor and slightly bent. Support yourself with your left arm. Hold a dumbbell in your right hand with your upper arm against your side and your palm facing inward.

As you inhale slightly, extend your arm backward until it's straight. Hold your elbow close to your body.

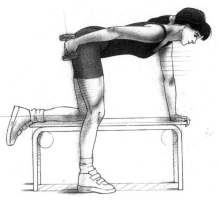

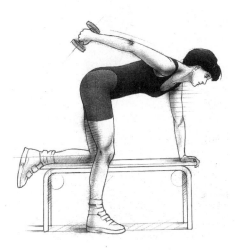

Pause for a moment. Then, keeping your arm as straight as possible, continue to move your arm backward and upward in an arc. Your reach should be well above the level of your back. Don't swing the dumbbell. Slowly lower your arm back to the starting position while exhaling. It's important to keep your back in a horizontal position during this exercise to avoid injury and maximize effectiveness. Repeat, then switch sides.

Standing One-Legged Calf Stretch

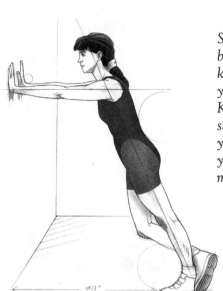

Stand facing a wall about 3½ feet back. Lean your body forward, keeping your arms outstretched until your hands are against the wall. Keep your head up, your back straight and your legs locked. Wrap your right foot around the back of your left heel. Do not let your hips move backward or forward.

Raise up on your toes as high as possible. Hold this position for a moment. Return to the starting position. Repeat the stretch with the opposite leg.

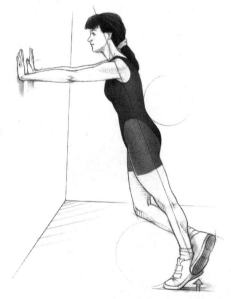

Raised Leg Sit-Up

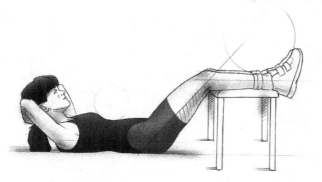

Lie on the floor with your lower legs on top of a padded bench. Your thighs should be at a 45-degree angle. Put your hands behind your head.

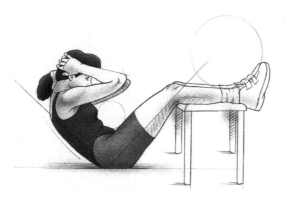

Exhale as you lift your upper body off the floor and raise yourself as high as possible. Return to the starting position, inhaling on your way down. Repeat.

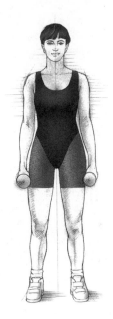

Side Lateral Raise

Stand with your shoulders back, chest out and lower back straight with a slight forward lean. Hold dumbbells down at your sides with your palms facing in. Bend your elbows slightly. Feet are shoulder-width apart.

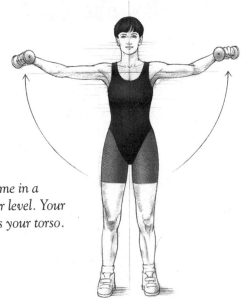

Raise both dumbbells at the same time in a straight line until they're at shoulder level. Your arms should be in the same plane as your torso. Lower your arms. Repeat.

Alternate Arm and Leg Lift

Lie on your stomach and rest your forehead on a rolled-up towel. Your arms are held straight and overhead. Slowly tighten your left arm and right leg. Raise your left arm and right leg approximately three inches off the floor. Hold this position for five seconds. Slowly lower your arm and leg to the floor. Repeat, then switch to the right arm and left leg.

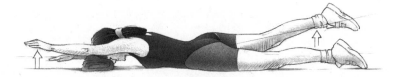

FINESSING YOUR FLEXIBILITY

It may seem like an afterthought in your fitness program, but stretching is the third major component in the exercise prescription, says Dr. Wilkinson. For one thing, stretching makes your joints more flexible, increasing the range of motion controlled by tendons, ligaments, muscles and bones. As you stretch, the muscle receives sensory information about the force and duration of the action. The muscle uses that information to relax, in effect "growing" like a rubber band. A longer, stretchier muscle enables you to move more freely with less pain.

Overall, the main benefit of stretching is to improve flexibility and coordination, says Dr. Wilkinson. More specifically, stretching is probably best known as a preventive strategy or an on-the-spot cure for muscle cramps—painful, involuntary muscle contractions—that you get during exercise and while resting, especially in the calves. By stretching them, you gradually warm your muscles, which helps prevent cramping.

But stretching is also a remedy for severe menstrual cramps—the kind that can leave women curled into a fetal position. Cramps are thought to be caused by excessive secretion of prostaglandins, substances that trigger contractions of the muscles in the wall of the uterus. The result is pain. Stretches that increase blood flow to the pelvis and uterus can provide relief. (To perform stretches for the pelvis, see the illustrations on page 325.)

As a therapeutic tool, stretching can also help prevent injuries such as muscle strains and pulls, soothe lower-back pain and limber up arthritic joints.

A WHOLE-BODY STRETCHING ROUTINE

Performed daily, the stretching exercises illustrated beginning on page 104 can keep you limber and pain-free. Here are a few tips from experts to help you stretch without soreness.

Warm up first. Doctors say that it's best to stretch when your muscles are somewhat warm and pliable, not after they have been inactive for some time. A cold muscle does not benefit from stretching and is more prone to injury or strain. To get the blood flowing and warm up muscles that should to be stretched, says Dr. DiNubile, first break a light sweat by doing three to five minutes of light exercise—like walking, cycling, jumping jacks or running in place.

Stretch s-l-o-w-l-y. Don't bounce when you stretch. Fast, jerky stretches can tear muscles, says Dr. DiNubile. "If you bounce, you momentarily stretch farther, but if the muscle is injured, it scars and you eventually lose flexibility.

"You want a slow, sustained stretch so that the muscle can elongate," says Dr. DiNubile. It's especially good to stretch for about five minutes before aerobic exercise—a warm-up and natural remedy that helps get blood circulating in any stiff or sore areas, he adds.

Hold that stretch. "You should hold each stretch for 15 to 30 seconds, to the point of feeling muscle tension but not pain," says Dr. Wilkinson.

Cool down with a stretch. Follow up your exercise routine with five to ten minutes of stretching, says Dr. Wilkinson.

Pick and choose. If you're pressed for time, the four areas to concentrate on are the lower back, hamstrings, calves and the fronts of the shoulders, says Dr. DiNubile. "Those are important areas to warm up before you exercise, especially if you've had back, leg or shoulder injuries. Not everybody is a Gumby—so don't compare yourself to someone with tremendous flexibility. Just focus on your own daily improvement," he notes.

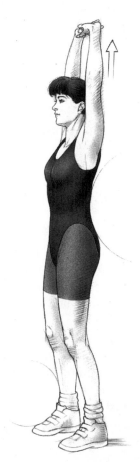

Overhead Arm Stretch

Stand with your arms held overhead, your fingers interlaced and your palms facing up. Knees are slightly bent. Push your arms slightly back and up. Hold for 15 seconds. You may also do this in a sitting position.

Shoulders, Triceps and Upper-Back Stretch

Stand with your arms overhead. Bend your right arm and hold your right elbow with your left hand. Pull your right arm behind your head gently until you feel a stretch in your arms and shoulders. Repeat with the other arm.

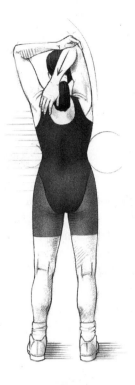

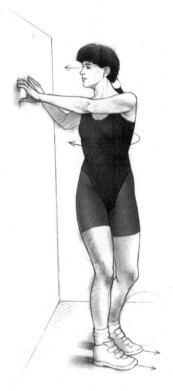

Upper-Body Stretch

Stand one to two feet away from a wall or a fence, with your back toward it. Your feet are shoulder-width apart and your toes are pointed straight ahead. Your knees are slightly bent. Slowly turn your upper body toward the fence and place your hands on it at about shoulder height. Hold for 10 to 20 seconds. Turn in the opposite direction and again place your hands on the fence. Do not force this stretch. Turn only as far as you comfortably can. If you have problems with your knees, do this move very slowly and cautiously.

Pelvic Tilt

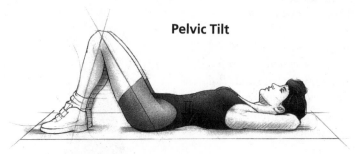

Lie on the floor on your back with your knees bent. Lace your fingers together and hold them behind your head. Pull your shoulder blades together. Flatten your lower back against the floor and tighten your buttocks. Hold this position for five seconds and then relax. Pull your head forward to stretch your neck and back. Repeat three or four times.

Groin and Back Stretch

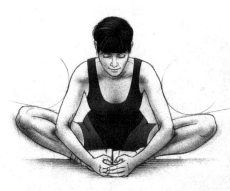

Sit on the floor and put the soles of your feet together. Wrap your fingers around your toes. Contract your stomach muscles while bending at your hips and pull yourself forward. You should bend forward until you feel a mild stretch in your groin. You may feel a stretch in your back as well.

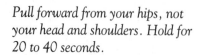

Pull forward from your hips, not your head and shoulders. Hold for 20 to 40 seconds.

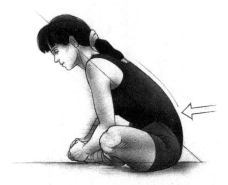

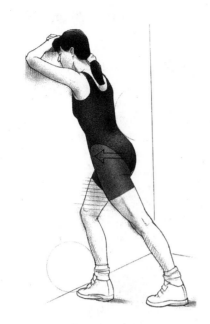

Upper-Calf Stretch

Stand closely in front of a wall and lean forward, placing your forearms against it. Rest your head on your hands. Place your right foot on the floor in front of you and bend your knee. Extend your left leg straight behind you. With your lower back flat, slowly move your hips toward the wall. Hold for 15 to 30 seconds without bouncing. Be sure to keep your left heel on the floor and your left foot pointed straight ahead or slightly turned when you hold the stretch. Repeat with the other leg. If you are an extreme pronator, you should not do this stretch.

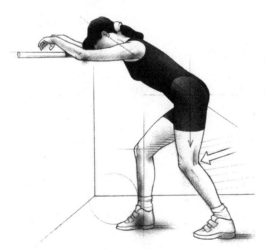

Lower-Calf Stretch

Holding on to a stable support, extend your left leg behind you. Lower your hips, bending your left knee slightly. Be sure that your back is flat. The toes on your left foot should point straight ahead or slightly inward and your left heel should be on the floor. You should feel only a slight stretch in the Achilles tendon area. Hold for 25 seconds. Repeat with the other leg.

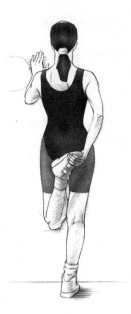

Quadriceps and Front-Thigh Stretch

Placing your left hand on a wall for support, hold the top of your left foot behind you with your right hand. Your foot should be held from the inside. Pull your foot gently toward your buttocks. Make sure that your knees are together and that you are standing tall to avoid leaning forward. Hold for 30 seconds. Repeat with the other leg.

Hamstring Stretch

Sit on the floor and extend your right leg straight out in front of you. Your right foot should be upright and your ankle and toes relaxed. Place the sole of your left foot

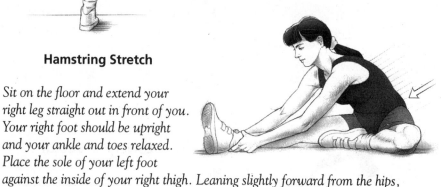

against the inside of your right thigh. Leaning slightly forward from the hips, gently wrap your hands around your right ankle. Be sure to keep your leg relaxed. Hold for 30 seconds. If you can't reach your ankle comfortably, you can use a towel to help you stretch. Repeat with the other leg.

Lower-Back, Hamstring and Buttocks Stretch

Lie on your back and pull your right leg toward your chest. Keep the back of your head on the floor without strain and your lower back flat. Hold for 30 seconds. Repeat with the other leg. After stretching both legs, bring both knees up to your chest and hold.

FELDENKRAIS METHOD

Master the Art of Awareness

When you go for a Feldenkrais session, don't expect wild theatrics or table-shaking, to-the-bone manipulation. The process is much more subtle than that—so subtle that as you're moved about on the table, gliding through a sequence of movements, you'll barely realize that you're being touched.

Here's how a session may go. You lie on a cushioned table as the practitioner begins manipulating various parts of your body. She touches your stockinged foot as gently as if it were made of blown glass, lightly pressing, turning it ever so slightly. She does the same to your leg, lifting it from the table and bending it gingerly at the knee, then slowly setting it down.

The session's not over yet. The practitioner will use foam pieces and styrofoam rollers to help support your body and allow you to be as comfortable as possible. The practitioner will then gently guide you through a series of custom-tailored movements to help you learn new motion possibilities.

Among the many goals in Feldenkrais, two are especially important: One is to help you become aware of habitual body positions and movements, which, unbeknownst to you, may be causing discomfort and fatigue. The second is to help you discover new ways of moving that are more compatible with your body's natural design and potential. It's a learning experience.

Sometimes the impact of a 45-minute session is immediate. When you rise to your feet, you'll feel like a free woman: You may feel taller. The movement of your arms and legs may seem fluid and flowing. Your range of motion may be greater. Sometimes the impact is felt later. You suddenly find that you can reach that jar on the top shelf without a stool. Dancing all night doesn't give you a creak in your neck anymore.

BEING AWARE

The Feldenkrais Method was developed by Israeli scientist Moshe Feldenkrais in the early 1950s after he suffered a crippling sports-related injury. Through studying how movement of the body influences the natural power of the brain, Dr. Feldenkrais was able to teach himself to walk again. He felt that people should reduce stress and fatigue and ease pain and stiffness through learning how to develop efficient and flexible movement.

More than just a few muscles are affected by rounding your shoulders or slumping your back. Over time, your entire body, from your feet to your head, will start to feel the strain of cramped movements and out-of-balance posture. It's not uncommon, proponents say, for this to lead to unexplainable chronic conditions such as headaches or lower-back pain.

It's not that we're unable to move our bodies in healthy, comfortable ways, says Amber Barbara Grumet, a Feldenkrais practitioner in New York City. It's simply that as we go through life developing habitual ways of moving to accommodate old injuries or traumas, we develop physical rigidities. Clenching our jaws, for instance, or favoring one leg after an old skiing accident may have served you well at one time, but those movements may be hindering you today without your realizing it, says Grumet.

After a single Feldenkrais session, says Bob Chapra, a Feldenkrais practitioner in Philadelphia, "I've had people say, 'I realized for the first time my habit of sitting with my shoulder up to my ears and clenching my teeth.'"

FEELING FOR PAIN

It's not surprising that Feldenkrais practitioners are as gentle as other body workers are vigorous. Their job, quite literally, is to feel what your body is trying to say. And often the messages are subtle: a little bit of stiffness here, a slight twinge there, a range of motion that's narrower than it used to be.

A Feldenkrais session isn't meant to solve your problems. The purpose is to help you become aware of your body's strengths. Once you discover your body's natural ability to move, you'll find more comfortable ways of standing, sitting, walking and so on.

Finding a balanced relationship in movement can have far-reaching effects. Not only will your body feel better, but so will you. And once your brain becomes aware of a more efficient way to move, your body can follow in that direction.

"We use our hands to bring movement into areas of your body that are not cooperating fully," says Grumet. "We try to allow people to learn to function in ways that are easiest for their systems and to help realize their human potential," she says.

Although many men attend Feldenkrais sessions regularly, it's an approach that's particularly appealing for women, says Sarnell Ogus, a certified Feldenkrais practitioner in East Hampton, New York.

"Women have very demanding lives these days, with children, jobs, husbands and parents who are getting older," she says. "This gives women an opportunity to take control of how they move, which can affect their lives and their health.

Indeed, Feldenkrais can also be a natural helpmate for pregnancy and childbirth. "Regular classes or lessons can help a pregnant woman adapt to the changes in her body and to her new relationship with gravity as she moves. A natural delivery is easier when you see yourself as a connected whole to push the baby," says Nancy Forst Williamson, a Feldenkrais practitioner in Lincoln, Nebraska.

A LONG-TERM PLAN

The Feldenkrais Method uses not one but two techniques: The first, known as Functional Integration, involves one-on-one sessions on a padded table. The second involves movement classes called Awareness through Movement. Each modality uses simple yet challenging move-

Getting**Started**

Feldenkrais Method

A Feldenkrais practitioner is trained in techniques meant to help you take charge of your emotional and physical health—techniques to improve posture and breathing and reduce stress and fatigue. Here's how to locate a Feldenkrais practitioner near you.

Number of practitioners in the United States: Approximately 800.

Qualifications to look for: Certification by the Feldenkrais Guild.

Professional associations: The Feldenkrais Guild, P.O. Box 489, Albany, OR 97321.

To find a practitioner: Contact the Feldenkrais Guild at the address listed above.

Approximate cost: $50 to $175 per session, depending on where you live.

Purchasing information: To order a copy of *Relaxercise: The Easy New Way to Health and Fitness* by David Zemach-Bersin, Kaethe Zemach-Bersin and Mark Reese, call 1-800-735-7950.

ments to gain new possibilities of functioning with comfort and ease at work and play. Some of the most important benefits of the Feldenkrais Method occur when you begin attending classes.

It's important to note what the classes are not. First of all, they are not dance classes. Music is never used. Nor are they aerobics or stretching classes. Instead, the point of each class is to introduce participants to movements that will help them move with greater freedom and acquaint them with new ways to function, says Marcy Lindheimer, director of the Feldenkrais Learning Center in New York City.

Each class focuses on different functions, which may include movements such as bending, arching, turning or reaching, says Lindheimer. The point is to introduce your body via your brain to new movement choices. Some of the movements you may never use outside of class; others will become part of your daily life. The goal, says Lindheimer, is to help you function more effectively in your life.

The movements that you'll practice in class are often quite simple—turning your head a few inches at a time, for example, or tilting your pelvis, says Williamson.

A Feldenkrais class will usually cover 12 to 15 movements built around a specific theme in each 45-minute session. Each movement is done gently and is generally repeated 10 to 15 times, explains Anat Baniel, a Feldenkrais practitioner and trainer in Greenbrae, California.

"Every movement variation in the lesson is one piece of the puzzle," she notes. "The variations are functionally connected from one to the other so that by the time you've done ten variations, all the movements of the lesson become easy and pleasurable, and your skill level increases."

WHAT TO LOOK FOR

Some Feldenkrais classes are designed for beginners, while others are more advanced. It's important to find a class and an instructor with whom you're comfortable. If you're just starting out, you should be able to join an ongoing class after three or four introductory lessons. If you've been involved in Feldenkrais for a long time, you will want to find an advanced class that will continue introducing you to new lessons.

If you stick with Feldenkrais for a while, you'll find that the movements gradually get more intricate and challenging—but are still safe. At some point, you may even find yourself doing somersaults and rolls, says Baniel. "Everything in Feldenkrais progresses. It helps people feel taller and lighter—more vital. It makes it easier and more enjoyable to walk, to breathe, to run, to move."

Most people experience meaningful changes within the first class. Attending class twice a week for ten weeks will bring about significant changes and improvements in flexibility, strength, vitality and self-awareness for almost everyone. After that, Baniel says that you can cut back to once a week, to keep yourself limber and in touch with your body. Or you may continue more intensely to get even more out of the method. Baniel notes that even weekend or weeklong seminars are offered, which provide an excellent opportunity for even more rapid learning, intensity and change.

Most people enjoy attending Feldenkrais classes because of the camaraderie and teamwork. But if classes aren't available in your area, or if you'd rather learn Feldenkrais techniques on your own, you can purchase illustrated Feldenkrais lesson books as well as audiotapes and videotapes in bookstores or from most practitioners.

WORKING ON YOUR OWN

Because the movements used in Feldenkrais are often quite subtle, it's a difficult program to master on your own. However, here are a few simple tips that experts say can make a big difference in your daily life.

Give your face a hand. In today's stressful world, it's often impossible to go a whole day without clenching your jaw, which is the body's natural reaction to stress. Over time this can lead to jaw pain as well as headaches.

While there's no easy trick for stopping stress, there is one for relaxing a tense jaw. Several times a day, take your left arm and fold it across your body, with your left hand holding your right elbow and your right hand pressing against your jaw, Jack Benny–style. "That automatically makes the jaw feel lighter and will make you less likely to clench your jaw," Chapra says.

Pay attention to your body. Awareness is where a sense of choice starts. It's helpful to spend a few minutes every day quietly sensing your body's movements and sensations, no matter how minute, says Williamson. For example, pay attention to how you're sitting. Some people tend to lean to one side much more than another, and over time this can affect the shape of their spines.

"It's difficult to change your movements unless you know what you're doing in the first place," says Williamson. "But many of us have never had the opportunity to learn to sense ourselves accurately."

Breathe easy. When you're exerting yourself—trying to wrestle the lid off a jar, for example—you may find yourself holding your breath. It's a bad practice, says Grumet. "Breathing helps with everything: your posture, your strength and how efficiently your body uses oxygen. You'll be surprised at how much easier everyday tasks become if you remember to breathe," she notes.

Here are some simple movements suggested by David Zemach-Bersin, Kaethe Zemach-Bersin and Mark Reese, authors of *Relaxercise: The Easy New Way to Health and Fitness*. These movements are designed to restore flexibility to your spine, improve your posture, loosen up your neck and back and help you bend with ease. Remember, these movements should be done slowly. Always make sure the movements are small and easy, and relax as much as you can.

Healthy Spine

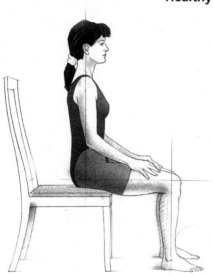

Starting Position

Sit on the front part of a firmly cushioned chair and rest your hands comfortably in your lap. Your feet should be shoulder-width apart and flat on the floor. They should be directly below your knees forming a right angle.

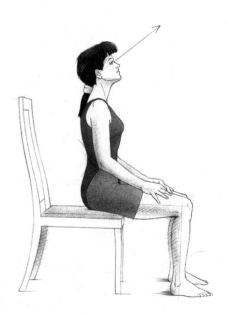

Position 2

Without straining your neck, slowly raise your head toward the ceiling. Your eyes should be looking toward the ceiling. Take notice of how far above your eyes you can see without feeling any strain. As you are looking up, let your back arch slightly. Exhale as you do this movement. Return to the starting position and relax.

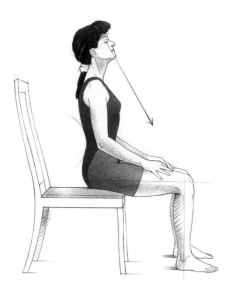

Position 3

Slowly raise your head and arch your back slightly while gazing downward. Relax your shoulders, neck and eyes. Because your eyes and head are moving in two different directions, you'll notice that the movement of your head and neck is limited. Exhale as you do this movement. Return to the starting position and rest briefly.

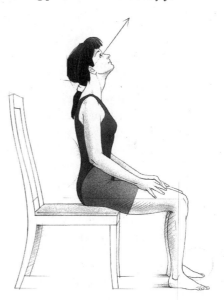

Position 4

Slowly raise your head and eyes toward the ceiling while arching your back. Your back may be arching with more ease, and at this point, you may notice that you can comfortably see a little higher above you. Exhale as you do this movement. Return to the starting position and rest briefly.

Position 5

Slowly lower your head and eyes toward the floor. Let your back round when you look down. Relax your shoulders, neck and chest. Exhale as you do this movement. Return to the starting position and rest briefly.

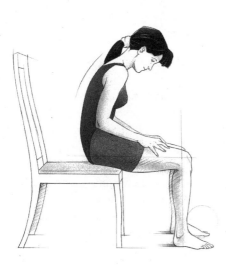

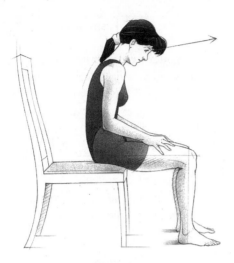

Position 6

Slowly lower your head and round your back. Raise your eyes toward the ceiling. Because your head and eyes are moving in two different directions, the movement of your chest and head is limited. Exhale as you do this movement. Return to the starting position and rest briefly.

Position 7

Slowly raise your head and eyes toward the ceiling while arching your back. You may notice that your middle and upper back are arching a little more without strain and your eyes can see a little farther above you. Exhale as you do this movement. Return to the starting position and rest briefly.

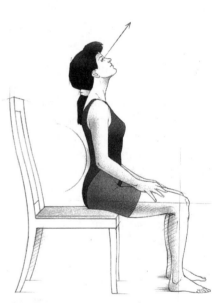

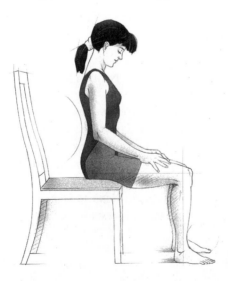

Position 8

Slowly hang your head down. Rest your chin comfortably close to your chest and slowly arch your back. Your pelvis may be tilting forward slightly. Keep your shoulders, stomach and neck relaxed. Exhale when you do this movement. Return to the starting position and rest briefly.

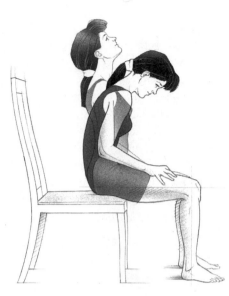

Position 9

While slowly raising your head and eyes toward the ceiling, arch your back. Make sure that your body is comfortable. You may notice that your pelvis tilts forward a little, your chest lifts and moves forward, your shoulder blades come together and your body stretches higher. Exhale when you do this movement. Then slowly lower your head and eyes toward the floor while rounding your back. You may notice that your pelvis tilts slightly backward, your chest flattens, your shoulders become rounded and your body is shorter. Exhale as you do this. Return to the starting position and rest briefly.

Position 10

Slowly turn your upper body to the right. Make sure that your body is comfortable. Then raise your head and eyes toward the ceiling while arching your back. Lifting your left hip up slightly may make this movement easier. Keep your legs, shoulders and neck relaxed. Exhale while doing this movement. Then lower your head and eyes toward the floor while making your back round. Continue to keep your legs, shoulders and neck relaxed. Exhale while doing the movement. Return to the starting position and rest briefly.

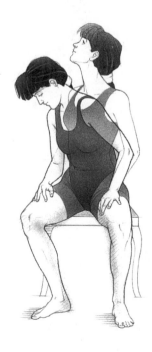

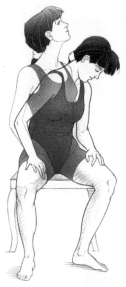

Position 11

Slowly turn your upper body to the left. Make sure that your body is comfortable. Then raise your head and eyes toward the ceiling while arching your back. Lifting your right hip up slightly may make this movement easier. Keep your legs, shoulders and neck relaxed. Exhale while doing this movement. Then lower your head and eyes toward the floor while rounding your back. Continue to keep your legs, shoulders and neck relaxed. Exhale while doing the movement. Return to the starting position and rest briefly.

Position 12

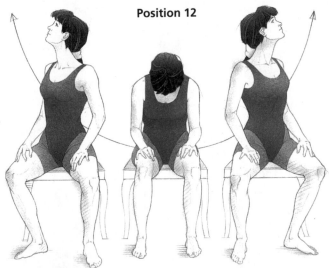

Slowly turn your upper body to the right while arching your back as much as you comfortably can. Raise your head and eyes toward the ceiling. You may notice that your left hip raises slightly and your shoulder blades move closer together. Then bring your body back through the starting position while lowering your head and eyes to the floor and rounding your back. Slowly turn your upper body to the left while arching your back as much as you comfortably can. Raise your head and eyes toward the ceiling. This time, your right hip may raise slightly as your shoulder blades come together. This movement should be continuous and smooth. Lower your head toward the floor and round your back while bringing your body back to the starting position. Exhale after each movement.

Position 13

This movement will allow you to see how your flexibility has improved. Lift your head and eyes toward the ceiling while arching your back. You may notice that you can comfortably see much farther above you than before and your spine bends with ease. Then relax. Your weight is equally balanced over your "sit bones," and your posture has improved.

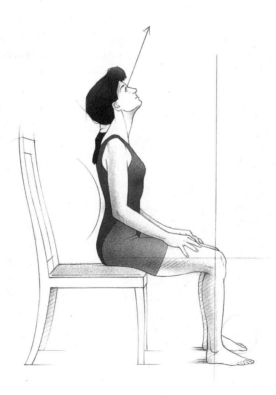

FOOD THERAPY
Healing Feasts and Other Dietary Tactics

At the Yat Chau Health Restaurant in Hong Kong, waiters don't ask, "What will you have?" but, "What *do* you have?" Your answer dictates what they suggest you order. Swollen glands? Try the chicken and sea horse stew. Feeling dizzy? Perhaps some rice with wolfberries. Menstrual cramps? The stir-fried celery is highly recommended.

Medicinal restaurants like Yat Chau are common, and popular, in Asia's ethnic Chinese communities. According to the tenets of Traditional Chinese Medicine, food has potent healing powers. Despite the availability of Western medicine, vast numbers of Chinese continue to seek the eating cure.

Food prescriptions aren't that foreign a concept, really. Think back to your childhood. Chances are, someone—probably your mother—told you that carrots could improve your vision. Or that eating fish would make you smarter. And of course, that eating prunes could cure constipation.

Scientific studies, in fact, find that food really is good medicine. Research shows, for instance, that leaner, nearer-to-vegetarian diets are linked to lower rates of heart disease and cancer—the top killers of American women—and diabetes and obesity. Studies suggest that a mostly meat-free diet can also help alleviate not-so-deadly but still troubling health problems such as arthritis, premenstrual syndrome (PMS) and headaches.

Sometimes a switch to a healthier diet can mean the difference between relying on medication or weaning yourself off it or between going under the knife or doing just fine without surgery. Compared with those alternatives, and the side effects that accompany them, food as medicine looks pretty attractive.

Take a quick glance at the bookstore shelves these days, and you'll see that there's no shortage of "therapeutic" diets out there. Truth is, some work, others don't. Still others work but are so strict that no real woman could follow them. Then there are the diets that restrict our choices so much that we run the risk of shortchanging ourselves on vitamins and minerals essential to our health, such as folic acid and calcium.

"You have to make sure that you meet your nutritional needs," says Adriane Fugh-Berman, M.D., former head of field investigations for the

GettingStarted

Food Therapy

Thinking of trying one of the food therapies? It's a good idea to check with your doctor or a nutritionist first, suggests Suzanne Myer, R.D., assistant professor and director of dietetics at Bastyr University in Seattle. A nutritionist can help you plan your daily fare so that you follow the diet's principles and get all the nutrients that you need. Depending on how you eat, she may recommend supplements, Myer says.

If you're pregnant or nursing, be sure to talk to an expert, says Joel Fuhrman, M.D., physician in Belle Mead, New Jersey, and author of *Fasting—And Eating—For Health*.

The effectiveness of the Ornish diet has been widely publicized, so if you want to try it, your physician is likely to be supportive. If you're taking medication for diabetes or heart disease, you should definitely check with her, says diet-originator Dean Ornish, M.D., cardiologist, assistant clinical professor of medicine at the University of California in San Francisco and director of the Preventive Medicine Research Institute in Sausalito. You may have to lower the dosage after a few weeks on the program. And she'll want to monitor your progress.

Same goes for the Pritikin plan, says James J. Kenney, R.D., Ph.D., nutrition research specialist for the Pritikin Longevity Centers in Santa Monica, California, and Miami Beach.

Number of practitioners in the United States: Approximately 69,000 registered dietitians and nutritionists.

Qualifications to look for: Registered Dietitian (R.D.). Some states require dietitians and nutritionists to be licensed. Also, M.D.'s, D.O.'s and Ph.D.'s in nutrition are qualified to give nutritional advice. Those with master's degrees in nutrition may also be qualified, depending on your state's licensing requirements.

Professional associations: American Dietetic Association, 216 West Jackson Boulevard, Chicago, IL 60606-6995.

To find a practitioner: Contact the American Dietetic Association at the address listed above.

Approximate cost: $50 to $100 for an initial consultation and $25 to $50 for shorter follow-up sessions, depending on where you live.

Office of Alternative Medicine at the National Institutes of Health in Bethesda, Maryland.

So it's important to check out a diet before you dig in. To make it easy, Here's an up-close look at a few of the more promising food therapies, from the most radical (no food at all) to the fairly familiar.

FASTING: FREEDOM FROM DIGESTION

In an old estate in the northern California woods, the Center for Conservative Therapy entices guests to change their lives for the healthier. Inviting walking trails spiral a scenic lake. Chefs prepare gourmet vegetarian meals with produce fresh from the center's organic orchards and gardens.

The center specializes in therapeutic fasting, however. So a good number of the guests—many of whom are women—eat nothing and spend their time lounging. For guests who fast, the prescription is: nothing to eat, only water to drink and plenty of rest.

"Fasting is not the only way to get well," says Alan Goldhamer, D.C., a chiropractor who co-founded the center in 1984. "Most of the people here do need to fast, but they can also improve by making changes in their diets and lifestyles. But some people don't get improvement quickly enough with those changes alone and really benefit from fasting first."

Advocates claim that fasting offers a wide array of health benefits. Forgoing food for a day or two allows your body to rest and heal itself, says Morgan Martin, naturopathic physician, licensed midwife and chairwoman of midwifery at Bastyr University of Naturopathic Medicine in Seattle. Freed from the heavy-duty job of digesting, your body can devote more energy to recovering from everyday illnesses, like colds, and dealing with stress, she explains.

Fasting for longer periods of time (one to three weeks) can help alleviate a range of chronic conditions, says Joel Fuhrman, M.D., physician in Belle Mead, New Jersey, and author of Fasting—And Eating—For Health. Fasting can, he says, reverse cardiovascular disease, shrink fibroids and other noncancerous growths and alleviate autoimmune problems (disorders in which the body turns on itself), such as rheumatoid arthritis, lupus, allergies and asthma.

Extended supervised fasts can also help correct insulin resistance in women and men with adult-onset diabetes, shrink ovarian and breast cysts and treat cervical dysplasia, says Dr. Goldhamer. (If you have diabetes, never consider a fast or other drastic change in eating habits without your doctor's consent and close medical supervision.)

"A variety of women's health problems respond well, too," he says. That's one of the reasons why women outnumber men at the center, he adds.

Why It Seems to Work

Fasting works in a number of different ways, advocates say. During a fast, your body goes through a wide range of physiological changes.

For starters, it begins breaking down and using stored fat, says Dr. Fuhrman. In the process, your body releases and eliminates pesticide residues and other toxins that have been stored in the fat, he says. Dr. Fuhrman claims that fasting can help control conditions that cause heart disease.

"Studies show that a very low fat diet can reverse arterial plaque buildup, and I'm finding that a fast can do it at an accelerated pace," says Dr. Fuhrman. "When you get malnourished, your body searches for nutrients wherever it can find them, including in plaques."

Getting**Started**

Fasting

Anyone considering a therapeutic fast should do so only with the guidance of a physician trained to supervise therapeutic fasting. Here's how to find a practitioner near you.

Number of practitioners in the United States: Approximately 25.

Qualifications to look for: A licensed physician (M.D., D.O., D.C. or N.D.) who has completed a six-month internship at a fasting facility and has been certified by the International Association of Hygienic Physicians (IAHP).

Professional associations: The International Association of Hygienic Physicians, 204 Stambaugh Building, Youngstown, OH 44503.

To find a practitioner: Contact the IAHP at the address listed above or the American Natural Hygiene Society (ANHS), P.O. Box 30630, Tampa, FL 33630, for a listing of certified fasting physicians. Or consult *Health Science* magazine, published by ANHS, which lists qualified practitioners in every issue.

Approximate cost: $85 for an initial 1½-hour consultation. In-patient fasting at a clinic or other facility will cost about $1,000 a week, which includes all examinations, counseling and accommodations. Prices vary depending on where you live.

Few studies on fasting, however, have been published in Western medical journals. One study, conducted by researchers in Norway, suggests that fasting can help some people suffering from rheumatoid arthritis. People with this type of arthritis showed measurable improvement after fasting for seven to ten days and then switching to a wheat-free vegetarian diet.

At the same time, fasting seems to stimulate appropriate immune system reactions, Dr. Goldhamer says. That may account for improvements that he has seen in women with cervical dysplasia (abnormal cells in the cervix, the neck of the uterus). A precursor of cervical cancer, dysplasia is usually caused by viral infection.

"It may be that fasting enables the body's immune system to react more aggressively to the virus," Dr. Goldhamer says. On the other hand, it's possible that the abnormal cells return to normal on their own, as happens in one of three women with cervical dysplasia.

Finally, fasting also causes weight loss, which helps to both lower blood pressure and stabilize blood sugar levels in women with diabetes, Dr. Fuhrman says. Nevertheless, neither he nor Dr. Goldhamer recommends fasting as a way to lose weight, since going without food slows down your metabolism, thus burning fewer calories and triggering weight regain once you start eating again. So after a fast, you must slowly work your way back to your regular eating habits.

Other Opinions

Experts in mainstream medical circles don't accept all the claims that advocates make for fasting.

"I haven't seen any evidence that fasting dissolves plaque in coronary arteries," says Dean Ornish, M.D., cardiologist, assistant clinical professor of medicine at the University of California in San Francisco and director of the Preventive Medicine Research Institute in Sausalito. A world-renowned cardiologist and author of *Dr. Dean Ornish's Program for Reversing Heart Disease*, Dr. Ornish was the first to prove that a combination of a very low fat diet, regular exercise and a stress-reduction regimen could shrink plaques.

"To the degree that you reduce your intake of dietary fat and cholesterol, your body can begin to heal itself," says Dr. Ornish. "But you don't have to fast to do that." (For details on following the diet recommended by Dr. Ornish, see page 132.)

In other cases, fasting may work, but it isn't the best treatment, practitioners say. Fasting may help correct insulin resistance in women with diabetes, says Alan J. Garber, M.D., Ph.D., professor of medicine at Baylor

College of Medicine and chief of endocrinology at Methodist Hospital, both in Houston. But it offers only temporary improvement, he notes.

In contrast, a low-fat diet and exercise offer more lasting improvement without the risk, which can be considerable. If you have diabetes and are taking drugs or insulin, fasting could cause your blood sugar to plummet, and even bring on a low blood sugar (or hypoglycemic) coma, Dr. Fugh-Berman says.

For their part, advocates of fasting acknowledge that women can achieve many of the alleged benefits simply by switching to a low-fat diet. In fact, Dr. Fuhrman insists that people who fast switch to a low-fat diet of mostly raw fruits and vegetables and cooked grains and legumes before they fast—and stay on it after. No matter how much your blood pressure or insulin resistance might improve on a long-term supervised fast, he notes, you'll lose the ground that you gained if you go back to your fatty food–eating, sedentary ways.

Nevertheless, Dr. Fuhrman and Dr. Goldhamer argue that some conditions simply won't respond to a low-calorie, low-fat diet alone, making fasting a viable option in their view.

"Certain diseases, such as asthma and lupus, are very hard to fix just with diet," Dr. Fuhrman says. "They usually don't change without the catalyst of the fast."

Proceed with Caution

Even advocates of fasting agree that, despite the potential benefits, some women shouldn't fast at all. If you're pregnant or nursing, or have nutritional deficiencies, you shouldn't do it, they say. Same goes if you are very malnourished due to the effects of a serious or chronic condition such as cancer or AIDS.

A one- to two-day fast is safe for most healthy people, says Dr. Fugh-Berman. Anyone with a medical condition should check with her doctor first, however. And if you take drugs or insulin for diabetes, she adds, you shouldn't fast.

All fasts that run longer than a couple of days should be medically supervised, ideally by a doctor trained in therapeutic fasting, Dr. Martin notes.

If you fast for more than a day or so, the levels of electrolytes—minerals that regulate heartbeat and other vital functions—in your body can go awry, Dr. Fugh-Berman warns. That puts your heart in jeopardy. So does another possible side effect: Fasting for a long time will cause your body to start consuming muscle, including heart muscle.

If you don't have any major medical problems and want to give fasting a try for a day or two, follow these guidelines.

Rest. The idea behind fasting is to give your body a rest, so take it easy, Dr. Fuhrman advises. Fast during a weekend when you have nothing else planned. Read, listen to the radio and watch TV or videos. Do some light stretching and walk around a bit to avoid stiffness, but avoid strenuous exercise.

Don't sweat it if you're not sleepy. Many people find that they need less sleep during a fast, Dr. Fuhrman notes. Nonetheless, you should still rest at night. Simply turn off the lights and lie quietly.

Bundle up. You may feel colder than usual during a fast, says Dr. Fuhrman, so wear an extra sweater or sleep with an extra blanket on the bed. Avoid hot baths, though, since they can dehydrate you.

Drink plenty of water. To further avoid dehydration, quaff at least eight eight-ounce glasses of water a day, Dr. Martin says. That's water only.

If you drink juice, says Dr. Goldhamer, you're on a juice diet, not a fast, and the physiological changes unique to fasting do not occur.

Consult an appropriate physician. Don't consider prolonging your fast for more than a couple of days without supervision. A doctor should monitor your electrolyte balance every day or two, says Dr. Fugh-Berman. Also, your blood pressure and pulse should be checked at least daily and tests to check your fluid levels should be done at least weekly, Dr. Fuhrman says.

THE RAW FOODS DIET: NO COOKING SKILLS NEEDED

Anna Maria Gahns Clement is no cook. Neither is her husband, Brian. On one typical night, the couple served their dinner guests a gourmet salad, an exotic nut loaf with nut gravy, and a colorful array of vegetables with a piquant sesame seed dip. The meal was delicious—but entirely raw.

"We eat mainly raw food because it's healthier," says Clement, who with her husband co-directs the Hippocrates Health Institute, an alternative health center in West Palm Beach, Florida.

Proponents of a raw-food diet (or living-food diet, as it's also known), the Clements eat mostly uncooked vegetables, fruits, nuts, seeds, sprouts, herbs and small quantities of cold-pressed vegetable oils. But other advocates of the raw-food diet have a wider choice: They'll include fermented plant food such as tofu and tempeh on their plates as well.

Either way, a raw-food diet is a strict, low-fat vegetarian diet—tartare. There's no meat, no poultry, no fish, no eggs, no milk and little or no cooking.

Why not? Cooking destroys many vitamins and other beneficial compounds in plants, says Dr. Fuhrman, who suggests eating a diet that emphasizes raw food when not fasting. Cooking also destroys the enzymes in plant food that help us digest and absorb nutrients, claims Brian Clement. Advocates theorize that by conserving nutrients and enzymes, a raw-food diet can improve your health in a variety of ways.

The Benefits to Women

For women, a short stint of eating mostly raw-food meals can help alleviate assorted gynecological problems, says Lisa Alschuler, naturopathic physician and chairwoman of the Department of Botanical Medicine at Bastyr University. She prescribes two to four weeks of a raw-food diet for chronic PMS, menstrual cramps and fibrocystic breast disease.

A couple of weeks on a mostly raw-food diet can also help you lose weight and clear out your digestive tract, says Kareen O'Brien, naturopathic physician and academic dean at Southwest College of Naturopathic Medicine and Health Sciences in Scottsdale, Arizona.

"I usually do it myself, for about two weeks, once or twice a year," Dr. O'Brien says. "The first few days, I feel a little tired and get headaches. But then I feel better and better. I wake up feeling more refreshed. I'm more alert. I usually lose a few pounds."

Eating mostly raw foods can give you more energy and boost your immunity, says Charito Bacaltos, M.D., assistant health administrator at the Hippocrates Health Institute. She says that raw vegetarian foods, especially when organically grown, are rich in oxygen and enzymes. She believes that these important elements are eliminated in cooked and highly processed foods. She maintains that raw, living foods are the best source of undiluted vitamins, minerals and proteins that are vital in promoting vibrant health. Dr. Bacaltos also says that raw foods help the body to clean out its toxins and strengthen the immune system, thereby effectively cutting down the risk of life-threatening conditions such as cancer, heart disease, high blood pressure and diabetes.

Some Scientific Merit

There's no shortage of evidence that plant food is good for you. Numerous scientific studies show that eating lots of vegetables and fruits— five to nine servings a day, raw or cooked—can lower the odds that you'll develop assorted chronic and debilitating illnesses.

Take cancer and heart disease, for example. Studies find that people who eat lots of produce run a lower risk of both. Why? Most vegetables and fruits are rich in nutrients such as vitamin C and folic acid, which protect your cells from cancer-causing toxins and help keep your coronary arteries clear of cholesterol-laden plaques, says Dr. Fugh-Berman.

Fruits and vegetables are also high in fiber. And because fibrous foods are filling—but relatively low in calories—they can help you lose weight. That, in turn, can lower your blood pressure.

Fiber also speeds food through your digestive system, easing constipation. And research finds that it may offer protection against colon cancer. One type of fiber, soluble fiber (found in fruits, some legumes and grains like oats, rye and barley), also helps lower cholesterol levels. These effects are additional dividends to women who run a higher-than-average risk of heart disease.

Some studies suggest that the fiber in plant food may lower a woman's risk of breast cancer and alleviate gynecological problems, notes Christiane Northrup, M.D., in her book *Women's Bodies, Women's Wisdom*. Research shows that diets high in vegetable fiber can lower the levels of estrogen circulating in your bloodstream, writes Dr. Northrup, who practices obstetrics and gynecology in Yarmouth, Maine, and is assistant clinical professor of obstetrics and gynecology at the University of Vermont College of Medicine in Burlington. Overproduction of estrogen seems to be related to the advent of not only breast cancer but also PMS, fibroids, breast and ovarian cysts and endometriosis.

That said, is a diet rich in raw vegetables and fruits better for you than a diet rich in cooked vegetables and fruits? Some research suggests that raw produce may offer greater protection on some fronts.

A study at the National Cancer Institute linked diets rich in raw fruits and vegetables to a lower risk of cancer of the esophagus. Since some vitamin C is destroyed by cooking, the extra vitamin C in the raw produce may have contributed an added measure of protection, speculates Linda Morris Brown, a researcher in the Department of Cancer Epidemiology and Genetics who headed the study.

While cooking destroys some vitamins in plant food, it also makes other nutrients more readily available, notes Robert S. Parker, Ph.D., associate professor of nutrition at Cornell University in Ithaca, New York.

Raw fruits and vegetables are more fibrous than their cooked counterparts, says Dr. Fugh-Berman. So it is possible that they're a better bet than cooked ones if you're trying to lose weight or prevent colon cancer. "But that's conjecture; there are no studies to back this up," she says. There's also no scientific evidence that the enzymes in raw food improve digestion and nutrient absorption, as raw-food advocates claim, says Dr. Parker.

The bottom line, Dr. Fugh-Berman concludes, is that a raw-food, or mostly raw-food, diet won't hurt you but probably isn't necessary. Lightly cooking your vegetables probably gives you the best of both worlds, she says.

Raw—Or Mostly Raw

If you want to give a raw-food diet a try, you have two options—a raw-food-only diet or a mostly raw-food diet.

According to the Clements, if you're recovering from a serious illness

---

A Typical All-Raw Diet Menu

If you'd like to try a raw-food diet, this sample menu will get you started. It's provided by Lisa Alschuler, naturopathic physician and chairwoman of the Department of Botanical Medicine at Bastyr University of Naturopathic Medicine in Seattle.

Breakfast
1 cup soaked almonds
1½ cups lentil sprouts

Late-Morning Snack
1 cup mixed juice (combine banana with orange and carrot juice)

Lunch
Large salad (chard and other dark, leafy greens; diced tomatoes and ½ cup seeds) with lemon juice or balsamic vinegar and 1 teaspoon cold-pressed olive oil

Afternoon Snack
1 cup mixed juices (combine carrot, celery, beet and ginger juice)

Early-Evening Snack
½ cup seeds with raisins or apple slices

Dinner
Large salad (avocadoes, dried seaweed, greens and garden vegetables) with lemon juice or vinegar and 1 teaspoon cold-pressed olive oil

Bedtime Snack
Carrot sticks
1 medium fruit

and your immune system needs recharging, a 100 percent raw diet is your best bet. Otherwise, they say, a mostly raw-food diet—75 percent raw and 25 percent cooked—should suffice.

For her part, Dr. Alschuler says that she has never recommended an all-raw diet to any of the women she treats—only mostly raw foods. Few people have a digestive system capable of handling all the fiber in an all-raw diet, she explains. And if you have digestive problems, like constipation, diarrhea or irritable bowel syndrome, you should definitely stay away from an entirely raw diet, she cautions. "Someone who feels tired after eating lots of carbohydrates shouldn't do it either."

No matter how good your digestion or your relationship with carbohydrates, an all-raw diet isn't for you if you're pregnant or nursing, says Dr. O'Brien. You'll be hard-pressed to get all the calories that you need. Ditto if you're underweight.

If you do go on an exclusively uncooked diet, Dr. Alschuler suggests that you stay on it for no more than a couple of weeks.

"It's hard for people to get enough nutrients eating only raw foods," she explains. And even if you eat lots of sprouted grains, nuts, seeds and sprouted beans, it's particularly hard to get enough protein, she says. Grains and beans are good sources of protein, but you can't eat them raw unless you sprout them to make them digestible. And you'd have to eat hefty servings of the raw stuff. One cup of dried grains or beans germinates into five to ten cups of sprouts.

Here's some more advice on going raw, or mostly raw.

Eat a rainbow. When you choose vegetables and fruits, go for the whole spectrum of color, advises Dr. Alschuler. Among fruits and vegetables, each pigment supplies unique and important nutrients. Deep yellow and orange fruits and vegetables (like carrots, cantaloupe and nectarines) are good sources of beta-carotene, which the body converts into vitamin A. Deep green leafy vegetables (like broccoli and romaine lettuce) supply the B vitamin folate, the mineral iron and, often, calcium.

Become a sprout farmer. To avoid missing out on protein, make sure that you eat plenty of raw and sprouted seeds and nuts as well as sprouted beans and grains, says Dr. Alschuler. Just keep the seeds moistened, covered with a damp paper towel, in a jar in a dark place for a few days. Aim for a total of a cup or two daily.

Eat often. A 100 percent raw-food diet is bulky and relatively low in calories, so unless you're trying to lose weight, it's hard to get all the calories that you need, Dr. Alschuler says. You'll probably need to graze all day rather than sit down for three main meals, she says.

Cook a quarter. If an all-raw diet is hard to follow, eat about a quarter of your food cooked, suggests Dr. Alschuler. Eat your oats and other grains cooked, instead of sprouted. Include some bread in your diet and steam half of the vegetables that you eat, she says.

Select organically grown produce. If your diet consists mostly of plant foods, Dr. Alschuler suggests choosing organically grown produce whenever possible, to minimize exposure to pesticides and other chemicals used to grow fruits and vegetables.

Add a supplement. Women following a raw or mostly raw diet need to take vitamin and mineral supplements to get the Daily Value of certain key nutrients, Dr. Fugh-Berman says.

Milk and milk products are a primary source of vitamin D and calcium, essential for strong bones. But milk, cheese, yogurt and other dairy products are off-limits on a raw-food diet. So getting all the vitamin D and calcium that you need gets tricky, says Dr. Fugh-Berman. To keep your bones strong, take a 1,200-milligram calcium supplement daily if you're still menstruating, or 1,500 milligrams daily if you're past menopause, she says. And look for a multivitamin/mineral supplement with vitamin D.

A Typical Mostly Raw Diet Menu

If an all-raw diet is inconvenient or hard on your digestion, experts suggest that you consider a menu of mostly raw rather than all-raw food. Here's a sample menu.

Breakfast
Fruit (unlimited)
1 handful of nuts or seeds

Lunch
Main-course salad—snow peas, sliced peppers, carrot sticks, tomatoes, red cabbage, beets, carrots, apples and any other vegetables or fruits that you can eat raw—topped with cooked beans or sprouts (unlimited) and dressed with lemon juice or balsamic vinegar and up to 1 teaspoon of cold-pressed olive oil
Fresh fruit

Dinner
Large salad with any combination of raw fruits and vegetables that you like, dressed with lemon juice or balsamic vinegar and 1 teaspoon of cold-pressed olive oil
1 cup steamed green vegetables or ½ cup cooked corn, mashed or diced sweet potatoes or mixed peas and carrots
Tofu or beans (unlimited) or 1 handful of nuts or seeds

Look out for vitamin B_{12} and zinc, too. Found only in animal products, B_{12} plays a role in the production of blood and DNA and helps keep your nervous system clicking. Your multi should also give you the zinc that you need. A mineral dear to your immune system, it's also harder to come by in plant food.

Have your iron levels checked. To make sure that you don't develop iron-deficiency anemia, Dr. Alschuler suggests that you get tested for anemia before starting a raw or mostly raw diet and every three to six months after. If your doctor recommends it, take a multivitamin with iron, she says.

THE ORNISH PROGRAM: GOOD FOR YOU AND FOR YOUR HEART

Miriam Leefe, a veteran horticulturist, has heart disease, but she's taking steps to avoid drastic measures such as bypass surgery.

Leefe's method? A very low fat, low-cholesterol vegetarian diet combined with walking, cycling, yoga, daily meditation and support group meetings, along with a mild cholesterol-lowering drug. It's all part of a program designed by Dr. Dean Ornish.

Four years after Leefe ditched her old diet and sedentary, stressed-out ways and started following the dietary and lifestyle advice of Dr. Ornish, tests show that she has progressively less cholesterol-laden plaque lining the arteries to her heart. Translated, that means that the results she's getting from this diet are bigger benefits than she could get from any conventional medical procedure alone. While bypass surgery and angioplasty improve blood flow to the heart, neither cleans cholesterol from arteries, as the Ornish program does. With the Ornish program, Leefe is effectively *reversing* heart disease.

"I'd never go back to my old eating habits," Leefe says. "I'm too greedy about all the things that I want to do to give them up. Some people say that this kind of change is too difficult. Well, it's not hard if you value life."

Excellent Results in Women

In the books that he's written, at his research institute, in the classes that he teaches and in the retreats that he runs for people who want to change their lifestyles, Dr. Ornish makes a very convincing case for eating and living the way Leefe does.

At the core of the Ornish program is the diet—one that gets a mere 10 percent of calories from fat. The standard American diet, by contrast, is 36 to 37 percent fat.

The Ornish diet consists of mostly vegetables, grains, fruits, beans and peas—no meat, poultry or fish; no whole-fat dairy products and no egg yolks. Egg whites, which are fat-free, are allowed. The diet also allows up to two servings of skim milk, nonfat cheese or other nonfat dairy foods. And you can have small amounts of sugar (the amount that you'd get in two fat-free cookies), salt (about a teaspoon a day, tops) and some alcohol (one drink only), if you like. Caffeinated drinks such as coffee are out, as is butter, margarine and added oil.

You'll probably find the Ornish diet less extreme and more palatable than the raw-food diet. It's still austere by American standards, but the benefits are clearer. Dr. Ornish has hard data to justify his recommendations. In fact, he was the first to provide hard scientific evidence that following such a diet, and making other lifestyle changes, could reverse heart disease, the number one killer of American women.

To test his hypothesis, Dr. Ornish recruited 48 volunteers with heart disease in 1989. He put half on the very low fat vegetarian diet and had them exercise and practice stress management daily. He had the other volunteers follow a standard diet that met the American Heart Association's guidelines—no more than 30 percent of calories from fat—and exercise.

After one year, people in the second group were worse off than they had been. Sophisticated tests showed that the plaques that had built up in their arteries were thicker than before. And members of the group complained more often of chest pain, a sign that less blood was reaching their hearts.

In contrast, the same kind of test revealed that 82 percent of the people in the first group had cleaner arteries than when they started. Their blood cholesterol levels and blood pressure (two risk factors of heart disease) had dropped. And nearly all said that their chest pain had disappeared. Four years later, a follow-up study showed that significantly more blood was reaching their hearts—a key finding, since a cutoff in blood flow to the heart is what causes heart attacks.

For people with heart disease, it seemed, the news couldn't get better. But for women, it did, says Dr. Ornish. "Our data showed disease reversal occurred earlier in women."

And that's just one of many benefits of the Ornish program. "The people we studied experienced an average weight loss of 25 pounds in the first year," says Dr. Ornish.

Moreover, people with diabetes who followed the program were better able to control their blood sugar. "Some were, under their doctors supervision, able to reduce or even discontinue their use of insulin or other drugs," he says.

A Diet Backed by Research

Dr. Ornish has plenty of solid scientific research to back up the do's and don'ts of his brand of food therapy.

Don't eat meat, period. Meat is, as a rule, high in saturated fat, and rafts of studies show that saturated fat is a prime culprit in the advent of heart disease. Not only does saturated fat increase levels of bad, artery-clogging cholesterol (low-density lipoprotein, or LDL) in the blood, it also lowers the levels of so-called good, artery-cleaning cholesterol (high-density lipoprotein, or HDL). Research suggests that the iron in red meat makes it especially pernicious, Dr. Ornish notes, since iron converts bad cholesterol into a particularly sticky form that's more likely to clog arteries.

Do eat more grains, beans and peas. The Ornish diet relies on grains and legumes for protein. Aside from being essentially fat-free, vegetable protein also lowers cholesterol levels. Also, research shows that grains, legumes, vegetables and fruits are packed with fiber, vitamins and other nutrients that lower cholesterol levels, aid weight loss and help prevent cancer.

Don't go overboard with sugar. Since they deliver lots of calories in a small package, sugar and sugar-laced foods and beverages contribute to obesity. And studies suggest that sugar can stimulate production of both cholesterol and triglycerides, two fats that contribute to heart disease, says Dr. Ornish.

Do limit salt and sodium. Though only a quarter of people with high blood pressure are salt-sensitive—that is, their blood pressure shoots even higher when they eat sodium, the main constituent of salt—large doses can raise anyone's blood pressure, Dr. Ornish explains.

Don't add caffeine. In Dr. Ornish's words, caffeine "shortens your fuse," and research finds that volatile, stressed-out people run a higher risk of heart disease. So caffeine isn't allowed.

Do have a drink, if you like. Several studies have found that moderate drinkers are slightly less likely to die from heart disease than nondrinkers. So alcohol is allowed in small quantities.

The Ornish Diet Shopping List

The following is a shopping list of what you need to buy to follow the Ornish diet, along with the number of servings that Dr. Ornish recommends you should have every day.

Whole-grain cereals and breads, pasta, brown rice, corn and potatoes. Two servings per day. (One serving equals 1 slice bread; ½ cup rice, pasta, cooked cereal, corn or potatoes; or 1 ounce dry cereal.)

Vegetables, including dark leafy greens and red and yellow vegetables for vitamin C and calcium. Three or more servings per day. But no avocados, olives, coconuts, nuts or seeds, since they're too high in fat. (One serving equals ½ cup raw or cooked vegetables or 1 cup leafy vegetables.)

Fruit. Two to four servings. (One serving equals ½ cup cooked fruit or juice, 1 whole piece fruit, ¼ cup dried fruit or 1 melon wedge.)

Protein-rich foods, such as soy milk or tofu (preferably calcium-fortified), soy burgers, beans, peas or egg whites. Two to four servings per day. (One serving equals 1 cup soy milk, ½ cup cooked beans or peas, 1½ ounces tofu or 2½ ounces meat substitute.)

Nonfat dairy, like milk, yogurt, cottage cheese or cheese. One to two servings per day. (One serving equals 1 cup nonfat milk or nonfat yogurt, 1 ounce nonfat cheese or ½ cup nonfat cottage cheese.)

A Typical Ornish Diet Menu

If you decide that the Ornish diet merits consideration, this menu will get you off to the right start.

Breakfast
½ medium banana
2 slices whole-wheat toast
1 shredded-wheat biscuit
1 cup nonfat milk

Morning Snack
1 apple

Lunch
1 cup chopped fresh spinach
½ cup sliced raw mushrooms
1 cup navy bean soup
2 slices whole-wheat bread
½ cup sliced strawberries

Afternoon Snack
1 orange

Dinner
1 cup whole-wheat pasta
½ cup tomato-basil sauce with ½ cup chopped cooked zucchini
2 slices whole-wheat bread
½ cup fresh blueberries
½ cup nonfat yogurt

Nonfat sweets, like honey or hard candy. Two servings or fewer per day.

If you're pregnant or nursing, add one or two servings of nonfat dairy or calcium-fortified soy and additional grains, vegetables and fruits, says Helen Roe, R.D., nutritionist at Dr. Ornish's Sausalito institute and chief nutritional consultant for his research studies.

Big Changes, Fast Results

Any woman who has tried the Ornish diet—and there are plenty of them—will tell you that the plan requires a lot of big changes. Nonetheless, people seem to have an easier time making big changes than making smaller ones, Dr. Ornish says. That's because the big changes get results, and relatively quickly. If you make small changes, like limiting fat to 30 percent of calories, you don't get quick results, he says. On the Ornish program, "People start feeling better after just a couple of weeks," he says.

In any event, you don't have to give up good food to eat à l'Ornish, promises Roe. If you master a few low-fat cooking techniques and know what to look for in the supermarket, you can do well by your taste buds and the rest of your body. Here's how.

Clean out the pantry. To get started, Roe suggests that you get rid of anything in your refrigerator or pantry that's not allowed on the Ornish diet: high-sodium canned goods, fatty chips, fatty and sugary desserts, meat, coffee and tea. To ease regrets, Roe suggests that you donate nonperishable no-no's to your local food bank.

Cook with less fat and more flavor. In his book *Everyday Cooking with Dr. Dean Ornish*, Dr. Ornish recommends these tricks and techniques.

- Replace oil-and-vinegar dressing with flavored vinegars or bottled fat-free Italian dressing.
- Sauté vegetables in a small amount of vegetable broth, wine or water instead of oil.
- Cook with a wider array of herbs and spices.
- Add dried herbs a few minutes before you finish cooking, so they have time to rehydrate and impart their flavor.
- Add fresh herbs at the last minute.
- Dress salads with a mixture of tofu or yogurt and herbs like dill, basil or cilantro and whole-grain mustard and vinegar.
- Add pungent ingredients like mustard, horseradish, soy sauce, miso (fermented soybean paste), hot-pepper sauces, sun-dried tomatoes, shiitake mushrooms and capers to dishes.

Revamp your favorites. You won't have to forgo your old standbys, Dr. Ornish says in his book. Here's how to make over your favorites.

- In baked goods, replace whole eggs with either egg substitute or egg whites.
- Replace the fat in baked goods with prune puree or unsweetened applesauce. (Use ¼ cup prune puree or applesauce for every ½ cup butter that the recipe calls for.)
- Substitute nonfat yogurt, mayonnaise or sour cream for the full-fat versions.
- Substitute fat-free cheese, such as nonfat ricotta, for whole-fat cheese in cooked dishes.
- Replace the cream in pasta sauces with nonfat sour cream or skim milk thickened with cornstarch (a tablespoon of cornstarch will thicken 1 cup of milk).

Take a multivitamin/mineral supplement. As with other diets that omit animal foods, you'll need a nutritional supplement that supplies vitamin B_{12}, found only in food from animals, says Dr. Ornish. Don't choose a multi with iron, though, unless your doctor tells you to. If you're not menstruating, you probably won't need it, he points out. (For guidelines on the roles of individual nutrients in preventing heart disease and other health conditions, see page 416.)

Work out, chill out. Diet is just one part of the Ornish program. Although diet is very important, it's the combination of exercise, stress reduction *and* diet that seem to reverse heart disease, says Dr. Ornish. So while you're on the diet, don't neglect other aspects of the total program. (For practical ways to work exercise into your life, see page 90; for guidelines on other relaxation techniques, see meditation on page 233, yoga on page 309 and breath work on page 67.)

THE PRITIKIN PLAN: MULTIPLE BENEFITS

To eat the Pritikin way, you have to learn certain table manners. These go beyond the usual no-elbows-on-the-table variety. There are other things that aren't allowed on the table, either. Butter, margarine, mayonnaise, excessive amounts of salt, and caffeine are out. Meat is allowed, as long as you only eat one serving a day and that one serving is very lean and limited to a 3½-ounce portion—the size of a deck of playing cards. Dairy products are acceptable, but only if they're nonfat, and even then, you shouldn't have them more than twice daily.

"Going to the Pritikin Longevity Center was an education, like going back to college," says Linda Melrose, an Indianapolis art dealer who abandoned her old diet five years ago and embraced Pritikin's low-fat, high-fiber program instead.

Engineering Good Health

Researchers first turned their attention to the low-fat eating and exercise plan, known as the Pritikin diet, back in the mid-1970s, when an engineer named Nathan Pritikin started promoting lifestyle changes for people with heart disease.

Diagnosed with heart disease at age 40, Pritikin refused to accept the conventional wisdom of the day—that surgery and drugs were his only options. With the same zeal that he brought to solving engineering puzzles, Pritikin turned to medical literature and started looking for alternative solutions. Intrigued by a handful of largely ignored studies that hinted at a link between diet, exercise and heart disease, he decided to change his lifestyle. He cut nearly all the fat out of his diet; gave up salt, sugar and caffeine and began exercising regularly.

Back then, the sophisticated tests that Dr. Ornish later used to prove that diet and lifestyle changes could clear the plaque out of arteries didn't exist. But treadmill stress tests and electrocardiograms showed that Pritikin's heart was getting progressively stronger—he could run longer and faster. Though they didn't prove it, the tests strongly suggested that he was, remarkably enough, beating heart disease by eating right and exercising.

That and subsequent successes led Pritikin to publish the first book on the plan, *The Pritikin Program for Diet and Exercise.* And in 1976, he opened the first Pritikin Longevity Center in Santa Monica, California. Later, a second center opened in Miami Beach.

Thousands of Converts

Every year, thousands of women (and men) check into Pritikin Longevity Centers in California and Florida or pick up copies of *The New Pritikin Program* to learn this new eating etiquette and make other healthy changes in their lifestyles.

Why? For two decades, it's been getting results.

Though best known for its success in treating heart disease, Pritikin's program has an enviable record against an assortment of other chronic and life-threatening diseases.

"If you want to lose weight without getting hungry; if you want to reduce your risk of high blood pressure, heart disease, diabetes and osteoporosis; if you want to avoid cancer, this is the way to eat," says James J. Kenney, R.D., Ph.D., nutrition research specialist for the Pritikin Longevity Centers in California and Florida.

On the heart disease front, studies find that the plan can lower blood pressure and cholesterol levels. In a study conducted at the University of California at Los Angeles (UCLA), 4,587 men and women who followed the plan for three weeks saw their cholesterol levels drop 23 percent. (Women in the study also saw their weight drop an average of 4.4 percent.)

For her part, Melrose says that her cholesterol levels dropped 25 percent. "And I lost 35 pounds without dieting!" she boasts.

Additional research shows that like Dr. Ornish's diet, the Pritikin plan can improve blood flow to the heart in people who already have coronary artery disease. In another UCLA study, tests showed that blood flow improved measurably after six weeks on the program.

The diet and exercise program has also been proven to help bring diabetes under control. In a UCLA study that followed 652 men and women with adult-onset diabetes, 71 percent of those taking drugs and 39 percent of those taking insulin were able to stop taking the medications after three weeks on the program. Not only did their blood sugar levels stabilize, their weight, blood pressure and cholesterol levels dropped significantly.

Finally, research suggests that the plan may also cut the risk of various types of cancer, including colon and breast cancer. Reducing fat, Dr. Kenney says, reduces the amount of bile acid, a product that the digestive system secretes. That is believed to lower cancer risk, in part, because certain bacteria in the colon convert those acids into cancer-causing compounds.

In another UCLA study, researchers found that women had lower levels of the female hormone estrogen in their bloodstreams after 22 days on the plan. That's significant, since evidence suggests that estrogen plays a key role in the genesis of breast cancer. Though it wasn't clear why the women's blood estrogen levels dropped, it's a good bet that the diet's low fat content played a key role, says R. James Barnard, Ph.D., professor of physiological science and medicine at the University of California in Los Angeles, who headed this and several other studies of the Pritikin plan. "Research is showing that societies who consume high-fat diets have a higher incidence of breast cancer than those where people eat a low-fat, high-fiber diet," he adds.

A Lifetime Eating Plan

Like the Ornish diet, most of the foods that you eat on the Pritikin plan are plants—vegetables, whole grains, fruits and legumes. The following are the basic tenets of the diet.

Allow yourself some dairy and meat. You can have up to two servings of nonfat dairy and, unlike the Ornish plan, modest portions of lean meat, poultry or fish, daily.

The truth is, most of us would be better off skipping the meat, poultry and fish, Dr. Kenney says. But if you can't imagine living the meatless life, stick with small portions of "fatty" fish, like salmon and mackerel. This may sound like strange advice, when the goal is to cut fat. But research shows that such fish are good sources of a special type of fat, omega-3 fatty acids, which seems to help protect the heart by reducing the tendency of blood clots when these acids are consumed in small doses.

"You don't benefit from eating more than four to six ounces a week, though," Dr. Kenney says. "If you eat it every day, evidence suggests that you'll have a higher cholesterol level and may be worse off in the long run."

Nix the sugar and fat. On the Pritikin plan, sugar, high-fat vegetables like avocados and olives, unsalted nuts, alcohol and most vegetable oils are considered "caution" foods—they're off-limits except on special occasions, and in limited amounts.

Avoid animal fats and other saturated oils. Like the Ornish plan, the Pritikin diet limits fat to 10 percent of total calories. So there's really no room for added oil, butter or margarine. Same goes for full-fat dairy products (like whole milk), egg yolks, tropical oils (such as coconut oil) and hydrogenated oils (often found in baked goods).

Say no to salt. The Pritikin diet prohibits salt, including salted nuts and high-sodium prepared foods, for a couple of reasons, Dr. Kenney says. Even if you're not the salt-sensitive type, whose blood pressure rockets when you eat the stuff, excess salt makes your body excrete extra calcium, raising your risk of osteoporosis.

What You *Can* Eat

Basically, the Pritikin plan is built around the following amounts of "go" foods, which you can eat every day.

Complex carbohydrates or starches, such as whole-grain cereals and breads, pasta, lentils and brown rice. Eat five or more servings a day. (One serving equals 1 slice of bread; ½ cup cooked rice, pasta or cereal; or 1 ounce dry cereal.)

Vegetables. Aim for four or more servings a day. (One serving equals ½ cup raw or cooked vegetables or 1 cup leafy greens.)

Fruits. Eat three or more servings a day. (One serving equals about ½ cup juice or cooked fruit, 1 whole fruit, ½ cup dried fruit or 1 melon wedge.)

Nonfat milk, yogurt or cheese. Allow yourself two servings per day. (One serving equals 1 cup nonfat milk, 6 ounces nonfat yogurt or ½ cup nonfat ricotta cheese.)

High-protein foods, such as lean meat, poultry or fish. Include one 3½-ounce serving per day. (Vegetarians can substitute ⅔ cup beans, 4 to 6 ounces tofu or 1 ounce nuts or seeds.)

A Typical Pritikin Diet Menu

This sample menu, adapted from *The New Pritikin Program*, will make it easy to get started on the Pritikin diet.

Breakfast
½ cup cooked oatmeal
½ medium banana
1 cup nonfat milk

Morning Snack
½ cup low-sodium vegetable juice
1 cup assorted chopped raw vegetables

Lunch
½ cup chopped steamed vegetables with lemon juice and salsa
2 ounces nonfat ricotta cheese
1 cup tossed salad with 1 to 2 tablespoons fat-free dressing
1¼ cups sliced fresh strawberries

Afternoon Snack
3 cups air-popped popcorn
1 cup raw green and red pepper strips
1 cup cherry tomatoes

Dinner
3½ ounces broiled fish
1 medium baked potato
1 cup chopped steamed broccoli
1 cup tossed salad with 1 to 2 tablespoons fat-free dressing
1 medium peach

There's no need to count calories on the plan, Dr. Kenney says. "The way that you determine how much you eat is simple. You eat the minimum recommended number of servings, and if you're still hungry, have more complex carbohydrates, vegetables or fruits, but no more dairy or protein. If you're eating this way, your appetite is a good guide to how much you should be eating," he explains.

If you're pregnant or nursing, add two servings of nonfat dairy, at least three extra servings of carbohydrates and more fruits and vegetables, says Diane Grabowski-Nepa, R.D., nutrition educator at the Pritikin Longevity Center in California.

Starting Out

All told, the Pritikin diet is very similar to Dr. Ornish's, just a little more liberal with meat, poultry and fish and a bit more restrictive with salt. Still, if you've been eating the average American diet, Pritikin is going to be a departure. Give it a try, though, and your palate will adjust quickly enough, promises Grabowski-Nepa. Here's how to make it work.

Set your own pace. There's no "right" pace when you're changing the way you eat. "Whether you want to make these changes in your diet gradually or all at once depends on your personality," says Grabowski-Nepa.

"But if you have a serious health problem, such as advanced arteriosclerosis, diabetes or blood pressure, or are very overweight, your doctor may recommend that you go 100 percent and jump right in," says Dr. Kenney.

Eat natural foods. Look for foods in their natural state, since they're less fatty, says Grabowski-Nepa. "Oatmeal, for instance, is a better, lower-fat bet than an oat bran muffin," she says.

Eat more soup. Grabowski-Nepa suggests bean and vegetable soups in particular, since they're filling, low in fat and calories and highly nutritious.

Seek out fat-free versions of your favorites. Take advantage of the proliferation of nonfat foods and convenience produce at the supermarkets, urges Grabowksi-Nepa. "This has really simplified the process of eating healthy. You can find nonfat cheeses, dressings and all sorts of prewashed, precut vegetables and fruits in bags."

Scope out sodium. There's a lot of salt hidden in processed foods like canned soups and vegetables, frozen entrées and prepared sauces, says Grabowski-Nepa. So read labels at the supermarket and opt for low-sodium versions, she advises.

Season sans salt. The Pritikin plan encourages use of salt-free seasonings such as garlic, herbs and horseradish.

Don't forget to exercise. "We advise people to walk at least two to four miles, at least five or six days a week," Dr. Kenney says. You can also get the same benefits by playing tennis, jogging or biking as often. Exercise will help lower your blood pressure, keep your blood sugar levels on an even keel, promote weight loss, improve cardiovascular fitness and give you more stamina, he adds. (For advice on designing your own custom exercise program, see page 85.)

TRADITIONAL CHINESE MEDICINE DIET: USED BY MILLIONS

In China, doctors regularly exhort their patients to eat "a balanced diet." But they mean something quite different than American physicians dispensing the same advice.

According to Traditional Chinese Medicine, a balanced diet isn't one that includes selections from four basic food groups. Rather, it's a diet that balances yin and yang, universal complementary opposites. (For an illustrated explanation of yin and yang, see page 278.)

"To enjoy good health, you must balance yin and yang," says Henry C. Lu, Ph.D., doctor of Traditional Chinese Medicine, principal of the International College of Traditional Chinese Medicine in Vancouver and author of *Chinese System of Food Cures*.

Think of yin and yang as two complementary sets of qualities. While yin is cool, watery, dark and contracting, for instance, yang is warm, dry, light and expansive. In the traditional Chinese view, everything in the universe—including you and every bite of food you eat—is yin or yang, to a greater or lesser degree.

Since yang is warm, foods that have a warming effect on the body, such as chili peppers, are predominantly yang. Watermelon and other foods that cool the body are predominantly yin, because yin is cool, explains Maoshing Ni, Ph.D., vice-president of Yo San University of Traditional Chinese Medicine and author of *The Tao of Nutrition*. Foods that neither warm nor cool the body, like brown rice, buckwheat, peas and lettuce, are neutral—no more yin than yang.

A balanced diet can include foods that are predominantly yin and yang as well as foods that are neutral, says Dr. Ni. But it includes them in such proportions that the yin and yang foods balance one another—and keep you in balance.

"Generally speaking, such a diet is heavy on grains and vegetables; uses a lot of beans and soy products; includes some fruits, nuts and seeds; and uses protein, like red meat, poultry and fish as a condiment," says Dr. Ni. In essence, it's the diet that most Chinese have been eating for thousands of years.

A Different Balance

Have the flu? Painful menstrual periods? Hemorrhoids? PMS? High blood pressure? Trouble conceiving? A Traditional Chinese Medicine doctor would advise you to check your plate.

According to the Traditional Chinese Medicine theory, diet not only contributes to but can also help alleviate virtually any health problem.

Most women with PMS, for instance, are too yang, Dr. Lu says. Cooling yin foods, such as celery, can help alleviate their symptoms. Hemorrhoids

Telling Yin from Yang, the Chinese Way

Not sure what's yin and what's yang? To help sort things out, refer to these basic guidelines from the *Chinese System of Food Cures*, by Henry C. Lu, Ph.D., doctor of Traditional Chinese Medicine and principal of the International College of Traditional Chinese Medicine in Vancouver.

Yin: Bamboo shoots, bananas, clams, crabs, grapefruit, kelp, lettuce, muskmelons, persimmons, salt, seaweed, star fruit, sugar cane, water chestnuts and watermelons

Somewhat yin: Apples, barley, bean curd, button mushrooms, cucumbers, eggplant, egg whites, hops, mandarin oranges, mangoes, marjoram, mung beans, pears, peppermint, radishes, sesame oil, spinach, strawberries, tangerines, tomatoes, wheat and wheat bran

Neutral: Abalone, adzuki beans, apricots, beef, beets, black sesame seeds, black soybeans, carp, carrots, castro beans, celery, Chinese cabbage, corn, duck, eggs, egg yolks, figs, grapes, honey, kidney beans, kohlrabi, licorice, milk, olives, oysters, papayas, peanuts, pineapple, plums, polished rice, pork, potatoes, pumpkin, rice bran, saffron, shiitake mushrooms, string beans, sugar, sunflower seeds, sweet potatoes, sweet rice and yellow soybeans

Slightly yang: Asparagus and malt

Moderately yang: Basil, brown sugar, cherries, chestnuts, chicken, chives, cloves, coconut, coffee, coriander, dates, eel, fennel, fresh ginger, garlic, ginseng, green onions, guavas, ham, kumquats, lamb, leeks, nutmeg, peaches, raspberries, rosemary, shrimp, spearmint, squash, star anise, sunflower seeds, vinegar, walnuts and wine

Yang: Black pepper; cinnamon; dried ginger; green, red and white pepper and soybean oil are usually associated with excess yang as well and respond to cooling yin foods like ripe bananas, he says.

While proper nutrition alone won't prevent every illness, good health is pretty much impossible without it, Dr. Lu explains. And while dietary change is rarely enough to treat severe illness—traditional Chinese doctors usually use acupuncture and herbs with hard-core cases—there's no curing someone who won't eat properly.

Yin Women Need Yang Foods

In keeping with the tenets of Traditional Chinese Medicine, everyone should eat a balanced diet. But that's not to say that everyone should eat exactly the same diet, Dr. Ni points out. That's because everything in the universe—every person, climate, lifestyle, season—is yin or yang to some degree.

To maintain balance, you need to fine-tune your diet, taking into account whether you're constitutionally more yin than yang; what your gender, age and activity level is; what kind of climate you live in; what you do for a living and what season it is, Dr. Ni explains. "If you tend to be more yin, eat more yang foods, and vice versa."

Women, who are generally more yin than yang, should choose more yang foods like yams, green onions and chicken, to even things out, Dr. Ni advises. When it's cold (yin) outside, we should all eat more of these warming (yang) foods. And if your job requires a lot of physical exertion or yang energy, you should also eat more yang foods to replenish that energy. That's for everyday maintenance. If you're sick, you'll need to adjust your diet again.

"Let's say that you have high blood pressure," Dr. Lu says. "There are different types with different causes, but one type is due to the liver being too yang." In that case, Dr. Lu might recommend eating more eggplant, which is not only yin but also can prevent arteriosclerosis.

Firsthand Research

Studies find that the traditional Chinese diet—mostly grains and vegetables; smaller quantities of legumes and fruit; occasional servings of meat, poultry and fish; and very little fat—is extremely healthy. The China-Cornell-Oxford Diet and Health Project, a research undertaking that has been gathering information on the eating habits and health of 10,000 Chinese since 1983, finds lower rates of heart disease, cancer, diabetes and obesity in China than in the United States.

So the diet seems to prevent health problems. But can it cure them?

There are no Western-style clinical studies to answer the question definitively, says Dr. Ni. Thousands of years of success stories, however, suggest that the diet has therapeutic power. "Each food has been researched for its therapeutic value for several thousand years," Dr. Ni says.

Customize the Diet

If you want to give Traditional Chinese Medicine's nutrition a try, experts suggest these steps.

Determine whether you're more yin than yang. People who are predominantly yang are usually outgoing, sometimes aggressive. They're more likely to feel warm and suffer from yang-type illnesses, such as stress, congestion, musculoskeletal pain, constipation, headaches, high blood pressure and heart disease, Dr. Ni says.

Yin people, on the other hand, are more collected and contemplative. They're more sensitive to cold and more vulnerable to problems such as fatigue, overweight and diarrhea.

A Traditional Chinese Medicine Diet Menu

In Traditional Chinese Medicine, there's no "right" diet for everyone. In general, the menu shown here is an Americanized version from *The Tao of Nutrition* by Maoshing Ni, Ph.D., vice-president of Yo San University of Traditional Chinese Medicine, appropriate for spring and summer in areas with temperate climates like the United States. Beyond that, say experts, you'll need to modify this sample diet depending on your body type and what you do for a living.

Breakfast
Cream of rice or wheat, with raisins and cinnamon
Steamed apples

Lunch
Winter melon soup with tofu
Rice cake with nut butter

Dinner
Stir-fried vegetables with tofu and gluten, a meat substitute made
   from wheat (available at health food stores)
Brown rice

Consider your lifestyle. If you run around a lot, you use up a lot of yang energy, so you need extra yang food, like beans and ham. If you sit at a desk, you'll want a more yin diet, with extra vegetables and grains, Dr. Ni says.

Accommodate the climate. "In tropical places where the weather is typically more hot and humid, you want to eat foods that are more cooling and foods that regenerate body fluid. You'll also want foods that are a little drying, so that the humidity and dampness does not accumulate in your body," Dr. Ni says. Extra fruits and vegetables are good choices.

In northern climates where the weather is cool, windy and dry, you should eat foods that are warming and hydrating, he says. You'd eat more chicken soup, for instance, than you would in the tropics.

Change menus with the seasons. By the same token, summer months are warm, or yang, so you should eat more cooling, yin foods during the dog days, Dr. Ni says. And winter months are yin, so choose more yang foods, like lamb and shrimp.

Eat less than you'd like. Unlike Western therapeutic diets, Traditional Chinese Medicine doesn't specify how much food you should eat. A good rule of thumb, says Dr. Ni, is to eat 80 percent of what you'd like to eat. That way you won't overdo it. When you sit down to eat, fill 70 percent of your plate with grains and vegetables; 25 percent with "condiments" like meat, nuts, seeds and legumes; and 5 percent with fruit.

A Typical Traditional Chinese Medicine Meal

The Traditional Chinese Medicine diet doesn't specify exact portions of specific foods. Instead, guidelines suggest that your meals should typically consist of 70 percent grains and vegetables; 25 percent meat, nuts, seeds and legumes; and 5 percent fruit. The menu should also change with the seasons.

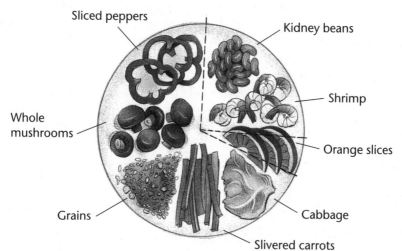

Sliced peppers

Kidney beans

Shrimp

Whole mushrooms

Orange slices

Grains

Cabbage

Slivered carrots

Talk to your doctor or consult a nutritionist. For complicated health conditions, such as infertility, you're better off seeing a professional, fully qualified Traditional Chinese Medical doctor (T.C.M.). Chinese nutritional theory is extremely complicated, and doctors take into account all sorts of variables beyond your constitution, lifestyle and locale when prescribing a diet for a particular problem. If the symptoms are severe, you may need herbal remedies and acupuncture as well, Dr. Lu says.

MACROBIOTICS: THE JAPANESE PRESCRIPTION

For breakfast one winter morning, Beth Saito is having miso soup with seaweed, brown rice with adzuki beans and greens, and pickled fermented cabbage.

She doesn't always eat this way. When the weather is warmer, she might have some steamed whole-grain bread and cold fermented soybeans with grated radishes for breakfast. Not your average coffee-and-muffin morning routine.

Saito follows a macrobiotic diet, a carefully prescribed, low-fat, nearly vegetarian regimen that aims for balance amid constant change. Depending on the season, where she is and how she feels, she adjusts the menu for optimal health.

"I feel much better eating this way," says Saito, a New York restaurant manager who has been following a macrobiotic diet for over a decade.

Like Traditional Chinese Medicine and the philosophy on which it's based, macrobiotics seeks a healthful balance of yin and yang. The idea is to steer clear of extremely yin foods like sugar and extremely yang foods like red meat and eat a combination of moderately yin or yang ones, like brown rice and vegetables. Overall, your diet might be slightly yin or yang, depending where you live, the season and how you're feeling, since all those things are either yin, yang or somewhere in between.

In temperate climates like the United States, brown rice and other whole grains—considered the most balanced of foods—make up about 50 percent of a macrobiotic diet. Vegetables, which are moderately yin or yang, make up 25 to 30 percent. Sea vegetables and beans, also moderately yin or yang, make up another 5 to 10 percent, as do soups made with vegetables, grains and beans.

Seasonal fruit and small quantities of roasted nuts and seeds are included in the diet several times a week. Lean white fish, such as cod, is included one to three times a week, if desired. A small amount of vegetable oil may be used in cooking.

Flexibility Rules

Macrobiotics made a name for itself in the United States in the 1960s when the counterculture made the diet its own. Unfortunately, macrobiotics got noticed for all the wrong reasons. Some people who adopted the diet, then known as Zen Macrobiotics, developed severe nutritional deficiencies. A few died.

Yin and Yang, Macrobiotic-Style

Macrobiotics defines yin and yang slightly differently than Traditional Chinese Medicine. According to the basic tenets of macrobiotics, yin is cooling, light, wet and expanding, while yang is warming, heavy, dry and contracting. Yin foods tend to be light and juicy; sour, bitter, very sweet or hot in taste; cool in color and grow up out of the ground. Yang foods, on the other hand, are usually heavy and dry; salty, slightly sweet or pungent in taste; warm in color and grow down into the earth, like garlic.

Why the divergence from Traditional Chinese Medicine?

"In Chinese history, the classification of yin and yang varied from philosopher to philosopher and from age to age," says Michio Kushi, founder of the Kushi Institute, a macrobiotics center in Becket, Massachusetts. Macrobiotics, he explains, adopted the definitions that were most comprehensive, dynamic and easiest to grasp.

For the record, here's a list of extremely yin, extremely yang and centrally balanced foods, according to macrobiotic thinking.

Strong yang foods: Eggs, fish, poultry, red meat, refined salt, salty, hard cheese and seafood

More balanced foods: Barley malt; beans and bean products; whole cereal grains and grain products; leafy greens; round and root vegetables; sea salt; sea vegetables, such as nori (dried seaweed); vegetable oil; spring and well water; decaffeinated or herbal teas and beverages; temperate zone fruit, such as apples and pears; seeds and nuts; rice syrup and other grain-based sweeteners, available at health food stores

Strong yin foods: Alcohol; aromatic and stimulating beverages like coffee and black tea; foods containing chemicals, preservatives, artificial colors or pesticides; frozen and canned foods; honey, sugar and other refined sweeteners; milk, cream, ice cream and yogurt; refined oils; spices; tropical fruits and vegetables; white rice and white flour

"It was very easily misunderstood—and in a very drastic way," says Michio Kushi, who introduced macrobiotics to the United States from Japan after World War II. To distinguish the new version from the old, he clarified the basic principles of macrobiotics and dropped the "Zen" from the name.

Contrary to popular belief, macrobiotics was never meant to be, and isn't, rigid, says Kushi, who has also published dozens of books on macrobiotics and runs the Kushi Institute, a macrobiotics center in Becket, Massachusetts. "The macrobiotic way of eating is not a set pattern. It's flexible, depending on climate, season and personal need."

Extremely yin or yang foods—red meat, sugar, dairy products, animal fats, caffeinated drinks, chocolate, alcohol, eggs, processed foods, poultry, hot spices and tropical fruits—are usually off-limits, for example. But if you're hankering for ice cream on your birthday or a slice of turkey at Thanksgiving, you should enjoy it, Kushi says.

And, while tropical fruits such as pineapple are considered too yin for temperate climates like the United States, they're allowable in the tropics, where they grow naturally. Similarly, red meat, which is very yang, is per-

Getting**Started**

Macrobiotics

With macrobiotics, how you prepare food is as important as what you eat. So adherents say that it's a good idea to invest in a macrobiotic cookbook—especially one that will show you how to make macrobiotic versions of familiar favorites, like apple pie and cornbread. Or try macrobiotic cooking classes.

Note: Strict macrobiotics, such as fasting and raw-food diets, may not be appropriate for children.

Number of practitioners in the United States: Unknown.

Qualifications to look for: Look for someone who has trained at the Kushi Institute, the founding center of macrobiotics, or who has trained with one of their instructors.

Professional associations: The Kushi Institute, P.O. Box 7, Becket, MA 01223.

To find a practitioner: To locate a macrobiotics counselor or cooking instructor in your area, contact the Kushi Institute at the address listed above.

Approximate cost: $225 for a 1½-hour session. Special weeklong sessions at the Kushi Institute, designed specifically for women, average about $1,200, including meals, programs and accommodations.

mitted in cold climates like Alaska, which is very yin. Again, it's a matter of balance.

Achieving balance means making other adjustments on a regular basis. In summer, when the weather is hot, or yang, in most of the United States, you should eat more raw vegetables, which are yin, Kushi says. In the dead of winter, which is more yin, you should eat more yang foods—a little more white fish, for instance. If you have menstrual cramps (usually a sign that you've been overdoing it with yang food), you should forgo the fish for a month or two until things come back into balance.

Of course, simply adjusting your diet isn't always enough to establish balance, Kushi notes. You need to strike a balance among work and relationships, relaxation, exercise and meditation, too. But diet is an important part of the equation.

Curative Powers?

According to macrobiotic theory, a diet that balances yin and yang can help prevent and relieve illness.

Headaches, skin problems, allergies, fatigue, menstrual problems and sexual and reproductive problems can all be averted and usually alleviated with a macrobiotic diet, says Kushi. In many cases, so can heart disease, diabetes, arthritis and cancer, he adds.

Like the Pritikin plan and Traditional Chinese Medicine diet, the macrobiotic diet is essentially a low-fat, high-fiber vegetarian diet very similar to what most rural Chinese people eat. And Chinese population studies have shown that people who eat this way have lower rates of heart disease, obesity, diabetes and cancer, including breast cancer.

"It's a very healthy diet, and it reflects the dietary traditions of countries that tend to have much better health profiles than we do here," says Neal Barnard, M.D., president of Physicians' Committee for Responsible Medicine in Washington, D.C., and author of *Eat Right, Live Longer*.

Some studies have investigated macrobiotics' power, but not as many have been done as for other types of diets, Dr. Neal Barnard says. But research has shown that the diet can lower blood pressure and blood cholesterol levels profoundly.

In her book *Women's Bodies, Women's Wisdom*, Dr. Northrup recounts the story of a woman who found relief from fibroid tumors after switching to the diet. An adherent of macrobiotics herself, Dr. Northrup notes that such low-fat, high-fiber diets may also lower your risk of other women's health problems—notably breast cancer and other gynecological problems, such as PMS and endometriosis.

Whether the diet can treat cancer isn't yet clear. Some cancer patients who have pulled through after making the switch to macrobiotics, including baby doctor Benjamin Spock, credit the diet with their recoveries. Anecdotal evidence suggests that those who switch to the diet live longer than those who eat standard American fare.

When you're talking about something like breast cancer, these examples make a lot of sense, says Dr. Neal Barnard. "Low-fat diets are associated with longer survival in women with breast cancer," he notes.

A Typical Macrobiotic Diet Menu

On an average day, a macrobiotic diet menu might include 3 cups of whole grains or grain products, such as noodles or pasta; 1 to 2 cups of soup; 1½ to 2 cups of vegetables; ½ cup of beans and ¼ cup of sea vegetables, says Michio Kushi, founder of the Kushi Institute, a macrobiotics center in Becket, Massachusetts. You can also have 2 to 4 ounces of seafood once or twice a week, fruit two or three times a week and a small amount of nuts and seeds a couple times a week, he says.

The following starter menu is, in general, balanced for anyone in a temperate zone who is fairly healthy.

Breakfast
1 cup cooked millet
1 cup miso soup
½ cup chopped steamed cauliflower
1 sheet of nori (dried seaweed, available at health food stores), lightly toasted

Lunch
½ cup cooked kidney beans
1 cup cooked brown rice (cooked with a pinch of sea salt)
Corn on the cob
Squash soup (cook butternut squash, then puree)
½ cup chopped steamed broccoli

Afternoon Snack
½ cup roasted pumpkin seeds

Dinner
1 cup lightly sautéed tempeh with chopped vegetables
1 cup steamed barley
½ cup boiled collard greens
Stewed apples

If a woman has breast cancer that has spread to other parts of her body, her risk of dying from the disease increases 40 percent for every 1,000 grams of fat that she consumes monthly, according to a study from the State University of New York in Buffalo. While low-fat diets like macrobiotics contribute about 400 grams of fat a month, Dr. Neal Barnard points out, the typical American diet packs a whopping 1,500 grams a month. (A tablespoon of butter, lard, oil or other fat contains an average of 13 grams of fat.)

Macrobiotics Simplified

If you're pregnant or nursing, be sure to talk to an expert before switching to a macrobiotic diet, says Dr. Fuhrman. Whether macrobiotic diets are nutritionally adequate for children is a matter of debate, so check with your pediatrician or a nutritionist before changing your children's diets. If you get the green light, here's how to proceed.

Stock up. Certain foods that originated in Asia, like miso soup, are staples in a macrobiotic diet because they're considered well-balanced. So if you're going to go macrobiotic, you'll need to stock up on these perennial players in macrobiotic fare, available at your local health food store: short- and long-grain brown rice; millet; whole-grain barley; whole-wheat noodles; soy products like miso soup and tofu; lentils; chick-peas; adzuki, pinto and navy beans; split peas; seaweed; sea salt; barley-malt syrup; brown-rice syrup; brown-rice vinegar; sunflower, sesame and pumpkin seeds; grain teas; grain-based coffee substitutes and organically grown seasonal produce.

Take your time. A macrobiotic diet is a major departure from standard American eating. So take your time making the switch, suggests Gale Jack, macrobiotic counselor and cooking instructor at the Kushi Institute.

Phase out meat and prepared foods. First, wean yourself from extremely yin and yang foods. Over a period of two to three months, phase out meat, poultry, dairy products, sugary desserts and prepared foods, including frozen and canned stuff.

More rice, beans and veggies. While you're jettisoning meat and prepared foods, says Jack, phase in more brown rice, beans and fresh cooked vegetables to your diet. Try stir-frys and casseroles—dishes that include less meat and more grains and vegetables, she suggests.

Eat local fruits and vegetables. Unless you live in the tropics, fruits such as papaya and mangos are too yin for most areas of the United States, especially during the cold-weather months.

Forgo the microwave. To truly adhere to macrobiotic theory, you should cook over an open flame or a gas stove and avoid electric stoves and microwaves, says Jack, since the latter affects the food in a way that makes it more yin. Likewise, you should cook with wooden utensils.

Know when to see a pro. If you have a minor illness—a cold, for instance—you can try macrobiotic foods to alleviate the symptoms, says Kushi. But if you're seriously ill, you should see a macrobiotic counselor. Coming up with the appropriate dietary changes for complex health problems is a complex process and requires expertise, he says. If necessary, a counselor may refer you to a medical doctor.

THE ASIAN FOOD PYRAMID: A SMART OPTION FOR WOMEN

From piquant and spicy Tandoor to fiery Korean and complex, surprising Vietnamese, Asian cuisine includes a wide array of distinct culinary traditions. Even so, all of these traditions share some notable similarities: Most are low-fat, verging-on-vegetarian affairs. Typical meals are primarily grains, vegetables, beans and fruits, garnished with meat or dairy, nuts and seeds.

As a rule, Asian cuisines are also very healthy—healthier than the standard American diet.

"When you look at lung, breast and colon cancer rates, those are much higher in the United States than in countries like China," says Banoo Parpia, Ph.D., senior researcher with the China-Cornell-Oxford Diet and Health Project, centered at Cornell University in Ithaca, New York.

Obesity, diabetes and heart disease are also less common in countries like China than in the United States, notes Dr. Parpia. Among Chinese women ages 35 to 64, the heart disease rate is roughly 10 per 100,000. In the United States, The researchers calculated a staggering 56 per 100,000.

Would American women be better off eating like the Chinese or, for that matter, the Thais?

Absolutely, says Lawrence Kushi, Sc.D., associate professor of public health, nutrition and epidemiology at the University of Minnesota School of Public Health in Minneapolis. And it's easy enough. Just follow the Asian Diet Pyramid, shown on page 157.

An Alternative to the USDA Food Guide

The brainchild of a group of internationally known nutritionists, chefs and epidemiologists, including Dr. Lawrence Kushi and Dr. Parpia, the Asian Pyramid is a simple-to-follow guide to Eastern gastronomy.

It bears a passing resemblance to the U.S. Department of Agriculture's

(USDA) Food Guide Pyramid—the familiar triangle-shaped eating guide that shows up on the backs of cereal boxes, bread wrappers and produce bags. But a closer look reveals some major differences.

Have less meat, less often. The Asian Pyramid relegates red meat to the smallest possible space, limiting it to once a month. The rationale: Studies show that Asians eat about one-tenth as much meat as we do, using it as a condiment in dishes that are mostly grains and vegetables. If you eat according to the Asian Pyramid, you can have poultry roughly once a week.

Enjoy fish or dairy, not both. Fish, which is lower in fat than poultry and meat and is a more common accompaniment to Asian meals, is okay on a daily basis. But the Asian Pyramid asks you to make a choice between fish and dairy. You can't have both high-protein foods every day. Dairy isn't part of traditional Asian cuisines, except in India, where many people don't eat meat.

Though most Asians consume very little dairy, osteoporosis is less common in Asia than in the United States, notes Dr. Lawrence Kushi. The reasons: Asians are more likely to get bone-strengthening exercise than Americans, and they're less likely to eat excessive amounts of protein, which prompts your body to excrete calcium.

Serve yourself more grains, legumes and seeds. Instead of meat, the Asian Pyramid suggests that you get your protein from grains, legumes and seeds. In combination, they provide sufficient but not excessive protein. And they add fiber, which may help account for the lower rates of obesity, diabetes and colon cancer in Asia, says Dr. Lawrence Kushi.

Like vegetables and fruits, which also figure prominently in the Asian Pyramid, legumes and grains are rich in vitamins, minerals and phytochemicals. This broad group of substances have been shown to protect against heart disease and certain types of cancer.

Use less oil, less fat. The Asian Pyramid diet gets a mere 15 to 20 percent of calories from fat, mostly from polyunsaturated sesame oil, Dr. Lawrence Kushi says. By comparison, the typical U.S. diet gets about 36 percent of calories from fat, much of it from animal sources, which are saturated. The lower fat content in the Asian diet helps account for the lower incidence of heart disease and obesity in Asia.

Sip, don't swig, tea and alcohol. The Asian Pyramid also suggests moderate amounts of tea and allows wine, beer or sake, a rice liquor that's common at Japanese tables. Tea contains flavonoids, natural compounds believed to protect against cancer. In studies, tea drinking has been linked to lower risks of bladder, kidney and urinary tract cancer.

The same phytochemicals appear to help prevent blood clots, thereby reducing the risk of heart attacks and strokes. Since modest amounts of alcohol may be associated with a small drop in heart disease risk, its place in the Asian diet may also help explain the lower heart disease rates in the East. Nevertheless, individuals who don't usually drink alcohol or need to avoid it for social or religious reasons shouldn't feel compelled to start.

Be stingy with sodium. With its reliance on soy sauce, Asian cuisine might seem a high-sodium proposition. But it really isn't, if you season the traditional way, which is sparingly, and avoid high-sodium processed foods, Dr. Lawrence Kushi says.

Get regular exercise. "In Asia, there's much less dependence on automobiles," says Dr. Lawrence Kushi, who links higher activity levels with lower rates of both osteoporosis and obesity in Asian countries. "People walk, ride bikes or take the train."

No Pu Pu Platters

The diet that the Asian Pyramid depicts isn't what you're used to eating at your local Chinese restaurant. That's because ethnic restaurants in this country cater to the American taste for more meat and more fat. And as countries like China become more affluent, adopting higher-fat, higher-protein diets like our own, they're starting to chalk up higher disease rates, Dr. Parpia notes.

An Asian Diet Pyramid Menu

Unlike the Ornish diet, the U.S. Department of Agriculture's Food Guide Pyramid and other Western food plans, the Asian Diet Pyramid doesn't call for specific quantities of each type of food.

Basically, a typical day's menu will look like this.

Breakfast
Cooked cream of rice or cream of wheat
Soy milk
Peanuts, as garnish

Lunch
Miso soup
Spring rolls stuffed with cabbage, carrots, bean sprouts and a small
    amount of tofu or shrimp
Plums

Dinner
Large serving of rice
Tofu stir-fried with broccoli, carrots, onions, mushrooms, peppers
    and water chestnuts, in a little sesame oil

Asian Diet Pyramid

When combined with regular exercise, the typical Asian diet scores high points for health benefits. A daily diet based on the Asian Pyramid consists mostly of grains, fruits, vegetables and legumes. Fish, shellfish and dairy should be consumed only as a daily option. Sweets, eggs and poultry, likewise, should be consumed only weekly. Meats are to be eaten most sparingly, eating only on a monthly basis. If used, alcoholic beverages should be consumed in moderation, primarily with meals.

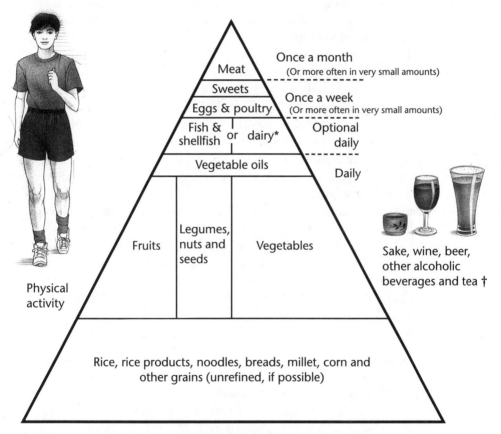

Meat — Once a month (Or more often in very small amounts)

Sweets

Eggs & poultry — Once a week (Or more often in very small amounts)

Fish & shellfish or dairy* — Optional daily

Vegetable oils — Daily

Fruits — Legumes, nuts and seeds — Vegetables

Physical activity

Sake, wine, beer, other alcoholic beverages and tea †

Rice, rice products, noodles, breads, millet, corn and other grains (unrefined, if possible)

*Except for the cuisine of India, dairy foods are generally not part of the healthy, traditional diets of Asians. In light of current nutrition research, if dairy foods are consumed on a daily basis, they should be used in low to moderate amounts, and preferably low in fat.

†Wine, beer and other alcoholic beverages should be consumed in moderation and primarily with meals and avoided whenever consumption would put an individual or others at risk.

That trend, in fact, helped inspire the international conference where the Asian Pyramid took shape.

"We want to look at ways to preserve the old, healthy culinary traditions before they get wiped out," says K. Dun Gifford, founder and president of the Boston-based Oldways Preservation and Exchange Trust. An educational organization dedicated to promoting healthy, environmentally friendly dietary traditions, Oldways organized the International Conference on the Diets of Asia and, before that, the International Conference on the Diets of the Mediterranean. Our idea, Gifford says, is to encourage Asians to keep eating a traditional diet and to encourage Americans to give that way of eating a try. If you want to try the Asian Diet Pyramid, experts offer these helpful hints.

Focus on grains and vegetables. Unlike the Ornish Diet and other Western diets, the Asian Pyramid doesn't specify serving sizes. More like Traditional Chinese Medicine and Macrobiotics, it's meant to be flexible. Once you've served yourself, though, your plate should resemble the Asian Pyramid, Dr. Lawrence Kushi says. Reserve about half of your plate for grains, a quarter for vegetables and a bit less than a quarter for legumes, nuts and seeds. An eighth of the plate is plenty of space for fish, poultry or meat. Then treat yourself to fruit, with a serving that's about the same size as your vegetable serving.

Sample soybeans. In much of Asia, the soybean is the legume of choice. And a healthy choice it is, says Mark Messina, Ph.D., nutritionist in Port Townsend, Washington, participant in the Asian food conference, author of *The Simple Soybean and Your Health* and co-author of *The Vegetarian Way*. Research suggests that soy offers added protection against osteoporosis, heart disease and certain types of cancer. It may also help soothe menopausal symptoms. Dr. Messina suggests a serving of soy a day. Here are some tips.

- Look for tofu, a mild soybean curd sold in supermarkets and Asian grocery stores. Scramble a couple of ounces of soft tofu instead of eggs at breakfast, suggests Dr. Messina.
- Spice up tofu by marinating it in a mixture of rice vinegar and soy sauce, advises Jerianne Heimendinger, R.D., Sc.D., research scientist at the American Medical Center's Cancer Research Center in Denver.
- Try low-fat, calcium-fortified soy milk with your morning cereal, says Dr. Messina.
- Indulge in a steaming bowl of miso soup, made from soybean paste.

Measure your oil. "Minimize it," Dr. Parpia says. If you're stir-frying, use one to two tablespoons of vegetable oil, just enough to coat the pan and impart some flavor, suggests Dr. Parpia. Use oil only while cooking foods. Don't add it at the table.

Spice things up. Fat heightens flavor, but you have other alternatives—like herbs and spices. Curry powder and Chinese five-spice seasoning can make dishes more flavorful and exotic, says Dr. Heimendinger. Just sprinkle them on during cooking. Or use black mustard seeds to flavor your vegetables. Add a small amount of sesame oil to a skillet, then add the mustard seeds and allow them to "pop" before adding diced cabbage, mushrooms or other vegetables. Finally, cover and steam for five minutes. Other spices, such as tumeric and cumin, can also be added for more flavor.

Go easy with the soy sauce. If you don't limit your use of soy sauce, you'll go overboard on sodium. Add soy sauce to some dishes, but not to everything that you eat. If you can't taste anything but soy sauce when you sample a dish, you've added too much, says Dr. Lawrence Kushi.

Consider calcium insurance. Since calcium-rich dairy products don't make regular appearances in the Asian diet, you may need to take a daily supplement for insurance, says Doris Derelian, R.D., Ph.D., former president of the American Dietetic Association and president of Health Professions Training in San Diego. Aim for 1,500 milligrams a day, she suggests.

THE MEDITERRANEAN DIET: CARDIO-HEALTHY CUISINE

While researching the diets of the people of the Mediterranean in the early 1950s, Ancel Keys, Ph.D., then a visiting professor of public health at Oxford University, compiled a description of the traditional Italian cuisine.

"Homemade minestrone; pasta in endless variety served with tomato sauce and a sprinkle of cheese, only occasionally enriched with some bits of meat or served with a little local seafood; a hearty dish of beans and short lengths of macaroni; lots of bread, never more than a few hours from the oven and never served with any kind of spread; great quantities of fresh vegetables; a modest portion of meat or fish perhaps twice a week; wine and always fresh fruit for dessert."

It wasn't just the wonderful flavor of the food that made an impression on Dr. Keys. It was the cuisine's effect on health.

During that visit and subsequent others, Dr. Keys noted that heart disease was extremely uncommon in rural parts of Italy and other Mediterranean countries like Greece and Spain. Other researchers found lower rates of certain cancers, including breast cancer, and other diet-related conditions, such as diabetes, along the Mediterranean.

"Every indication says that we would all be better off eating the Mediterranean way," says Dr. Keys, now professor emeritus of public health at the University of Minnesota in Minneapolis.

To make it easy, Dr. Keys and other leading scientists joined forces at the International Conference on Diets of the Mediterranean and came up with the Mediterranean Pyramid.

Like the Asian Pyramid, the Mediterranean Pyramid is an alternative to the USDA Food Guide Pyramid. It's a blueprint for eating the way that most rural Mediterranean people did in the 1950s and 1960s—before their diets started to resemble Americans' diets and, not coincidentally, before their rates of heart disease and chronic illness started to soar.

A Mediterranean Pyramid Diet Menu

Traditionally, women in Greece, Italy, Spain and other Mediterranean countries don't compulsively measure their food. It takes away from the joy of eating. And you won't have to starve yourself, either, if you limit fats and get plenty of exercise along with your Mediterranean diet.

Remember, in Mediterranean climates, a plate of grapes, plums and other fruit is a respectable way to end a meal. That takes the place of the usual American dessert that's laden with heavy doses of sugar, fat and calories.

So, to get started, pretend you're vacationing in a villa on the Adriatic Sea and start with this one-day sampling.

Breakfast
Toasted bread with quince jam
Orange
Yogurt

Morning Snack
Figs

Lunch
Pasta with vegetables

Dinner
Large salad with endive, escarole, arugula and plum tomatoes, sprinkled with olive oil and red-wine vinegar
Rice with vegetables and a small amount of seafood, such as calamari (squid) or shrimp
Fresh fruit with a small piece of cheese, such as feta, provolone or scamorze (similar to mozzarella)

"The traditional Mediterranean diet is much more plant-based, with more whole grains and fresh vegetables," says Dr. Lawrence Kushi, who worked on the both the Mediterranean and Asian Pyramids. He notes that the Mediterranean diet also has much less meat than the traditional American one.

A Friendlier Fat

The Mediterranean Pyramid shows a diet that's higher in fat than you might expect. But it's in keeping with Mediterranean culinary tradition. In the 1950s and 1960s, Mediterraneans got 25 to 35 percent of calories from fat.

Even with that much fat, heart disease was uncommon, probably because olive oil was the primary source of fat in the traditional diet, Dr. Lawrence Kushi explains. Olive oil consists mostly of monounsaturated fatty acids, the kind that have been shown to lower levels of "bad," artery-clogging cholesterol in the blood, while raising levels of the "good," artery-cleaning stuff. By contrast, the saturated fatty acids in butter, margarine and animal fat raise the levels of bad cholesterol while lowering levels of the good kind.

Fruits and vegetables shine, too. Like a backyard garden in the Mediterranean region, the Mediterranean Pyramid devotes a lot of space to fruits and vegetables, which helps to explain the lower rates of heart disease as well as cancer and certain birth defects that researchers found in the region in the 1960s.

Fruits and vegetables are good sources of antioxidants—cancer-fighting vitamins such as beta-carotene and vitamin C that provide protection against the oxidation within cells, linked to cancer, aging, heart disease and other health conditions. And they're a good source of folate, a B vitamin linked to a lower risk of heart disease and birth defects. Lack of folate has also been associated with cervical dysplasia, the precursor to cervical cancer.

Pasta and beans figure heavily. The Mediterranean Pyramid also sets aside a good chunk of space for grains and legumes. Like fruits and vegetables, they're good sources of fiber, which lowers cholesterol and fights colon cancer. Together, grains and legumes supply protein in the diet, without supplying the saturated fat that accompanies meat, poultry and fish.

Beef is a rarity. Like traditional Mediterranean cuisine, the Pyramid includes red meat only once or twice a month. If eaten more often, red meat is only a small part of a dish that's mostly grain and vegetables, like pasta with meat sauce.

Mediterranean Diet Pyramid

Praised for its many health benefits, the typical Mediterranean diet centers around potatoes, breads, pasta and other grains, along with fruits, vegetables, legumes, cheese, yogurt and olive oil as daily mainstays. Fish, poultry, eggs and sweets are enjoyed less regularly, and red meat is served only occasionally— just a few times a month. Alcohol, usually wine, is enjoyed in moderation only. Exercise is also an essential part of the Mediterranean lifestyle.

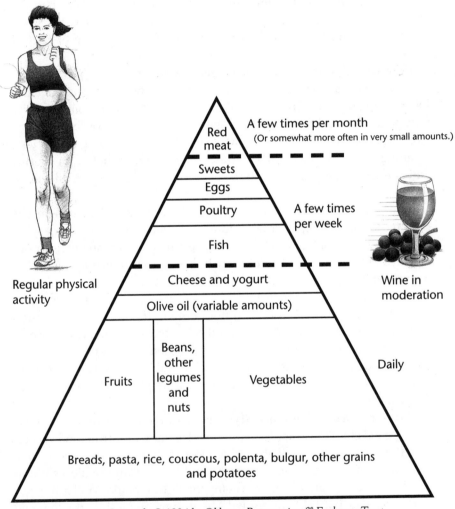

Regular physical activity

Red meat — A few times per month (Or somewhat more often in very small amounts.)

Sweets

Eggs

Poultry — A few times per week

Fish

Cheese and yogurt

Olive oil (variable amounts)

Wine in moderation

Fruits

Beans, other legumes and nuts

Vegetables

Daily

Breads, pasta, rice, couscous, polenta, bulgur, other grains and potatoes

Dairy is a condiment. Cheese and other milk products get little space on the Pyramid, since dairy products were used pretty much as condiments—Parmesan sprinkled on a plate of pasta, for instance. Though Mediterraneans didn't eat much dairy in the 1960s, hip fractures due to osteoporosis were rare. That's probably because protein consumption was adequate but not excessive, says Dr. Lawrence Kushi.

Wine is a regular. Alcohol gets some ink in the Mediterranean

Garlic, the Healing Bulb

In Mediterranean cuisine, it seems, even the seasonings are healthy.

Consider garlic, the quintessential Mediterranean herb. Studies find that this flavorful bulb can protect against heart disease and various types of cancer, including breast cancer, says Robert I-San Lin, Ph.D., executive vice-president of Nutrition International in Irvine, California, and chairman of the First World Congress on the Health Significance of Garlic and Garlic Constituents. The active ingredients in garlic and garlic preparations—sulfur compounds including an amino acid derivative called alliin and allicin—appear to offer protection in several different and complementary ways.

How much garlic should you eat for maximum protection? Dr. Lin suggests that you shoot for two to five cloves' worth daily. Here are three ways to get your garlic.

Dine like a true Mediterranean. For lunch, spread some pita bread with hummus (chick-pea and garlic puree) and serve with garlic soup and pasta puttanesca (garlic is a key ingredient). For dinner, bake chicken breasts with roasted garlic.

Spike your food with garlic powder. According to Dr. Lin, dehydrated, ground garlic offers the same benefits that fresh garlic does. Try mixing it into tomato juice and sauce, Dr. Lin suggests. (A teaspoon of garlic powder is the equivalent of 2½ cloves of garlic or half the ideal daily dose.)

Supplement with capsules. If garlic powder sounds unappetizing, you can pick up garlic supplements at most health food stores. There are three types of garlic supplements—garlic powder tablets and capsules, aged garlic extract liquid and powder capsules, and garlic oil capsules. These supplements differ substantially in potency, safety and ability to produce body odor. Eight capsules or tablets of garlic powder will also give you the equivalent of three cloves of the fresh stuff, Dr. Lin says.

Pyramid, as it did in the Asian. Traditionally, wine accompanied the evening meal in most Mediterranean countries.

A healthy dose of work and exercise. As with the Asian Pyramid, regular exercise is part of the Mediterranean Pyramid. Obesity was relatively rare in most villages, in large part because people got plenty of exercise working in the fields and the home, Dr. Lawrence Kushi notes.

The Best of Both

Of the two diets, Asian and Mediterranean, researchers say that it's hard to determine which is healthier.

"The big difference is in fat content," Dr. Lawrence Kushi notes. "Whether a predominantly plant-based diet with a moderately high olive oil content, like the Mediterranean, is healthier than a low-fat, predominantly plant-food diet, like the Asian, isn't clear. There's evidence that both are healthy. They have disease patterns that look very similar—low rates of cancer and heart disease when compared with the United States."

For his part, Gifford suggests alternating between the two diets, eating Asian for a couple of days each week, then Mediterranean for a couple. Here's how to do the Mediterranean part.

Size up your plate. Like the Asian Pyramid, the Mediterranean Pyramid doesn't specify serving sizes. Make the proportions of grains, vegetables, legumes, fruit and meat on your plate match the proportions of those same foods in the pyramid, and you'll be okay, Dr. Lawrence Kushi says.

Your plate should be roughly half grains, a quarter vegetables, a quarter legumes and one eighth dairy or meat. For dessert, treat yourself to some fresh fruit.

Eat plants on every occasion. "It's easy to eat more fruits and vegetables," says Dr. Heimendinger, who also developed the National 5-a-Day for Better Health program. She offers these tips.

- In the morning, add raisins or banana slices to your cereal. Or have some fresh figs, berries or an apple and half a glass of orange juice.
- Enjoy grapes or other fruit or carrot sticks for a snack. "Or have those mini-carrots—they're really easy (require no preparation) and they're crunchy. And one thing people look for in a snack is crunchiness." These carrots also travel well in the car and can be an after-work snack.
- At dinner, add a vegetable or two—squash and kale, or asparagus and grilled red peppers, for instance.

- When you're serving more vegetable-based main dishes, think pasta with marinara or pasta e fagioli (pasta and garbanzo beans).

Substitute olive oil, don't add it. Use olive oil in place of, not in addition to, other sources of fat in your diet. And try not to get carried away.

Some studies have linked breast cancer with diets high in total fat. Yet despite the relatively high fat content of the Mediterranean diet, a study in Greece found breast cancer rates were relatively low in that country. It's not exactly clear why. But it's possible that the incidence was different in the Mediterranean because the type of fat in the diet was monounsaturated fat instead of saturated or polyunsaturated.

In the United States, where breast cancer rates are higher than in Mediterranean countries, women get more of their fat calories from saturated fat. Until researchers know more, says Dr. Lawrence Kushi, "going overboard on the olive oil isn't a good idea."

Limit the booze. The pyramid suggests a moderate amount—which, for the average woman, would mean 4 to 5 ounces of wine, 12 ounces of beer or an ounce of liquor, Dr. Lawrence Kushi says. Research suggests that while modest amounts of alcohol may be associated with a small drop in heart disease risk, for women, drinking alcohol is also associated with a small increase in the risk of breast cancer and osteoporosis.

So, should you drink or not? Your decision may depend in part on whether you run a higher risk of breast cancer or heart disease. If you do imbibe, red wine or red grape juice may be of particular benefit because they contain a substance called resveratrol, found in grape skins, says Dr. Fugh-Berman.

Garnish with calcium supplements. If you eat by the Pyramid, you may get less calcium than the American Dietetic Association and the Food and Nutrition Board of the National Academy of Sciences suggest that women get to protect against osteoporosis.

The traditional Mediterranean diet seems to have provided adequately for most Mediterranean women, since osteoporosis has been pretty uncommon in those countries. But perhaps the problem has been less common since Mediterranean women tended to be smaller and generally more active than the typical American woman is today, says Dr. Derelian. To be on the safe side, she suggests that you take a calcium supplement. Shoot for about 1,500 milligrams of this bone-friendly mineral daily.

Exercise. You don't have to labor away hand-harvesting saffron threads in Spain to get the kind of exercise that makes the Mediterranean healthy. Pounding the pavement in search of the perfect pair of Italian shoes will do, as will other forms of walking, running, swimming, skating or doing whatever you like best.

HELLERWORK
Smoothing Out the Rough Spots

Your husband is driving you nuts—not only because he won't hang up his shirts but because he acts like the entire bedroom floor is his personal laundry basket.

Yet you know, even when your pique has peaked, that it's not really his housekeeping skills (or the lack of them) that's making your blood pressure rise. What's really ticking you off is his lack of consideration.

Pain can be like that, too. What you think is causing pain—a sore neck, for example—might actually be a symptom of a problem somewhere else.

Take Laura Lindahl, a homemaker in Los Gatos, California. She hurt her back in a toboggan accident over 30 years ago. And for much of that time she was also plagued with neck and shoulder pain. But until she had a Hellerwork session several years ago, she never realized that the neck and shoulder pain and the earlier back injury were connected.

"I learned during my session that your whole body is interconnected," she says. "Everything affects everything else, and one problem can cause another one somewhere else."

Hellerwork is a program that uses bodywork, an important part of which is massage, to help uncover and straighten out structural imbalances in the body. According to Hellerwork practitioners, vigorous bodywork helps loosen areas of the body that have become tense, compressed or twisted—the body's way of compensating for a variety of physical and emotional hurts.

"The tension in the muscles is relieved and, when the session's done, you feel like a million bucks: relaxed, straightened, almost like they've ironed out your tissues. It's wonderful," Lindahl says. "They can look at your body and see what area needs to be unrotated or realigned. It's amazing."

HELP FOR BODY AND SOUL

Hellerwork was developed in 1978 by Joseph Heller, an aerospace engineer who had studied with Ida Rolf, founder of the form of deep tissue massage called Rolfing. Heller patterned his method on the ten-session Rolfing program. But whereas Rolfing focuses on the physical aspect of bodywork, Hellerwork also takes emotional stresses and strains into account.

The basic Hellerwork program consists of 11 sessions. Each 1½-hour session focuses on a different area of the body. Bodywork plays a big part, of course, but so does talking—what practitioners call dialogue. In order to relieve the problem, it's essential that you understand what's going on emotionally that might be causing or contributing to it. So don't be surprised when you're asked a lot of questions and encouraged to share your experiences. It's all part of the process.

Suppose, for example, you frequently get backaches, says Don St. John, a certified Hellerworker and trainer in Seattle. It may be that you're frequently repressing anger, which causes the back muscles to tense up. Someone who's under constant stress may clench her jaw a lot, which could cause temporomandibular problems.

It's not uncommon for muscles to get increasingly tense over time. Since this occurs so slowly, however, you may not even realize that you've lost the ability to completely relax, says St. John. "It's like how water in a freezer gets real cold before it turns into ice. Your muscles tighten very gradually and get very tight before you're in agony. We attempt to relax them and to connect the client's awareness to her body," he explains.

Getting**Started**

Hellerwork

Hellerwork practitioners conduct a series of 11 sessions combining vigorous bodywork and dialogue to align your body, ease a variety of ailments and almost always improve posture and bearing. To locate a Hellerwork practitioner in your area, follow these guidelines.

Number of practitioners in the United States: Approximately 250.

Qualifications to look for: A Certified Hellerwork Practitioner (C.H.P.); certification in Hellerwork requires a minimum of 1,200 hours of training.

Professional associations: Hellerwork International, 406 Berry Street, Mt. Shasta, CA 96067.

To find a practitioner: Contact Hellerwork International (listed above); Northwest Hellerwork, 3814 Densmore Avenue North, Seattle, WA 98103; or Hellerwork Institute of Washington, Seattle Branch, 3027 NW 59th Street, Seattle, WA 98107.

Approximate cost: $90 to $125 for each 1½-hour session.

A CONVERSATIONAL APPROACH

The verbal interplay between the Hellerworker and her client is a vital part of the program, especially for women, says Douglas Drucker, Ph.D., a clinical psychologist and certified Hellerworker and trainer in Los Gatos.

Traditional health care, he says, revolves around an authority figure (the doctor) who tells you what to do. "Women have been very frustrated because they want to create a system based on participation, communication and relationships."

Hellerwork does just that. All Hellerwork practitioners are trained to listen carefully, says Donna Bajelis, a physical therapist and certified Hellerworker in Seattle.

"We ask people to look at the relationship between their attitudes and beliefs and the tension in their bodies," she says. "If you think life is hard, your body will look like it—all hunched over, your shoulders forward and down, like you're carrying a burden."

Indeed, teaching people how to use their bodies better is an essential aspect of Hellerwork, says Dr. Drucker. Each session includes movement education—teaching people to stand, walk, sit and bend to avoid putting unnecessary stress on their bodies.

"You can't put Band-Aids on the problem," says Dr. Drucker. "A cortisone shot in the back won't get to the pain. It blocks it out for a little while, but you're not getting to the cause. That's why people are so frustrated. They're looking for solutions and want to get to the root of it."

Generally, people seek out Hellerwork practitioners for relief of musculoskeletal problems: back, neck and shoulder pain, headaches, foot problems, arthritis, carpal tunnel syndrome and fibromyalgia (painful "trigger points" in the muscles), says Dr. Drucker. He says Hellerwork has also been helpful for such physical and emotional problems as anxiety, depression, irritable bowel syndrome and weight gain.

MAKING THE PIECES FIT

Just as the shinbone's connected to the knee bone and the knee bone's connected to the thighbone, the sessions in Hellerwork progress from one body part to another. The connections aren't just physical, either. Hellerworkers believe that each area of your body connects with a specific emotion or problem in your life.

Here's a quick rundown of what each session includes.

Session 1. The emphasis is on breathing, says Bajelis. Bodywork targets your rib cage, and you could be asked to describe what inspires you and to make connections between your emotions and how you breathe. Practitioners say that this session could help asthma, allergies, depression and grief.

Session 2. Bodywork focuses on your legs, and the dialogue focuses around support systems such as your family or networks of friends. This session could help with knee problems, osteoarthritis, muscle strains and ligament pulls, says Bajelis.

Session 3. Bodywork focuses on your arms, legs, shoulders and sides of your rib cage. The theme of the session is reaching out in life. The discussion will concentrate on how you give and receive in life and also on issues of anger and self-esteem. This session helps with tension in your shoulders, neck and arms, says Bajelis.

Session 4. Bodywork focuses on the insides of your legs and your pelvic-floor muscles. The dialogue focuses on themes of control and surrender, shame and guilt. According to practitioners, this session could help you with incontinence, constipation, hemorrhoids, distended colon and sexual dysfunctions.

Session 5. Bodywork focuses on your abdominal muscles. You will talk about intuition, gut feelings and how you express emotion. This session could help you with lower-back problems, constipation and restricted breathing, practitioners say.

Session 6. Bodywork focuses on your back, all the way from your buttocks to the back of your neck. You will talk about how you are repressed or afraid of expressing feelings in your life. This session could help you with back problems, says Bajelis.

Session 7. Bodywork focuses on your neck, face and mouth. You will discuss how you communicate, how well you talk about emotions and how well you speak your mind. This session helps with temporomandibular (jaw) pain, says Bajelis. It's also used to help relieve sinus infections, with the Hellerworker using a gloved pinkie finger to work on loosening up the nasal passage, she adds.

Sessions 8 to 11. These are open sessions, in which bodywork and dialogue are targeted to those parts of the body that need additional attention. The themes focus on integration of the masculine and feminine parts of your personality.

While each session in the Hellerwork program is sequential—practitioners advise completing all 11 sessions—you can go back and repeat sessions as often as necessary, Bajelis says.

Hellerwork can improve posture and bearing in just about everyone, says St. John. "The common assumption is that after age 25, it's downhill physically," he says. "Or that you get more stiff and hunched over with age. But it doesn't have to be that way. I'm finding at age 54 that my body is more aligned than at 25."

Indeed, the treatments have been known to add a quarter-inch or so of height to folks whose muscles have had the kinks ironed out, notes Dr. Drucker.

BRINGING YOURSELF IN LINE

Although you need to see a certified Hellerworker to get the full benefits of the program, they also teach and empower you to do things for yourself to help bring your body back into alignment.

Let it hang out. When walking or standing, it's a natural tendency to pull back your pelvis and hold in your stomach to make it flat. Unfortunately, this can put your body out of balance and lead to back pain, Bajelis says. "It makes you hold your breath and your energy gets held in. The best body stance is to have your weight evenly distributed over both whole feet."

Let your head go down. When bending to pick something up, don't force your head to stay up, says St. John. "With your head up, you contract the back of your neck muscles instead of allowing the head to drop down and the spine to lengthen, which is much healthier," he says.

Let 'em swing. When walking, allow your arms to hang down and don't hold your shoulders up, says St. John. "You're always told to keep your shoulders up, but we teach you to sense the weight of your arms being down along the sides of your rib cage. This helps your shoulders stay down," he says.

The Right Way to Sit

Sit forward on your pelvis so that you are sitting on top of your "sit bones." Using a pillow to raise your sit bones above your knees may make it easier to sit correctly. Your back is in an uncurved, natural position.

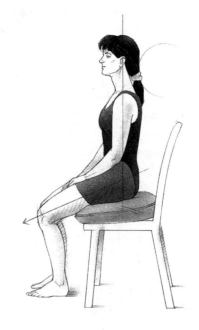

The Right Way to Stand

Whether standing or walking, the best way to position your body is to shift yourself so that your weight is balanced over the spot where your heel and arch meet. As if joined by an imaginary line, your ear, shoulder, hip and the middle of your knee and ankle should be aligned. Look down at your ankles. If you can see them and your weight is still distributed over the juncture of your heel and arch, you're probably in good alignment.

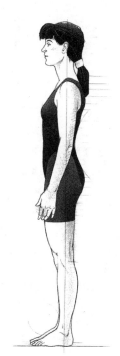

The Wrong Way to Bend

Even if you remember to bend your knees to pick up a small object off the floor, forcing your head to stay up and look straight ahead will needlessly tense the back of your neck.

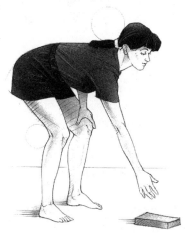

The Right Way to Bend

The healthy way to bend is to lengthen your spine. Let your head drop down and look toward the object as you bend. You may want to use one hand to balance yourself on your knee.

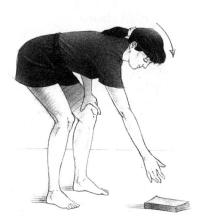

HERBAL MEDICINE
A Woman's Garden of Natural Healing

Long before science created today's powerful pharmaceuticals, Mother Nature had a mighty arsenal of her own to treat the ills and injuries that affect us all from time to time. That arsenal? Herbs.

Examples? Valerian root eased the nerves of anxious women 1,000 years before the advent of sedatives such as Valium. Native American women relied on black cohosh tea to soothe menopausal problems for centuries. And women have been using feverfew leaves to combat migraine headaches since A.D. 78.

What's more, few people realize that some of the most widely used drugs available to women are derived from herbs. Examples include digitoxin, originally derived from the foxglove plant and used for congestive heart failure; the antimalarial drug quinine, from Peruvian bark; and reserpine, a blood pressure medication made from Indian snakeroot.

And today, medical researchers are unearthing new revelations about medicinal herbs, says Ethan Russo, M.D., a neurologist at the Western Montana Clinic in Missoula, academic adjunct professor in the Department of Pharmacy at the University of Montana and clinical assistant professor in the Department of Medicine at the University of Washington School of Medicine.

Dr. Russo believes that yet-to-be-discovered herbs may one day play a pivotal role in human healing. "We have yet to tap the enormous potential of our rain forests' herbal resources," he says. For example, says Dr. Russo, the sap from the jungle-growing croton tree, known as dragon's blood, contains taspine, a substance that seems to increase wound healing.

"NEW" MEDICINE WITH OLD ROOTS

What is a medicinal herb? Simply, any plant whose seeds, berries, roots, leaves, bark or flowers are used for medicinal purposes.

The exact moment when humans discovered that herbs had the power to heal is lost in time. One theory is that our earliest ancestors took a botany lesson from even earlier ancestors: Primates use herbs as an antiparasite medicine.

Whether it's instinct or observation, of this we are certain: We have used herbal remedies to treat ourselves and our families since the dawn of humanity. As soon as we began recording history, it seems, we began recording our use of herbal medicine.

Babylonians carved herbal prescriptions into clay tablets dating from 2600 B.C. Egyptians inked their herbal remedies into the *Papyrus Ebers* nearly a millennium later. And in China, the *Shang Han Lun*, written 1,800 years ago, ranked the 365 herbs that formed the backbone of Chinese herbology and is still used today.

Use of medicinal herbs is old. Scientific study of their use began in the eighteenth century, but in the United States it fizzled out during the 1960s. Though it has been making a comeback in the United States, interest remains small in comparison to some other countries. Of the 42 small grants awarded by the Office of Alternative Medicine in the National Institutes of Health over a two-year period, only 5 focused on herbs. Europe is another matter: Researchers in Germany, for example, have published 300 scientific reviews of the use of herbs. Experts hope that someday the Food and Drug Administration will adopt standards for the use of medicinal herbs based on German research now applied in that country.

For women, medicinal herbs may present a distinct advantage over standard medications, say advocates. "For certain health concerns such as fibrocystic breast 'disease' (harmless breast growths) or heavy menstrual bleeding, herbs are a far better choice than conventional prescription drugs," says Adriane Fugh-Berman, M.D., former head of field investigations for the Office of Alternative Medicine at the National Institutes of Health in Bethesda, Maryland.

"That's because the drugs that we use for problems like these—drugs such as tamoxifen or danazol for fibrocystic breasts—are very powerful and wreak havoc with a woman's delicate hormonal balance. But herbs used for these problems are relatively mild. They work *with*, not against, a woman's system."

FOOD, TONIC OR DRUG?

Medicinal use of most herbs takes know-how. The following descriptions categorize medicinal herbs from mildest to potentially toxic, according to Susun S. Weed, an herbalist, teacher and author of the *Wise*

Woman herbal series from Woodstock, New York, who speaks widely on the medicinal use of herbs at medical gatherings.

Nourishing herbs. Leafy herbs such as calendula flowers, fennel seeds, lemon balm, nettles, oatstraw, raspberry leaves and violet leaves are some of "nature's safest herbs," says Weed. Like leafy, dark-green vegetables, they're highly nutritious, and they may be used daily for long periods of time.

Tonic herbs. Herbs such as burdock, chaste tree, dandelion, Dong Quai, ginseng, hawthorn, motherwort, wild yam and yellow dock nourish a particular organ or system, says Weed. They act slowly and have a cumulative, rather than immediate, effect. "It's best to take tonic herbs in a broken pattern, like three days on, four days off, rather than daily," she explains.

"Herbal tonics have benefits as preventive medicine," says Marcey Shapiro, M.D., a family practitioner in private practice in Durham, North Carolina, who lectures widely on herbal medicine. "They were once widely used but have been lost to us in modern Western medicine."

Herbs that sedate or stimulate. Herbs such as catnip, hops, poppies, wild lettuce, wintergreen, passion flower and valerian, among others, are sedating. Others, such as cayenne, ephedra, primrose, ginger and guarana, are stimulants. Herbs that sedate or stimulate must be used carefully. They're powerful and can produce side effects or other unwanted reactions. Long-term use of sedating or stimulating herbs can lead to addiction, says Weed. "These herbs should be used in small doses for fairly short periods of time," she continues, suggesting that you rely on expert guidance when it comes to this class of herbs.

Potentially toxic herbs. More powerful herbs, such as blue cohosh, black cohosh, goldenseal and rue, among others, are potent medicines that must be used with caution, says Weed. While these herbs can stimulate powerful healing effects, taking too much of them will, almost always, produce side effects, she adds. "For example, goldenseal has become very popular lately, but it can cause liver and kidney damage."

At the same time, potent herbs can be extremely useful. So Weed suggests seeking the guidance of an experienced herbal practitioner rather than self-treatment with these herbs.

HERBS EVERY WOMAN SHOULD KNOW

If you were to ask leading herbal healers to list the most important herbs for women, none of their lists would be identical.

Nevertheless, the herbs that follow include nourishers, tonics, sedatives and other medicinal herbs that experts frequently recommend for women. Herbs that can be easily garden-grown are noted. Herbs are used medicinally as teas, infusions (a water-based solution stronger than tea), decoctions (concentrated infusions), tinctures (herbs in a vinegar, glycerin or alcohol base) and poultices and ointments (topically applied mixtures).

Black Cohosh: Nature's Hormone?

Healers have long used the dried roots and rhizome (woody stem) of the black cohosh (*Cimicifuga racemosa*) to treat the spectrum of women's discomforts, and now we know why. Research shows that black cohosh helps

Getting**Started**

Herbal Medicine

Medicinal herbs have a lot to offer. But, like any medicine, that doesn't mean you can use them with abandon or forgo proper diagnosis.

"It's always a good idea to seek an herbal practitioner's guidance," says Sandra McClanahan, M.D., executive director of the Integral Health Center in Buckingham, Virginia. Here's some basic information to assist you in your search.

Number of practitioners in the United States: 15,000 to 20,000.

Qualifications to look for: Traditional Chinese Medical practitioner, licensed naturopathic doctor (N.D.) or an herbalist approved through the peer-review process of the American Herbalist Guild (AHG).

Professional associations: American Herb Association, P.O. Box 1673, Nevada City, CA 95959; American Herbalist Guild, 3051 Brown Lane, Soquel, CA 95073; American Association of Naturopathic Physicians, 2366 Eastlake Avenue, Suite 322, Seattle, WA 98102.

To find a practitioner: Contact one of the professional organizations above for a listing of practitioners in your area. Or, ask your family doctor to recommend an herbal practitioner.

Approximate cost: $45 to $75 for an initial consultation and $35 to $55 for follow-up visits.

Purchasing information: You can find herbs in the form of capsules, teas, loose leaves, tinctures, extracts, poultices and ointments at most local health food stores. Some supermarkets carry herbal teas. Costs range from less than $1 for about one ounce of tea to $20 for more expensive preparations like evening primrose oil. Herbal plants and seeds can be purchased at an herb farm or at some greenhouses and nurseries. They cost about the same as other annuals and perennials.

ease hot flashes by suppressing the secretion of luteinizing hormone (LH). It may be an alternative to estrogen-replacement therapy: One study showed that following hysterectomies (surgical removal of the uterus and ovaries), there was no significant difference in menopausal symptoms among women treated with estrogen and those treated with black cohosh extracts.

In addition, researchers consider black cohosh to be effective for treating PMS, menstrual cramps and emotional problems associated with menopause. "Black cohosh is excellent for hot flashes," says Dr. Fugh-Berman. Use black cohosh only in consultation with a health care practitioner familiar with herbs.

Calendula: Nature's Band-Aid

This herb reduces inflammation and helps wounds heal. Shown to be effective against staphylococcus germs, calendula (*Calendula officinalis*) is used externally for cuts, bruises, rashes and other skin irritations. It's most commonly applied to the skin in the form of poultices, ointments or infusions.

Calendula makes a hardy addition to your flower or herb garden. Sow fresh seeds directly into a sunny flower bed in April or May and enjoy the creamy yellow to brilliant orange floral display until fall.

Chamomile: Tension and Tummyache Tamer

Chamomile (*Matricaria recutita*) is so popular and well-regarded for its healing benefits that in 1987 it was declared "the medicinal plant of the year" in Germany.

Among the healing herbs, chamomile has been extensively studied and is an effective remedy for stomachaches and other gastrointestinal upsets. The volatile oil of chamomile, which is blue in color, contains anti-inflammatory and antispasmodic substances—namely the terpenoids and matricin. The flower also contains other compounds, known as flavonoids, that scientists say make chamomile an effective digestive aid.

Chamomile has tiny daisylike flowers and a distinctive sweet-apple fragrance. A natural sedative, chamomile works gently and safely, says Dr. Fugh-Berman. If you are allergic to ragweed, however, you may want to avoid it.

In Germany, chamomile is designated as safe and effective for treating everything from skin problems and topical bacterial infections to bronchial irritations.

If you decide to try chamomile, experts advise that you look for whole, dried flowers, purchased from reputable sources. Avoid powdered or pulverized chamomile—it may not be pure. If you decide to grow your own, chamomile will tolerate most soils and likes lots of sun and moisture.

Dandelion: The Good-for-You Weed

So you thought dandelions were only weedy, yellow lawn-wreckers. Wrong! Dandelion, says Weed, is a dandy—and the perfect first herb for beginners to try.

Young, tender dandelion greens (*Taraxacum officinale*) are even more nutritious than spinach and make great salad additions. "Like spinach, dandelion is loaded with nutrients that women especially need, including calcium, vitamins A and C, folate, iron and potassium," says Weed. "I encourage women to eat two raw pesticide-free dandelion leaves a day."

Evening Primrose Oil: Hot-Flash Cooler

Evening primrose oil and the similar, but less widely available, oils of borage seed and black currant seed are excellent for painful fibrocystic breasts and hot flashes, according to Dr. Fugh-Berman.

"These conditions aren't serious, but they certainly are uncomfortable for many women," notes Dr. Fugh-Berman. "One out of two women has harmless breast lumps, yet the only medications that we have to treat these problems have serious side effects."

Evening primrose oil (*Oenothera biennis*), from the seed of a Native American wildflower, is a good source of gamma-linolenic acid (an essential fatty acid), and it's also useful for rheumatoid arthritis and eczema, says Dr. Fugh-Berman. "Doses range from two 500-milligram capsules twice a day for breast pain to 8 to 12 capsules a day for eczema or arthritis." Start with the minimum dose and proceed cautiously, she warns. Some people experience nausea, diarrhea or headache when taking this oil. If you experience side effects, discontinue its use.

Feverfew: Migraine Mediator

"I see a lot of women with chronic headaches and migraines, and I tell them to start chewing a feverfew leaf every single day and work up until they get the relief they need. And for a significant percentage of them, it works," says Dr. Russo.

For 2,000 years, feverfew (*Tanacetum parthenium*) has been used to reduce fever. Lately, science has resoundingly proven its value against headaches, particularly migraines, and the nausea and vomiting that often accompany them.

Scientists have identified parthenolide as the active component responsible for feverfew's ability to knock out a headache. In Canada, authorities recommend that feverfew products contain a minimum of 0.2 percent parthenolide.

Dr. Russo recommends purchasing a plant or growing feverfew plants from seeds. British feverfew seeds are preferred for their quality. High-quality feverfew seeds can be purchased from two British companies: B and T World Seeds, Whitnell House, Whitnell, Bridgewater, Somerset, TA5, 1JE, United Kingdom and Chiltern Seeds, Bortree Stile, Ulverston, Cumbria, LA12, 7PB, United Kingdom.

But be prepared, Dr. Russo warns. "Feverfew tastes terrible, and it gives a small number of people—perhaps 5 percent of those who use it—mouth sores. Aside from that, I haven't noticed any side effects."

Feverfew has small, white daisylike flowers and grows like a weed. It needs very little cultivation to survive happily in most gardens.

Note: Bees hate the smell of feverfew and will avoid the entire garden that it grows in, so be sure not to plant it anywhere you have flowering plants that need pollination.

Garlic: Nature's Infection Fighter

"Garlic is so good for you," says Dr. Fugh-Berman, "that I wish everyone would eat a lot of it, every day. Then none of us would have to worry about having 'garlic breath.'"

Garlic (*Allium sativum*) fights viral and bacterial infections. Its active ingredient, allicin, is a potent antibiotic, though easily destroyed by heat. Consumption of garlic and onions has been linked with a lower risk of developing stomach cancer, says Dr. Fugh-Berman.

Scientists say that garlic is also effective for reducing risk factors for coronary artery disease and arteriosclerosis (hardening of the arteries) and may be helpful in treating digestive problems, bacterial and fungal infections and high blood pressure.

The difficulty with garlic is knowing how much to take—and in what form. "To lower cholesterol," suggests Dr. Fugh-Berman, "you need to take 12 capsules of raw garlic oil or eat 10 to 12 cloves, daily. Unfortunately, some of its activity may be lost when garlic is cooked."

Ginger: The Tummy-Settler

Don't swear off sailing because of your seasickness until you've given ginger a try, says Dr. Russo. "For motion sickness and dizziness with nausea, ginger is my remedy of choice. The only drugs available for this problem cause sedation or other serious side effects. I've taken ginger to prevent seasickness, and I can tell you that it works for me."

But ginger's real value is in its proven power to treat nausea of all kinds, including morning sickness. "Pregnant women can stave off morning sickness with ginger," says Mary Hardy, M.D., clinical instructor at the University of Southern California School of Medicine and an associate at the Huntington Medical Foundation in Los Angeles. "I tell women to grate one-quarter to one-half teaspoon fresh ginger into a cup of tea, steep for five minutes, strain and drink first thing in the morning to prevent morning sickness," she adds.

One study also indicates that ginger (*Zingiber officinale*) can reduce the nausea and vomiting that can follow major surgery. In addition, there is some scientific support for ginger's use against migraine headaches, and it may even help ulcers.

"I find that ginger is excellent for cramps, because it is an antispasmodic and it encourages menstrual flow," says Dr. Shapiro. "I also recommend ginger for women who have acute sinus problems with clear mucus."

Dr. Russo's favorite way of taking ginger is in its candied, crystallized form (available in Oriental food markets). "Just eat a hunk before you board the boat to prevent seasickness," he says. You can also chew on a slice of fresh ginger or grate a small amount, to taste, into tea, notes Dr. Russo. Ginger capsules are also available. Each piece or capsule of ginger is equal to 500 to 550 milligrams of ginger, the standard dose.

Hawthorn: A Tonic for the Heart

Researchers believe that hawthorn (*Crataegus laevigata*) relaxes the smooth muscles of the coronary blood vessels, which increases blood flow and may reduce angina—that is, chest pain resulting from decreased blood supply to the heart. "Hawthorn makes a good heart tonic—it supports cardiac function," says Dr. Fugh-Berman. "And in Western medicine, we don't have much in the way of preventive drugs."

While few healthy women under the age of 50 should have immediate concerns about heart disease, it happens to be the number one cause of death among older women. So hawthorn may be useful as a preventive medicine, especially for people with a history of heart disease or who have a family history of heart disease, suggests Dr. Fugh-Berman. She is quick to note that if you're being treated for existing heart disease, hawthorn can't replace the conventional cardiac therapy recommended by your doctor, which might include medications such as digitoxin, drugs known as beta-blockers or nitroglycerin.

Purple Coneflower: Cold and Flu Foe

Scientists say that echinacea (*Echinacea purpurea*) sparks the production of two protein substances—interferon and properdin—which fight off bacteria and viruses. In Germany, it's approved for use to help heal infections, wounds and inflamed skin conditions.

"There's lots of scientific evidence to support our use of echinacea," says Dr. Fugh-Berman. "It's a proven immune-system stimulant, and it's antiviral. That's important, because we don't have effective Western drugs that combat viral infections such as colds or the flu. Now if I'm exposed or feel the first symptoms of a cold, I take echinacea for a few days and can usually avoid a full-fledged infection."

Taken in tinctures, echinacea will make your mouth feel a little numb, says Dr. Fugh-Berman. "If it doesn't, then you don't have fully potent echinacea. Genuine echinacea always has a slight numbing action."

"Take echinacea in divided doses," she continues. "To ward off colds, take the lowest recommended dose twice a day. If you have a cold or flu, take a larger dose three or four times a day. Don't use it every day; it will lose its effectiveness."

Echinacea is a handsome, hardy perennial that looks like a purple black-eyed Susan. Sown from seed or transplanted, echinacea will thrive in most gardens. Wait till several hard frosts have passed before you harvest echinacea for medicinal purposes; then clean and dry the root. You can replant the crown after you harvest the root, but it won't be as potent as it was before.

OTHER HERBS IN BRIEF

In treating health problems, herbalists choose from among hundreds of other plants. Here are short takes on a few more herbs that experts consider especially useful.

Cranberry. A glass of cranberry (*Vaccinium macrocarpon*) juice a day might keep urinary tract infections away, according to physicians who treat women with herbal medicine.

Hops. In beer, hops (*Humulus lupulus*) acts as a natural preservative, keeping the brew fresh. Dr. Fugh-Berman suggests drinking hops as a gentle, relaxing tea, which is especially effective for insomnia. (Don't worry—you won't get drunk.)

Oatstraw. The green parts of the same oats that you eat for breakfast make a supernourishing infusion that's rich in calcium and B vitamins, says Weed. Oatstraw (*Avena sativa*) calms nerves, reduces cholesterol and helps you sleep restfully, she says.

Psyllium. Also known as plantago seeds, the cleaned, dried, ripe seeds of psyllium (*Plantago psyllium*) "help lower cholesterol and provide the roughage that keeps things moving through the lower intestine," says Dr. Fugh-Berman.

Stinging nettle. Nettles (*Urtica dioica*) are extremely rich in vitamins and minerals and make a valuable nourishing infusion for women during pregnancy and menopause, says Weed. An excellent diuretic, nettles are also good for women who retain water. And don't worry—despite the name, when dried, nettles don't sting.

Valerian. Tea made from dried valerian (*Valeriana officinalis*) root has been used as an effective minor tranquilizer and sleep aid for more than 1,000 years. One caution, though: "Valerian can easily become addictive," says Weed. To avoid dependency, she advises using it for less than a month—and not daily. Otherwise, you'll find it hard to fall asleep without the herb.

MORE M.D.'S PRACTICE HERBAL MEDICINE

As consumer interest in herbal medicine has grown, so has the number of herbal practitioners, says Roy Upton, president of the American Herbalist's Guild.

"Herbs range from safe nourishers like nettle to useful but dangerous plants such as pokeroot," says Weed. Many plants can heal us, but only a few can hurt us. Although herbs are natural, some can occasionally have side effects. Most herbs are safe to use even if you only have a little knowledge, while others are best left to experts, she explains.

"The problem is, in the United States, anyone can hang out a shingle and call himself an herbalist," cautions Penny King, research and education coordinator for the American Botanical Council.

"Conservatively, I'd estimate that there are between 15,000 and 20,000 healers in this country who prescribe medicinal herbs," says Upton, noting that the numbers encompass naturopaths, Traditional Chinese Medicine practitioners and midwives, in addition to a growing number of conventional medical doctors.

"Now, medical schools are starting to incorporate herbal studies into their curriculums," says Upton. "Harvard, Columbia, Cornell and the University of California in Los Angeles all have programs that provide at least some level of herbal instruction," he continues.

At the University of Arizona College of Medicine in Tucson, medical students can study herbalism with Andrew Weil, M.D., professor of herbalism and director of the Program of Integrative Medicine and best-selling author of *Spontaneous Healing* and *Health and Healing*.

For details on what credentials and training to look for when locating a qualified herbal practitioner, see page 175. For information about finding a naturopath or doctor of Traditional Chinese Medicine trained in herbal medicine, see pages 251 and 284.

USING HERBS WISELY AND SAFELY

Should you decide to try a mild herbal remedy for minor complaints, Weed offers this advice.

Pay attention to the botanical names of herbs. Every plant has an official botanical name, and that includes herbs. "What's sold as eyebright (an

Pregnancy Alert

If you're pregnant, cooking with herbs is fine. Medicating with herbs is not.

"I'm going to take a hard line on this: Pregnant women shouldn't use nonfood herbs," says Adriane Fugh-Berman, M.D., former head of field investigations for the Office of Alternative Medicine at the National Institutes of Health in Bethesda, Maryland.

Used in normal seasoning amounts, food herbs like ginger (good for morning sickness), garlic, chilies, mint leaves and culinary herbs such as sage, rosemary and thyme are safe.

A few herbs—namely, pennyroyal, black and blue cohosh, goldenseal and possibly cotton root bark and tansy—are known to induce miscarriages, says Dr. Fugh-Berman.

Certain herbs, such as red raspberry leaf, can promote and even ease labor and are safe to use during the last month of pregnancy and during labor—if you're under the care of a qualified midwife or herbalist, says Dr. Fugh-Berman. "Prescribing them is best left in the hands of someone with lots of herbal expertise," she says.

herb used for eye conditions) in one store may be sold by another name elsewhere. But *Euphrasia officinalis* means eyebright everywhere," says Weed.

Use one herb at a time. "Don't buy herbal combinations—you won't know which herb will work best for you. Instead, learn about one herb before trying others," says Weed.

Start small. "Begin by using gentle, nourishing tonic infusions and vinegars and watch for side effects or reactions (such as headache, skin rash, hives or visual disturbances) for 24 hours the first time you try a new herb," cautions Weed. "Anyone can be sensitive to anything. Some people can be bothered by strawberries, chamomile, anything."

Start gently. Use tinctures only after you've gained an understanding of herbs, and then use the smallest recommended dose, says Weed. Build up slowly as needed.

Use herbs for minor complaints first. Learn about an herb's effectiveness for a minor problem (such as menstrual cramps or insomnia) before you try herbal healing for more serious concerns, suggests Weed.

Don't expect instant results. Using herbs can be as easy (and as familiar) as going to the local discount drugstore and buying some pills or capsules. Don't expect herbs to be as instantly effective as over-the-counter drugs, however. "That's not the way herbs work," says Dr. Hardy.

Dr. Hardy believes that the rituals surrounding herbs are an important part of the healing process. When you use herbs for self-care, she suggests, you might be actually growing or gathering them, chopping them, steeping or brewing them, eating them raw or cooking with them, bathing with them or applying them directly to your body. "You make a positive mental connection when you use herbs; the ritual aspects of their use are very powerful," she says.

HOMEOPATHY
Like Cures Like, and Less Is More

Homeopathy (from the Greek words *homeo*, meaning "like," and *pathos*, meaning "suffering") is based on the principle of similars: A substance that causes certain symptoms in a healthy person will *cure* those symptoms in a sick person.

Here's how one homeopath puts it: "If a healthy person takes a little taste of arsenic, it might cause vomiting, diarrhea, abdominal cramps, chills and clammy sweats," says Linda Johnston, M.D., diplomate in homeopathic therapeutics and founder of the Academy for Classical Homeopathy in Van Nuys, California, and author of *Everyday Miracles: Homeopathy in Action*. "So we'd use a homeopathic arsenic preparation to remedy an intestinal flu that produces exactly those symptoms."

Don't be alarmed by the mention of arsenic: The quantities used in homeopathy are so infinitesimal that otherwise toxic ingredients are harmless. Other substances commonly used by homeopathic practitioners include plants, such as *Arnica* (mountain daisy), *Calendula* (marigold) and *Urtica urens* (stinging nettle) and minerals such as copper, iron, zinc and sulfur, among others.

What's more, if you ask homeopaths to explain why their like-cures-like healing practice works, you're likely to hear, "We don't know."

PUZZLING BUT PROVOCATIVE

Homeopathy was developed during the late 1700s by medical rebel Samuel Hahnemann. A brilliant, well-educated German physician, Dr. Hahnemann grew disgusted with bloodletting and other ineffectual, barbaric eighteenth-century healing rituals. So he quit the practice of medicine and supported himself by writing and translating medical works.

While translating a medical text, Dr. Hahnemann read that Peruvian bark was effective against malaria. But the explanation for why it worked didn't seem to make sense. When, out of curiosity, Dr. Hahnemann dosed himself with the bark, which contains quinine, he found himself developing symptoms of malaria—the very illness that the bark was supposed to cure. Intrigued, he began testing quinine and other substances on other healthy people, carefully noting their reactions. He called his tests provings.

Dr. Hahnemann found that administering the similar medicine—a medicine that was capable of producing symptoms similar to those his sick patient was experiencing—could greatly relieve the patient's suffering. However, the patients sometimes suffered ill effects from the full-strength medicines. He therefore set about to develop a method of making the medicines safer. After much experimenting, he found that diluting and shaking the medicines could enhance their healing effects while reducing their harmful effects. In fact, the more he diluted and shaked, or succussed, the medicines, the more potent they became.

In 1796, Dr. Hahnemann published his essay "On a New Principle for Ascertaining the Curative Powers of Drugs," and homeopathy, as he called this healing system, was born.

In 1825, homeopathy was introduced to the United States, much to the dismay of conventional doctors who lined themselves up against the new practice as it gained popularity. In 1846, they formed an organization, the American Medical Association (AMA), whose members were sanctioned for merely associating with "irregular practitioners."

Eventually, the AMA won its battle against homeopathy. In 1890, one-sixth of all physicians were homeopaths. But by 1940 or so, homeopaths in America had become nearly as scarce as the bald eagle.

Interestingly, homeopathy never received such opposition elsewhere in the world. In other countries, it was—and is—a widely accepted medical practice. Around 40 percent of British, French and Dutch doctors use homeopathy, and one in five German doctors do. Other surveys indicate that 25 to 56 percent of Belgian, French, British, Dutch and Danish people use homeopathy, in addition to significant numbers of people in Sweden, Italy, India, Mexico, South America and the former Soviet Union.

In the United States, homeopathy is regaining popularity and is practiced by several hundred medical doctors, osteopaths, naturopaths, dentists, veterinarians and other health care professionals across the country. In a typical year, nearly five million Americans visit homeopaths. And sales of homeopathic medicines are estimated at $201 million per year and are growing at a rate of nearly 20 percent a year.

THE MYSTERY OF POTENTIZED REMEDIES

Homeopathic remedies are *potentized*. That means that a substance, which in its original form produces certain symptoms, will be added to water, then succussed 60 or more times. The mixture is then diluted again with water and the process can be repeated up to hundreds of times, until not a molecule of the original substance remains in the remedy.

The principle of potentized remedies gives even experienced homeopaths pause when it comes to explaining how their healing art works. But on one thing they all agree: It does.

"The bottom line is that no one really knows how homeopathic remedies work," says Dr. Johnston. "What I do know is that my patients get better. Unlike conventional medicine, homeopathy doesn't treat symptoms—it corrects whatever is disturbing your system and producing those symptoms."

"I don't know how homeopathy works either," admits Joyce Frye, D.O., an obstetrician/gynecologist and chairperson of the gynecology department at Presbyterian Medical Center and a clinical faculty member at Jefferson Medical College, both in Philadelphia. "But that doesn't mean it doesn't work. Scientists are making discoveries every day that shatter the laws of physics as we know them. A new kind of physics, one that we haven't even explored yet, may soon explain what now seems mysterious."

Ask Ellen Goldman, doctor of naturopathy and chairperson of the homeopathy department at Bastyr University of Naturopathic Medicine in Seattle, how such dilute solutions can possibly cure diseases and she replies, "We don't yet have instruments sensitive enough to measure this effect. Dr. Hahnemann, the father of homeopathy, said that homeopathic medicines stimulate the vital force, or the healing energies, in the body. My opinion is that the remedies affect the brain's limbic system, which governs certain aspects of our emotions, behaviors and physiology."

"Homeopathy stimulates the body's self-healing mechanism," says Jennifer Jacobs, M.D., assistant clinical professor in the Department of Epidemiology at the University of Washington School of Public Health in Seattle. "How can so dilute a remedy be effective? Just ask the luna moth. This beautiful insect finds her mate from a half-mile away when he releases just one molecule of a hormonelike substance called a pheromone."

To better accept the paradox behind homeopathy, it helps to consider other, more conventional medical treatments: If you take allergy desensitization shots, you regularly receive a tiny amount of the very substance that makes you sneeze, wheeze or itch. Eventually, your body will develop a tolerance to that substance and your symptoms will stop. Similarly, hyperactive children are sometimes given the stimulant Ritalin, but instead of making them more hyper, it actually calms them down. And finally, those vaccinations that prevent everything from chickenpox to smallpox are nothing more than dead or crippled germs that, in their potent form, would cause the disease for which they're given.

WHAT HOMEOPATHY OFFERS WOMEN

Homeopathy has many benefits to offer women, according to Dr. Johnston.

Some of those benefits, adds Dr. Jacobs, include relief for menstrual difficulties, childbirth, menopause difficulties and even breastfeeding. "I think the fact that homeopathy is nontoxic and has no side effects makes it very helpful for women's health problems."

Dr. Frye echoes those sentiments. "The real benefit of applying homeopathy to the problems of menopause or premenstrual syndrome (PMS) is that instead of taking a powerful drug on a regular basis, you can be given a remedy that you might only take a few times to regulate your system," she says. "The right remedy can end PMS symptoms entirely."

"Another plus is that, unlike other approaches that have you stick to special regimens or keep journals of your symptoms, homeopathy doesn't require that women change their lifestyles to eliminate PMS," says Dr. Johnston. "Instead, homeopathy will correct the physiological problem that causes PMS in the first place."

That doesn't necessarily mean that homeopathy is the answer to everything. Homeopathy may not be the appropriate solution for all the problems that many women face around the time of menopause, says Dr. Frye. "Vaginal dryness, for example, doesn't usually respond well to homeopathy."

Plus, each woman's menopausal problems will present themselves differently, suggests Dr. Frye. "Some women's faces will flush. Others will feel a flash of heat on their chests. Still others will wake during the night dripping with sweat. So each woman needs a homeopathic remedy individualized just for her. When individualized, homeopathy can make menopause a peaceful transition," she says.

A VISIT TO A HOMEOPATH

Visiting a homeopathic healer is likely to be a very different medical experience than any you've ever known. In a way, your encounter will more closely resemble a consultation with a psychiatrist, psychologist or other mental-health practitioner.

(continued on page 192)

Commonly Used Homeopathic Remedies and Their Uses

Healers who practice homeopathy choose from among thousands of possible homeopathic remedies derived from various substances—animal, vegetable and mineral. Some homeopathic remedies (such as silica, a mineral found in rocks and plants) are familiar substances from familiar sources. Others (like lachesis, derived from snake venom) are un-

AILMENT	SYMPTOMS
Headache from muscular tension in the neck	Headache at the top of the head; feeling of pressure at the top of the head; eye pain; stiff neck, spreading across the shoulders; neck spasms
Heartburn during pregnancy	Extreme thirst, but trembly after drinking; marked passing of gas; burning on the tip of the tongue; a craving for stimulants; a sinking feeling in the pit of the stomach
Indigestion with nausea and vomiting	Indigestion begins two hours after eating, especially in the evening; sense of pressure under the breastbone; pounding heart; bad taste in the mouth; maybe a headache around the eyes; depression, tearfulness and self-pitying attitude
Insomnia with an inability to relax	Overactive mind; eventually falls asleep, but tosses and turns in anguish; often brought on by receiving good or bad news
Morning sickness (constant nausea with vomiting)	Liquids and solids are vomited; nausea is not eased by vomiting; tongue feels clean rather than thickly coated; excessive saliva production; lack of thirst; possible fainting spells
Premenstrual syndrome with fluid retention and swollen, tender breasts	Painful joints, weakness and lack of energy; possible vaginal discharge or yeast infection; depression; indifference; tearfulness; irritability; loss of concentration; anxiety that symptoms have been observed; fear of insanity
Sinus congestion with facial tenderness	Facial bones are very tender, even to the slightest touch; excessive yellow mucus, with sneezing; irritability; subject to chills
Sprains, splinters, bruises, cuts, minor burns and insect stings	For wounds and injuries with moderate to severe bruising, swelling, pain and bleeding

familiar substances from sources found outside the United States. Strange as homeopathic remedies may be to the uninitiated, they're widely used.

A representative sampling of homeopathic remedies, from the ordinary to the exotic, are shown here, along with the types of health problems for which they're used.

REMEDY	SOURCE
Cimic	Black cohosh (*Cimicifuga racemosa*)
Capsicum	Chili pepper
Pulsatilla	Windflower (*Pulsatilla nigricans*)
Coffea	Coffea (*Coffea arabica* or *Coffea cruda*)
Ipecac	Cephaelis ipecacuanha (a rain forest shrub)
Calc. carb.	Oyster shells (calcium carbonate)
Hepar sulf.	Calcium sulfide (*Hepar sulfuris calcareum*)
Arnica (Arnica montana)	Fresh, flowering Leopard's bane (also known as mountain tobacco and sneezewort)

(continued)

Commonly Used Homeopathic Remedies
and Their Uses—Continued

AILMENT	SYMPTOMS
Anxiety with restlessness	Chills; fatigue; disturbed appetite; tendency to be meticulously tidy; clammy skin; rapid pulse
Candidiasis (yeast infection) with offensive discharge	Marked vaginal and vulval itching; soreness and burning in the vagina; possible ulcers on the labia; white discharge that is worse after intercourse; tearfulness, irritability and indifference toward loved one, associated with menopause or hormonal imbalance
Cold with irritability	Tendency to be overly critical of others; subject to chills; nose runs during day and is blocked at night; watery eyes; sneezing; headache; sore throat
Flu with a severe, throbbing headache	Violent headache that is made worse by coughing or by moving the eyes slightly; dehydration with a need to drink lots of fluids at infrequent intervals; irritability; a desire to be home
Heavy menstruation with faintness and irritability	Severe cramps; irregular menstruation; visual disturbances; itchy vaginal discharge; sweating during menstruation; tearfulness; indifference to loved ones
Menopause with suspiciousness and a tendency to talk too much	Overexcitement; congested feeling all over the body, as if something needs to come out; dizziness and a tendency to faint; headache that's worse upon rising and on the left side; constricted feeling in the abdomen; difficulty breathing; sleeplessness
Sore throat	Back of the throat is bright red and severely swollen; burning and stinging pains; depression and irritability

REMEDY	SOURCE
Arsen. alb.	Arsenic (*Arsenicum album*)
Sepia	Cuttlefish ink (*Sepia officinalis*)
Nux vomica	Seeds of the *Strychnos nux-vomica* tree
Bryonia	Bryony root (*Bryonia alba*)
Sepia	Cuttlefish ink (*Sepia officinalis*)
Lachesis	Fresh venom of the bushmaster snake (*Lachesis muta*)
Apis	Honeybees

That's because along with your physical examination, talking is just about all that occurs during your 60- to 90-minute (or longer) first visit. And you're going to be doing most of it.

Meanwhile, the homeopath will ask probing questions, take copious notes and consult her *Materia Medica of New Homeopathic Remedies*, the homeopathic handbook listing the 2,000 remedies and their corresponding symptoms. Be prepared: Some questions will fall way outside the scope of what you'd expect during a conventional medical exam.

You'll be closely questioned about your current symptoms. But you'll also be asked all about your childhood, your fears, your phobias and your sex life. And she'll want to know at what temperature you are most comfortable. What foods do you like or dislike? What kind of personality do you have? How do you spend your free time? Do you drink? Do you dream? How's your digestion?

You'll be asked how you express anger and how often. Would you describe yourself as driven? Some of the questions may stir up uncomfortable memories for you. In the words of one woman, "When the two-hour visit was over, I'd told the homeopath more about myself than I'd ever told anyone in my life."

Dr. Johnston says, "Don't be concerned if entire areas of information commonly asked by conventional medical doctors are ignored, and entirely different areas are given great attention and concern. Your doctor will ask questions that provide information that will lead her to the one correct remedy for your set of symptoms out of 2,000 possibilities."

The success of your homeopathic treatment depends on answering the doctor's questions to the best of your ability and then carefully following her suggestions about avoiding substances that can interfere with the action of homeopathic remedies.

Dr. Frye recalls the complex analysis that she used to select a homeopathic remedy for a 45-year-old woman that she treated for chronic sinus trouble. "Sinus problems are ubiquitous," says Dr. Frye. "But this woman also had a terrible spider phobia, a family history of breast cancer and diabetes and a caretaker personality—a cluster of traits that cancer specialists say is common to many women who develop breast cancer."

Instead of dismissing the spider phobia as irrelevant, Dr. Frye used it as a clue. "I find that with homeopathy, strange, rare and peculiar symptoms usually point the way to the right remedy," she says. "So, I looked up homeopathic remedies for arachnophobia—fear of spiders."

Of the six remedies listed, Dr. Frye chose Carcinosinum Burnett. "The personality profile for Carcinosinum well-matched the woman in question on many levels," she notes. "I prescribed a single-dose remedy of Carcinosinum Burnett and, months later, she remained completely free of sinus problems. As a bonus, she was able to accompany her son to a local pet shop and visit the tarantulas."

NOT A ROUTINE PRESCRIPTION

As the woman who consulted Dr. Frye for help with sinus trouble discovered, homeopathic remedies may not look like any medicine that you've ever taken before. Don't be surprised, for instance, if yours is a couple of dozen pinhead-size sugar drops, to be downed all at once, one time only. Remedies come in various concentrations, marked with a number and either a "c," for the centesimal scale, which means potencies are diluted 100 times each time that they are shaken, or an "x," for the decimal scale, which means that potencies are diluted 10 times each time that they are shaken. The higher the number, the more dilute the substance, yet the more powerful it is. Of the two units, c is more common.

And with your medicine might come instructions to avoid coffee and strong-smelling substances such as camphor, eucalyptus and peppermint, suggests Dr. Goldman.

Or, you just might leave the doctor's office without any remedy at all, says Dr. Frye. "Sometimes, it takes me a day or two to review the *Materia Medica of New Homeopathic Remedies* before I can prescribe a remedy. Searching through 2,000 remedies and sets of symptoms to find the right one can be very time-consuming." And therein lies the art of a good homeopath, she adds.

"I don't really do anything other than this matching process," says Dr. Frye. "If the symptoms are clear and we're able to identify the right remedy, a healing response should be expected."

But occasionally, even the most assiduous questioning and artful matching produces no results. "Rarely, I'll have someone for whom the appropriate homeopathic remedy can't be discerned," says Dr. Frye. "When that happens, I choose a different treatment or refer them to an appropriate specialist."

ONE REMEDY OR MANY?

The approach that Dr. Frye describes is what's known as classical, or constitutional, homeopathy. All of an individual's symptoms—physical and emotional—lead to the selection of a single remedy. And if it's the correct remedy, a healing response may occur on many levels.

With combination remedies, a common practice especially in France and Germany, remedies are blended and prescribed to treat the symptoms of a specific illness. In this country, mixed remedies are available over the counter in health food stores for colds, the flu and a variety of other conditions.

Treatments vary from highly individualized to the more general. "For injuries, for example, extensive questioning isn't necessary, and arnica is almost always the right remedy for first-aid problems such as cuts, burns, stings and sprains or acute injuries," says Dr. Frye.

For acute viral diseases, like colds and the flu, treatments must be more individualized. "If ten people are in an elevator and get coughed on by a sick person, not all ten will get sick," says Dr. Frye. "And those who do will likely have different symptoms. The homeopath has to match the treatment to the person by answering the question, 'Why did *this* person develop *these* symptoms?'

"In cases of chronic disease, how much healing ensues depends on the vital force of the prevailing problem as well as on how early in the process treatment begins," she says. "The ability of homeopathy to heal depends on how much damage the disease has done."

WHAT SCIENCE SAYS

If you ask your family doctor about the merits of homeopathy, you're likely to be greeted with skepticism. When a natural-healing technique produces results that are difficult to explain scientifically, as is the case with homeopathy, critics often write off the results as a placebo effect. In other words, if the doctor and patient expect a remedy to work, there's about a 30 percent chance that it will work, even if the remedy is an inactive substance, according to at least one medical report.

Advocates of homeopathy, however, point to a number of scientific studies that show positive results for homeopathic remedies.

Among 107 scientific studies of homeopathy reviewed over a number of years, 77 percent pointed to homeopathy's effectiveness, according to David Taylor Reilly, homeopathic researcher and physician at the Glasgow Homeopathic Hospital in Scotland.

HOMEOPATHY WITHOUT A HOMEOPATH

The National Center for Homeopathy states that homeopathic medicines are recognized by the Food and Drug Administration as drugs and that 95 percent of them are available over the counter—that is, without a prescription. Stroll through your local drugstore or health food store and you're likely to find dozens of homeopathic remedies for sale.

Note: If you use over-the-counter homeopathic remedies, be sure to see a physician if you do not improve quickly or if your condition worsens. See a medical professional for chronic, long-term conditions such as diabetes or high blood pressure.

But just because you can self-medicate with homeopathy, does that mean you should? The answer depends on whom you ask.

"You're not doing yourself any favors by self-medicating with homeopathic remedies, because you never address the problem causing the symptoms that you're trying to cure," says Dr. Johnston. She uses being in debt as a metaphor. "How you solve indebtedness depends on what caused your financial difficulties. Do you spend too much? Make too little? Max out your credit cards? Incur large bills? It's the same thing with your health. To use homeopathy effectively, you need to find out why you have colds so often, rather than continually fighting off symptoms," she explains.

Other practitioners differ. "If you're treating something mild, it won't hurt you to use homeopathic remedies," says Dr. Frye. "But it's better if you come to recognize your particular health pattern."

Homeopathy can be used successfully at home for minor first-aid problems, according to Richard J. Weintraub, M.D., consulting psychiatrist at the Spaulding Rehabilitation Hospital and assistant clinical professor of psychiatry at Tufts University School of Medicine, both in Boston. "I see no problem using homeopathy for black eyes or bee stings," he says. "Arnica, for example, is the most amazing plant. Take it right after you've been bruised, and you'll cut your healing time considerably.

"But I don't recommend that people attempt to self-medicate for anything more complicated than minor first-aid," he cautions.

FINDING A PRACTITIONER

It's easier than ever to consult a homeopathic practitioner if you have a health problem that needs attention. At last count, the number of homeopathic practitioners had grown from fewer than 200 in the 1970s to approximately 3,000 today, according to the National Center for Homeopathy (NCH). Of those, close to 1,000 are medical doctors or osteopaths. The rest are naturopaths, nurse-practitioners, physicians' assistants, dentists, licensed acupuncturists, chiropractors and veterinarians. Fewer than 5 percent are nonmedically trained, and many of those practitioners work with licensed practitioners.

The basics of homeopathy are being introduced to medical students in complementary medicine courses at many medical schools, including:

- Harvard, Yale and Tufts University in Boston
- Georgetown University in Washington, D.C.
- Emory University in Atlanta
- Jefferson Medical College in Philadelphia
- Mount Sinai School of Medicine, Albert Einstein College of Medicine and Columbia University, all in New York City
- the Universities of Arizona, California, Cincinnati, Indiana, Louisville, Maryland, North Carolina, Virginia and Washington

In-depth training programs offering 500 or more hours in homeopathic philosophy, methodology, materia medica and clinical training are offered by several organizations across the country. In addition, Bastyr University, the National College of Naturopathic Medicine in Portland, Oregon, and

Getting**Started**

Homeopathy

Although you can buy homeopathic remedies over the counter in most health food stores and at many drugstores, many practitioners say that for certain ailments, homeopathy is most effective when used under the guidance of a trained homeopath.

Number of practitioners in the United States: Approximately 3,000.

Qualifications to look for: Certification in homeopathy. Look for D.Ht. (Diplomate in Homeotherapeutics) added to the credentials of medical doctors and osteopaths. Naturopathic doctors who are certified in homeopathy use DHANP (Diplomate of the Homeopathic Academy of Naturopathic Physicians). Other practitioners of homeopathy use CCH (Certified in Classical Homeopathy).

Professional associations: American Institute of Homeopathy (AIH), 925 East 17th Avenue, Denver, CO 80218.

To find a practitioner: Write to the National Center for Homeopathy at 801 North Fairfax Street, Suite 306, Alexandria, VA 22314. Ask for their "Directory of Homeopathic Practitioners." Or you can purchase a membership directory from the AIH (address listed above).

Approximate cost: $140 for the first session, which lasts 60 to 90 minutes, and $55 for each follow-up visit, which lasts about 30 minutes.

Southwest College of Naturopathic Medicine in Scottsdale, Arizona, offer intensive homeopathic training.

"Homeopathy is an incredibly complex healing system, one that has a very steep learning curve," says Dr. Weintraub. "I'm still awed by how much there is to know."

HYDROTHERAPY
Water: The All-Natural, All-Purpose Healer

Have you ever iced a sprain? Draped a hot towel over a stiff neck? Soaked away tension in a hot tub? Then you've practiced the ancient healing art known as hydrotherapy.

Using water to help the body heal is a practice that's probably as old as time. Sanskrit writings dating from 4,000 B.C. mention water therapy. In the ancient Greek temples devoted to Asclepius, the god of medicine, water baths were used to treat the sick. And centuries before the Roman baths became a famed tourist attraction, residents of Crete used water therapy extensively.

But as a healing discipline, hydrotherapy was officially born in the early 1800s, when a German farmer named Vincent Preissnitz used cold wet compresses to heal his mangled hand and badly broken ribs.

Inspired by his own remarkable healing response to hydrotherapy, Preissnitz began using it to treat his friends and neighbors. Soon, word of his cures spread beyond his Prussian village, and because of Preissnitz's impressive record of clinical successes, the Crown of the Austro-Hungarian Empire set aside its customary regulations for medical training and permitted him to continue his practice despite the protests among practicing physicians of the time.

Hydrotherapy emigrated to America in 1840 with Robert Wesselhoeft, whom Preissnitz had cured of rheumatic fever. With medical studies under their belts, Wesselhoeft and his brother, William, settled in Vermont. In 1845, they founded the Brattleboro Infirmary, where the likes of Henry Wadsworth Longfellow and Harriet Beecher Stowe tried water's curative power.

And in 1876, the famed health reformer, John Harvey Kellogg, opened his sanitarium in Battle Creek, Michigan. Kellogg treated his patients with nutrition (he invented cornflakes) and hydrotherapy. Kellogg and his rather eccentric use of hydrotherapy, and other therapies, inspired the zany cinema satire *The Road to Wellville*.

SIMPLE BUT EFFECTIVE

"In general, one of the basic cornerstones of naturopathic medicine is hydrotherapy, which is used to trigger the basic healing mechanisms of the body," says Jared Zeff, naturopathic physician, licensed acupuncturist and professor of naturopathic medicine at the National College of Naturopathic Medicine in Portland, Oregon.

Some forms of hydrotherapy improve circulation, according to Dr. Zeff. For many conditions, improving the circulation is key to stimulating the body's healing process. Other illnesses, like common colds, coughs and sinus problems, respond well to steam treatments. When your head or chest is congested, breathing in steam's vapors provides relief because steam shrinks the swollen mucous membranes in your upper respiratory tract and promotes drainage.

Hydrotherapy that uses water in its solid form, ice, can provide potent pain relief in many situations. Ice slows down the ability of your nerves to transmit pain, says Irene von Estorff, M.D., assistant professor of rehabilitation medicine at New York Hospital–Cornell University Medical Center in New York City.

Moist heat hydrotherapy is known for its ability to ease muscle aches and cramps, according to Dr. von Estorff. "Many women rely on a moist hot pack to take care of their monthly cramps or their sore muscles after a stressful day at the office. If a soak in a warm bath feels good in such situations, then by all means do it," she continues. "The soothing effect of lying in a tub full of hot water—but not too hot—has been known for centuries. However, we still have much to learn about the specific changes that occur."

Hydrotherapy may be the easiest alternative therapy to master for at-home use. In fact, you've probably already used hydrotherapy for yourself or your family without even realizing it.

Each form of hydrotherapy—water, ice or steam baths, showers, hot towels, steam treatments or otherwise—creates a different physiological reaction. So how you use hydrotherapy to help you heal will depend on your own needs.

BATHS: HOT, COLD AND JUST RIGHT

You probably don't look at your bathtub and think "home health care device," but that's just what it is: a potentially useful vessel for treating everyday problems like skin irritations, insomnia, muscle spasms and congestion.

The basic therapeutic bath comes in three temperature ranges: cold (55° to 75°F), neutral (92° to 97°F) and hot (105° to 110°F). You can buy a small thermometer to check water temperature at stores that sell hot tubs or in the baby department of stores. But before you take a plunge, read on to see what Letitia Watrous, naturopathic physician in Spokane, Washington, and lecturer at Bastyr University of Naturopathic Medicine in Seattle, recommends for each type of bath.

Cold Baths for Hardy Souls

At a chilly 65°F or below, cold baths can give you a st-st-stimulating boost, to say the least. In Sweden, a plunge into cold water is de rigueur after a hot sauna; the sauna–cold bath combo is said to induce complete pleasure. Even at a temperature of between 65° and 75°, a bath can serve as a brisk tonic that strengthens circulation and digestion. Stay in the bath for 30 seconds to two minutes. But this chilly treatment isn't for everyone: Don't take a cold bath if you are ill or weak or have heart or digestive problems or high blood pressure without first seeking your physician's advice.

To get the pleasures of the Swedish treatment without the travel: First warm your body for ten minutes, either with a hot shower or bath, or in a hot tub or sauna, if available. Then end the treatment with a brisk cold shower or plunge into a cool swimming pool for up to two minutes, depending on your tolerance. The chilled feeling that you experience will be followed by one of comfort. Hop out of the cold water and rub yourself down energetically with a towel.

Neutral Baths Equal Instant Tranquillity

At body temperature (about 92° to 97°F), neutral baths have been called nature's finest tranquilizer and are perfect for easing your way into a sound sleep. Fill the tub with water so that you're covered to the neck; make sure the room is quiet, dim the lights and use a towel or bath pillow to cradle your head.

Skin irritations can be well-eased in a tepid bath; try adding 2 cups of finely pulverized oatmeal. Other additives, such as Aveeno or 1 or 2 drops of juniper berry oil (available at health food stores), are also soothing. Follow the directions on the label. You can also add 1 to 2 tablespoons of baking soda for a wonderful skin treatment or ½ to 1 cup of Epsom salts to relieve sore muscles.

Hot Baths for Pain or Tension

A long soak in a hot tub of water is a time-honored way to ease painful muscle spasms or just relax when you're keyed up.

The water should be between 105° and 110°F, or as hot as your body can comfortably tolerate. Keep a cool wet towel on your forehead to offset the rush of blood from the head.

Stay in a hot bath up to 20 minutes. As the water cools, let some out and replace with hot water to maintain the temperature. Be sure to end the hot bath with a cool shower to prevent fainting.

ICE: NATURE'S MOST EFFECTIVE PAINKILLER?

"Most people are surprised when I tell them to put ice on a muscle spasm," says Dr. von Estoroff. "Many assume that the soothing power of heat is the best way to relax a muscle. But for intense, immediate pain—when you wake up with a painfully stiff neck or suffer an intense muscle spasm, for example—ice is my treatment of choice."

Ice can be more effective than heat for decreasing the pain and swelling that accompany injuries, says Dr. von Estorff. When an injury first occurs, applying ice can slow down a nerve's ability to conduct painful stimuli. So ice breaks the vicious cycle of muscle spasm/pain/muscle spasm.

Ice also works on the blood vessels to reduce the swelling caused by the leakage of fluid into the surrounding tissues, says Dr. von Estorff. Blood vessels react to ice by narrowing, a reaction called reflex vasoconstriction. The surrounding muscles respond to all of these physiological actions by relaxing and thus breaking the spasm.

To take advantage of this inexpensive and convenient therapy, read on.

Try an ice massage. Although gel ice packs are widely available, Dr. von Estoroff says that nothing beats the healing power of real ice. She suggests filling several paper cups with water and storing them in the freezer till needed. When it's time for an ice treatment, tear the paper away from the top rim of the cup, but leave the bottom of the cup intact so that you have something to hold.

Slowly massage the injured area with circular or short, overlapping strokes. Keep the ice moving so that you don't freeze surface tissue and suffer frostbite. The area may start to feel numb as the pain signals slow down, and as the blood vessels narrow, the skin may look pale. When the blood vessels open up again, the skin will turn red. Discontinue the ice after three to four minutes. You can repeat the ice treatment as often as every hour. When using ice in a pack or bag, make sure to cover it with a thin towel to protect the skin.

Set a timer. Apply an ice pack to an injury for 15 to 20 minutes, no longer. Dr. von Estorff recommends keeping the ice pack on for a full 20 minutes to achieve the maximum effect. After 20 minutes, she says, ice is no longer beneficial. As with ice massage, this treatment may be repeated every hour, if needed.

STEAM-POWERED HYDROTHERAPY

Remember when you were a kid and Mom slathered your chest with Vicks VapoRub, turned the hot water on full blast in the bathroom sink, draped a big towel over your head and shoulders and made you breathe in the steam? Your mom was a hydrotherapist.

When you're fighting a cold, flu, allergies or sinus problems, steam is a powerful and effective ally, explains Barbara Yawn, M.D., associate professor of clinical family medicine and community health at the University of Minnesota in Minneapolis. When you inhale steam, the warm, moist air helps relieve coughs and reduces the inflamed mucous membranes in your nose and throat. And the steam helps drain your sinuses.

If you have a respiratory ailment, here's how Dr. Yawn recommends that you get steamed safely.

Turn your shower into a steam bath. Turn on the shower full force with hot water, close your bathroom door and sit on the toilet seat for 15 minutes. Breathing the steam will loosen the mucus in your upper respiratory tract and promote drainage. Or, just take a good, long hot shower.

Use a vaporizer, cautiously. An electric steam vaporizer is an easy, effective way to get steam's decongestant benefits, but hot-steam devices rely on boiling water to generate the steam. Use any vaporizer with care, especially around children. Cool misters add humidity with greater safety. But cool misters must be cleaned with bleach after use to prevent bacterial growth.

HOT TOWELS, COLD TOWELS

Constitutional hydrotherapy is a fancy way of describing a simple variation of water therapy: alternating applications of hot wet towels and cold wet towels. According to Dr. Watrous, constitutional hydrotherapy is an essential element of naturopathic healing.

"I use constitutional hydrotherapy for almost every condition," says Dr.

Watrous. "It's very gentle, and I've had much success with it. I find that everything from infections to premenstrual syndrome and menopausal problems responds well to constitutional hydrotherapy."

Dr. Zeff agrees. "Constitutional hydrotherapy lets you direct and improve blood flow to specific areas of the body that need attention," he says. "Combined with appropriate dietary changes, herbal medicine and other naturopathic treatments, you can achieve a very powerful healing effect."

If you visit a naturopathic physician who uses constitutional hydrotherapy, here's some of what you can expect: While you lie on your back in the naturopath's office, she will cover your bare chest and abdomen with two thicknesses of terry cloth dunked in comfortably hot water and wrung out. You'll then be covered with a woolen blanket to ward off chills.

After five minutes, the hot towels will be removed and replaced with a single thickness of towel dunked in cold water and wrung out, and you'll be re-covered with the blanket. The cold towel will be left on for ten minutes.

Finally, you'll then be asked to turn over, and the same treatment will be repeated on your back. From start to finish, a constitutional hydrotherapy session will last for about 30 minutes.

Dr. Zeff suggests trying the following constitutional hydrotherapy at home whenever you have a fever or want to ward off an illness. "It's a subtle yet powerful treatment," he says.

Take a hot five-minute bath or shower. Get out and towel-dry yourself quickly. Dunk a large bath towel in cold water and wring it out. Wrap the towel around the trunk of your body, from armpits to groin. Then lie down and cover yourself with a wool blanket to avoid getting chilled. Leave the towel in place for at least 20 minutes, until it is warmed.

IMAGERY AND VISUALIZATION
Using Your Mind's Eye to Heal

You can't take a laser gun and zap away cancer cells. And you can't sweep endometriosis out of your pelvic cavity with a broom. But setting aside time each day to *think* about doing those things could be the first step in getting better.

In a world of high-tech medical gadgetry and space-age technology, the best software in the world is still that gray matter between your ears, notes James S. Gordon, M.D., director of the Center for Mind-Body Medicine in Washington, D.C., and author of *Manifesto for a New Medicine*.

Using thoughts to deal with pain, control illness or reach goals is known as imagery or visualization. Strictly speaking, visualization uses the mind to concentrate on visual images, while imagery borrows from all the senses—mainly touch, sound, sight and smell. To use visualization to relax, for example, you might visualize a restful beach scene. Imagery, however, is more of a self-guided, multimedia event; you imagine hearing the waves, feeling the breeze and smelling the salt air.

MAKE THE PIZZA CONNECTION

To get an idea of how strong the mind-body connection is, try this exercise: Picture a big, gooey pizza. The smell of garlic, tomato and basil tickles your nostrils. The cheese is all bubbly and the crust is golden brown. Imagine that you pick up a slice and take a bite. Taste the tangy sauce, the chewy cheese stretching like a mozzarella rubber band from your mouth to the slice.

If your mouth waters just thinking of that tantalizing pizza, then you get an idea of how your thoughts can trigger physical reactions in your body. And it's no surprise that mental images can be used to treat everything from headaches to menstrual cramps, says Judith Green, Ph.D., professor of psychology and biofeedback in the Department of Behavioral Sciences at Aims Community College in Greeley, Colorado, and author of *The Dynamics of Health and Wellness*.

"With arthritis you might envision someone coming along with an oil can, and the rough edges of the joint smoothing out," says Dr. Gordon. "Or with headaches, I encourage people to imagine the size, shape and color of their pain and to see it disappearing."

Guided imagery occurs when someone else—most often a psychotherapist—shapes the images or kinds of images that you have, based on what kinds of images seem to have the strongest healing potential for certain conditions.

To help give reality to the image, therapists often show you medical text pictures or x-rays of what your disorder looks like in the body or even of what the body part looks like. That makes visualization much easier, says Dr. Green.

"Then you could see an arthritic joint as a beautiful ball bearing that's smooth and perfect, or a person with asthma can see all the little bronchial tubes open while breathing perfectly," she notes.

"It's the difference between telling someone with cancer to find her own image that helps strengthen her body and taking someone through her body, telling her to see the white cells move the cancer cells out," says Dr. Gordon.

TWO-WAY COMMUNICATION

To be sure, it's annoying to be told that a health complaint is "all in your head." That's an oversimplification. But how you feel really is largely dictated by mental outlook, says Dr. Green.

"Imagery is the primary language of the body," she notes. "The body understands English and you can talk to it directly, but it truly loves images."

The mind-body connection centers in the hypothalamus, the section of your brain that regulates the autonomic nervous system, which controls automatic processes such as blood pressure. The hypothalamus regulates two branches of the autonomic nervous system—the sympathetic, which responds to stress and gets the heart pumping, and the parasympathetic, which calms the body's responses, explains Dr. Green.

"These parts of the brain are set up so that they'll respond to our thinking and feelings," notes Dr. Green. So, if your brain regulates your body and your thoughts regulate your brain, it only makes sense that you can affect many of your physical responses, including illness.

The relaxation response that visualization and imagery create has a positive effect on the body, notes Howard Hall, Ph.D., assistant professor of pediatrics at Case Western Reserve University and psychologist at Rainbow Babies and Children's Hospital, both in Cleveland. "Stress causes hormones like adrenaline to flush through the body, which may cause physical symptoms," says Dr. Hall. "Imagery helps counterbalance stress."

After burning himself on a hot pan, Dr. Hall used the technique himself. "Thinking 'cool' and 'comfortable' actually helped ease the pain," he says. "That and applying ice, of course."

Another way that the technique works is by changing the rate of blood flow in the body. "If you or your child gets cut, a calming suggestion in a crisis will help stop the blood from gushing," he notes. In other cases, such as Raynaud's phenomenon, you can increase blood flow by achieving a relaxed state. Imagery specifically dealing with warming the hands, such as holding a cup of warm hot chocolate, or less specific images, such as picturing oneself on a beach, facilitate warming. Images should be tailor-made to suit each person's preference.

Doctors who employ imagery and visualization often combine them with other mind-body techniques, such as biofeedback, hypnosis and relaxation, notes Dr. Hall.

Many of the psychologists, psychiatrists and medical doctors who use visualization, for example, do so either in tandem with alternative treatments or with conventional therapy, notes Patricia Norris, Ph.D., clinical director at the Life Sciences Institute of Mind-Body Health in Topeka, Kansas. "I don't think of it as a stand-alone treatment," she says.

A MODERN USE FOR AN ANCIENT SKILL

Imagery was used by the ancient Egyptians, in East Indian Ayurvedic medicine and yoga as well as by the shamans (or healers) in American Indian tribes thousands of years ago, notes Archana Lal-Tabak, M.D., clinical psychoneuroimmunologist (who studies the mind-body connection) at the American Holistic Centers in Chicago. "So really, historically, we've been looking at a mind-body connection throughout time," she says.

It wasn't until the 1960s, however, that Western medicine stood up and took notice. Oncologist Carl Simonton, M.D., and psychologist Stephanie Simonton, Ph.D., developed a program for cancer patients using conventional treatment and visualization after Dr. Carl Simonton noticed that patients with spontaneous remission of cancer were usually the ones who said, "I always imagined myself as well."

The visualization involved four pictures: seeing the treatment destroy cancer cells that are too weak to repair the damage, seeing the white cells of the immune system swarm all over the cancer, seeing the cancer shrink and seeing a return to health.

In the early 1970s, the Simontons tested this procedure on 159 cancer patients who'd been given one year to live. Of these, 63 patients were alive two years after their diagnosis. Of those 63, 22 percent showed no evidence of cancer, while 19 percent saw their tumors get smaller and 27 percent had stabilized.

Later studies have shown visualization and imagery to be effective with less serious ailments as well. In a study of 15 women who suffered from menstrual or premenstrual problems such as pain, water retention and mood changes, for example, troublesome symptoms were cut roughly in half through the use of guided imagery.

Western medicine hasn't always considered the value of mind power in treatment of ailments, says Dr. Green. But that's slowly changing. Over a two-year period, for example, researchers have done at least 30 studies involving the use of imagery and visualization. These techniques are most commonly used for headaches, cancer, pain, colds, asthma, allergies, arthritis, gynecological problems (like heavy or painful menstrual periods), menopausal symptoms (such as hot flashes), infertility, ovarian cysts, lupus (an autoimmune illness in which the body attacks healthy tissue), fibromyalgia (painful "trigger points" in the muscles) and chronic fatigue, notes Dr. Lal-Tabak.

That doesn't mean that imagery or visualization is a panacea for every problem or that conventional medicine isn't also a good idea, notes Dr. Norris. "It's not necessarily a cure. It helps the immune system and eases pain," she says. "If you can get over a cold in three days instead of ten, then you're helping your body."

BELIEF CAN BRING RELIEF

An open mind is key to using imagery and visualization successfully, says Dr. Green. That's why children are especially good at it; they truly believe that it will work, she notes. "Children are successful because they have no preconceived notions that imagery will not work," she notes. "They are more 'tuned in' to using their minds than adults are."

Once grown, however, it's women who have the real edge when it comes to using the old noggin for healing, notes Dr. Gordon. "I think that women are much more open to anything that has to do with psychological aspects of illness and, in general, are more open to self-help," he notes. "Men are more oriented to a technological fix and to letting someone else do it for them."

In fact, being easily hypnotized, which indicates that you're open to suggestion, is another sign that visualization and imagery could come easily to you, says Dr. Hall. Hypnotizable people can focus and concentrate better, so they could also probably create images better as well.

But Dr. Hall stresses that, with practice, anyone can make visualization and imagery work for them. "The most important thing is that you just have to be motivated. It's constant practice that makes the headaches go away," he notes. "And other things, like exercise, diet and state of mind, can all have an effect on how well it works for you."

PICTURE YOURSELF WELL

Getting started with visualization and imagery is as simple as closing your eyes. In fact, a brain (as well as an open mind) is all the "equipment" that you'll ever need when using visualization to help the body heal. Say you have asthma. Picture your bronchial tubes opening and then cleaning them out with a vacuum cleaner. Do this for about ten minutes, twice a day.

Getting**Started**

Imagery and Visualization

Imagery and visualization can be useful tools in promoting healing. To take full advantage of these techniques, find a practitioner who can guide you.

Number of practitioners in the United States: Approximately 500 specialize in imagery and visualization; about 4,000 certified hypnosis professionals are also trained in imagery and visualization techniques.

Qualifications to look for: An M.D., D.O., Ph.D., psychologist or nurse with training in imagery and visualization from a state-accredited training program or certification in hypnosis.

Professional associations: American Institute for Mental Imagery, 351 East 84th Street, Suite 10D, New York, NY 10028; American Society of Clinical Hypnosis, 2200 East Devon Avenue, Suite 291, Des Plaines, IL 60018-4534.

To find a practitioner: Contact one of the professional associations listed above.

Approximate cost: $55 to $125 per session, depending on the region.

This visualization guides the body toward healing, says Dr. Green. (But don't stop using your asthma medications without close supervision by your health care provider.) Visualization can also be used as a preventive measure, she notes.

In general, though, it's probably best to learn how from a psychologist or psychotherapist who is trained in using imagery or visualization and can help you find images that best work for you, notes Dr. Norris.

If you want to try imagery or visualization for yourself, these guidelines can help get you started.

Sit quietly and comfortably. Then start deep breathing—that is, breathe in and out with your eyes closed and your stomach 'soft,' says Dr. Gordon. Let that softness spread from your belly into your legs and upper body, breathing deeply.

"At this point, I take people using guided imagery on a little trip—walking down a road, going off the road, crossing a meadow, stepping into a clearing," he says. "Or I ask them to mentally visit a place where they feel completely comfortable."

Imagine a bright white light. To utilize imagery for general good health, says Dr. Lal-Tabak, picture a bright light going through your body, surrounding and protecting you, keeping out negative energy. Do it for about 15 minutes twice a day—once in the morning and once at night—she says.

Do it daily. Whether you select a healing image from your mind's image gallery, follow imagery suggested by a professional or practice "maintenance" bright light imagery, experts say that you should practice regularly. "It's a skill that you really can sharpen," says Dr. Green.

Daydream at your leisure. Aside from doing visualization and imagery, you can daydream whenever you have a moment, says Dr. Green.

"Daydreaming is a way to learn how to get into the quiet state and let the images come to your mind," she notes. "So learn to be more creative by turning on your mental eye, relaxing and getting into a state of reverie." Then add the images that come to your "databank" of healing visions.

LIGHT THERAPY
A Safe, Simple Way to Lift Your Moods

The scenario is familiar: Cooped up in windowless meeting rooms all day, you suddenly have the urge to make a break for it and take advantage of the brilliant sunshine outside. Ah, that feels better. Fifteen minutes later, you return to work renewed and refreshed.

You've just treated yourself to a mood-elevating dose of light therapy. Though its roots are 2,000 or so years old—great Greek geniuses like Herodotus and Hippocrates recognized its healing power—light therapy is still considered a scientific frontier, says George Brainard, Ph.D., professor of neurology and director of the light research program at Jefferson Medical College in Philadelphia.

"The very best data we have for light therapy is for its ability to help relieve seasonal affective disorder (SAD)—a form of depression that many women experience during the fall and winter, when there are fewer hours of daylight," says Dr. Brainard. "Those studies date back to just 1982. And only a handful of medical schools in this country have full-fledged light research programs, including ours here at Jefferson," he notes.

A CURE FOR THE RAINY-DAY BLUES

Unfortunately, doctors who use light for therapy can't depend on the weather. When it's dreary or nasty outside, it's harder to take advantage of nature's free light treatment. But there is an artificial alternative. A light box that mimics the sun's natural rays has been shown to be effective against SAD.

Natural or artificial, light therapy need not be intense or prolonged to lift your mood. A study done in Switzerland showed, for example, that a daily 30-minute walk in the morning—even on a cloudy morning—is as effective for treating seasonal affective disorder as using a special light box, says Dr. Brainard.

"The brightest light box that we recommend for therapeutic use measures 10,000 lux at eye level," he says. "That's equivalent to daylight about a half-hour after sunrise." (Roughly translated, 10 lux equals the lighting power of a single candle at a one-foot distance from the eye.)

"So an early-morning walk may be exactly as effective as sitting in front of your light box," says Dr. Brainard. For the sake of comparison, he notes, the light at midday on a clear, sunny day measures 100,000 lux.

Experts know that light therapy works, but they don't exactly know why or how. They do know that light affects the secretion of melatonin, a hormone produced in the pineal gland. The pineal gland is controlled by the hypothalamus, the part of the brain that serves as the body's "clock."

Melatonin secretion occurs mainly at night, and light suppresses the release of the hormone, explains Norman E. Rosenthal, M.D., chief of the Unit of Outpatients Studies and staff psychiatrist at the National Institutes of Mental Health in Bethesda, Maryland. It's unclear whether SAD is related to melatonin. Nevertheless, Dr. Rosenthal and his colleagues have effectively treated SAD by exposing patients to bright light for several hours a day.

SHEDDING NEW LIGHT ON WOMEN'S HEALTH

According to Dr. Brainard, what researchers are learning about the therapeutic use of light has a great deal of promise—especially for women.

As a proven treatment for SAD, light therapy is good news for the millions of women who become clinically depressed during winter's shorter, darker days. "Perhaps as many as four times more women than men seek treatment for SAD symptoms," says Michael Terman, Ph.D., director of the winter depression program and the light therapy unit at Columbia-Presbyterian Medical Center in New York City.

But women may benefit in other ways. "A handful of small studies indicates that light therapy may be effective for easing the symptoms of premenstrual syndrome," says Dr. Brainard. And, he says, there's additional hope for women who are unable to conceive due to overly long menstrual cycles.

"As far back as the 1960s, researchers found that light therapy could normalize long menstrual cycles," says Dr. Brainard. "In recent years, a research team working with Daniel Kripke, M.D., at the University of California at San Diego repeated those studies with good results," says Dr. Brainard. In Dr. Kripke's studies, it was shown that exposure to light during the night for three days during the middle of the menstrual cycle significantly shortened and normalized long, irregular menstrual cycles.

And light therapy has been found to be helpful for women whose sleep is disturbed by jet lag and shift work. One group of researchers at the Biological Rhythms Research Laboratory at Chicago's Rush-Presbyterian–St. Luke's Medical Center concluded that controlling light and dark artificially can overcome the sleep problems encountered by shift workers.

LIGHT THERAPY DO'S AND DON'TS

Using a light box is pretty simple, according to Brenda Byrne, Ph.D., director of the Seasonal Affective Disorder Clinic affiliated with the light research program at Jefferson Medical College. All you have to do is plug it in, sit in front of it and follow the manufacturers instructions for proper light exposure.

For light therapy to work, explains Dr. Brainard, the light must illuminate your retina, the part of the eye that conveys light signals to the pineal

Getting**Started**

Light Therapy

Before using light therapy, it's important to get a professional diagnosis and work with a practitioner trained in this treatment. Talk to your doctor if you feel depressed or think you may have seasonal affective disorder.

Number of practitioners in the United States: Approximately 1,000.

Qualifications to look for: Practitioners with an advanced degree (M.D., Ph.D.) who are qualified to diagnose and treat psychiatric conditions or health conditions related to changes in daily body rhythm.

Professional associations: Society for Light Treatment and Biological Rhythms, 10200 West 44th Avenue, Suite 304, Wheat Ridge, CO 80033-2840.

To find a practitioner: Contact the Society for Light Treatment and Biological Rhythms (above); or write to the SunBox Company, 19217 Orbit Drive, Gaithersburg, MD 20879.

Approximate cost: $250 to $550, depending on which type of light box you buy.

Light-box suppliers: SunBox Company (address listed above); Bio-Brite, Inc., 7315 Wisconsin Avenue, Suite 1300W, Bethesda, MD 20814-3202.

gland. "But it's very important to get a specially designed light box from a reputable dealer," says Dr. Brainard.

Whatever you do, warns Dr. Brainard, don't confuse light boxes with tanning lights—you can't get safe light therapy at a tanning salon, even if you wear protective goggles. "Ultraviolet rays from tanning lamps can seriously damage your eyes," says Dr. Brainard. "For that same reason, never stare directly at the sun, either."

Dr. Byrne offers these other do's and don'ts for light therapy.

Get the go-ahead from your doctor. Depression can be a serious disorder. Don't buy a light box to treat your blues before talking to your doctor about your symptoms.

Let there be light before breakfast. Begin your day with a 35-minute walk or light-box session, says Dr. Byrne. Morning light treatment is especially helpful for people with seasonal affective disorder who find it hard to get up in the morning. If you can't arrange a morning session, pick a time that's not too late in the evening and stick to it, suggests Dr. Byrne.

Read the directions. The proper distance between you and the light will vary. Follow the manufacturer's directions.

Don't count on the light of a sunny window, says Dr. Byrne. "Daylight reflects off even clear glass, so it's hard to know just how much light you're getting through a sunny window."

Don't just sit there—do something! Use your 30-minute daily light-box session to your advantage, suggests Dr. Byrne. "Many women use their light-box time to meditate, eat breakfast, ride an exercise bike, read or put on makeup. Just make sure that you're sitting close to the box."

MASSAGE AND BODYWORK
The Power of Healing Hands

If you think massage is an indulgence of the very rich, think again. Therapeutic massage is now becoming recognized as a useful nondrug technique for alleviating a number of ailments or rejuvenating your stressed-out body, especially for women. And all you have to do is lie serenely on a padded table.

"Massage is a great way to recharge your batteries, especially for women who expend vast amounts of energy taking care of others at home, in the community or on the job," says Shawne Bryant, M.D., gynecologist and certified massage therapist in Virginia Beach, Virginia. "Massage fosters a woman's physical, mental and spiritual well-being in a way that few other therapies or stress-busting activities can." And, she adds, the benefits of massage begin the minute that your appointment begins.

"You've set aside an uninterruptible hour just for you. That alone is a powerful healing message, which for most women is too often denied," says Dr. Bryant.

A NECESSITY, NOT A LUXURY

"Massage clearly induces physiological changes that not only make you feel better but also reduce stress hormones and enhance immune function," says Tiffany Field, Ph.D., professor of pediatrics, psychology and psychiatry at the University of Miami School of Medicine. As director and founder of the Touch Research Institute at the school, Dr. Field has conducted extensive research on the physiological benefits of massage.

Massage can allow quicker recovery from physical stress and trauma and help eliminate the postworkout buildup of lactic acid, a byproduct of exertion that causes muscle aches, writes licensed massage therapist Thomas Claire, author of *Bodywork: What Type of Massage to Get—And How to Make the Most of It.*

Dr. Bryant says that more research studies need to be developed on the benefits of massage therapy. But massage may work because it increases circulation.

"When you increase the blood supply to the massaged area, you increase the delivery of oxygen and nutrients to the tissues, and you facilitate the removal of waste products," says Dr. Bryant. "In addition, increased circulation promotes healing by increasing the cells involved with fighting infection and disease."

"There are good studies showing that massage decreases the lymph-related swelling that many women experience following mastectomies," says Adriane Fugh-Berman, M.D., former head of field investigations for the Office of Alternative Medicine at the National Institutes of Health in Bethesda, Maryland. And, she says, studies showing that your urine output increases following a massage might mean that massage speeds your body's waste-removal process.

A NATURAL AID FOR EMOTIONAL HEALING

Other practitioners recommend massage for women under emotional stress.

"Just think about the act of stopping yourself from crying," says Ben E. Benjamin, Ph.D., muscular therapist and president of The Muscular Therapy Institute in Cambridge, Massachusetts. "It's physical as well as emotional. You contract muscles all over your body to make yourself stop crying, and those contractions can lead to stiffness and soreness over time."

"The same thing happens when you get angry, tense or scared," says Dr. Benjamin. "Eventually, these negative emotions are stored in your tissues. Massage—also referred to as therapeutic bodywork—can reduce tension formed in the body by these repressed emotions."

MASSAGE À LA CARTE

Strictly speaking, massage is a catchall term for more than 100 hands-on techniques, says Robert A. Edwards, licensed massage therapist and director of the Somerset School of Massage, in New Jersey.

Massage techniques fall generally under one of four widely accepted therapeutic approaches, says Gene Arbetter, certified massage therapist; co-director of Wellness Associates, a holistic family medical practice in Chicago; and former national information director and spokesman for the American Massage Therapy Association in Evanston, Illinois. These approaches are the traditional Swedish massage, contemporary Western massage, bodywork and Oriental forms of bodywork, such as shiatsu. (For details on shiatsu massage, see page 16.)

Anatomy of a Swedish Massage

As performed at resort spas, health clubs, day spas and massage clinics, the traditional Swedish massage is probably the massage style that most women know best, according to Arbetter. In a typical traditional Swedish

Getting**Started**

Massage and Bodywork

If you'd like to find a massage therapist or bodywork practitioner in your area, follow these guidelines.

Number of practitioners in the United States: For massage, estimates vary. About 1,000 practitioners are trained in Rolfing and Structural Integration, and nearly 600 practitioners are trained in the Trager Approach.

Qualifications to look for: For massage, look for an L.M.T. (licensed massage therapist) or a C.M.T. (certified massage therapist). For Rolfing, look for certification by The Rolf Institute or The Guild for Structural Integration; for the Trager Approach, practitioners should be certified by The Trager Institute. For Polarity Therapy, look for an A.P.P. (associate polarity practitioner) or R.P.P. (registered polarity practitioner), certified by the American Polarity Therapy Association.

Professional associations: American Massage Therapy Association, 1130 West North Shore Avenue, Chicago, IL 60626; American Polarity Therapy Association, 2888 Bluff Street, Suite 149, Boulder, CO 80301; The Guild for Structural Integration, P.O. Box 1559, Boulder, CO 80306; The Rolf Institute, 205 Canyon Boulevard, Boulder, CO 80302; and The Trager Institute; 21 Locust Avenue, Mill Valley, CA 94941-2806.

To find a practitioner: Contact one of the professional associations listed above.

Approximate cost: For a massage, $45 to $60 per session, which lasts 30 to 60 minutes; for polarity therapy, $40 to $85 per session, lasting about 60 minutes; for Rolfing or Structural Integration, $80 to $120 per session, which lasts about 60 minutes; for the Trager Approach, $45 to $90 per session, lasting 60 to 90 minutes.

massage, you are ushered into a quiet, dimly lit room that is furnished with a massage table covered in soft, clean bed linens. As she leaves the room, your massage therapist directs you to undress and slip between the sheets. (You can leave on your underwear if it makes you more comfortable, Arbetter says.)

Once you've settled onto the table as requested, the massage therapist re-enters the room and asks whether there's any specific area that you want her to work on. Your shoulders? Your back? Your neck? Do you have any medical conditions? She'll want to know. She encourages you to tell her whether the temperature in the room is comfortable and whether you prefer light or deep touch. And then your massage begins.

During your session, which can last 30 minutes to an hour or more, the massage therapist will ask whether there's too much or too little oil on her hands and whether her strokes are too light or too deep. She'll deftly drape and undrape your body as she works, uncovering only the part of you that she's working on, for modesty and warmth.

Then, each part of your body, unless you request otherwise, will be systematically massaged with some variation of the five classic Swedish massage strokes, shown here. By the time the session is completed, those knots in your shoulders, neck and back will have melted away and you will, in all likelihood, be left in a relaxed yet energized state of bliss.

Swedish massage is the root from which has sprung a variety of massage therapies, including medical massage, on-site massage, sports massage and pregnancy massage. All are in wide use today.

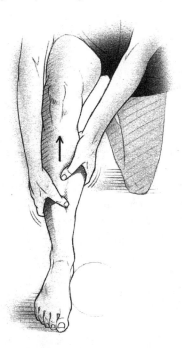

Effleurage

Effleurage is the smooth, gliding stroke used at the beginning of massage sessions to warm and relax the muscles.

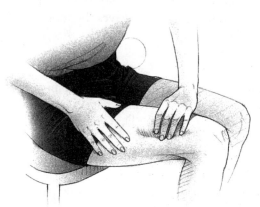

Petrissage

Petrissage means "kneading," and that's what your massage therapist does to you, with her hands, thumbs or fingers.

Friction

Effleurage and petrissage are usually followed by friction strokes and deep circular or back and forth motions made with the fingertips or thumb tips.

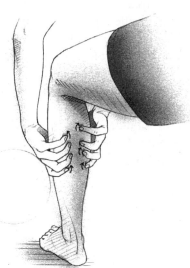

Tapotement

Tapotement is the pounding motion most often associated with Swedish massage. Your therapist may use the edge of her hands, cupped hands or her fingers to rapidly deliver these staccato strokes.

Vibration

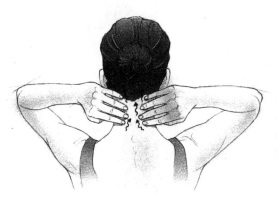

To perform vibration movements, your therapist spreads her hands down firmly and rapidly shakes them over an area with a trembling motion.

Medical massage is practiced by specially trained massage therapists and may be recommended by M.D.'s, osteopathic physicians and chiropractors in conjunction with other therapy. Massage therapy may be beneficial in providing temporary pain relief for arthritis, fibromyalgia (painful "trigger points" in muscles) and chronic back pain. Individuals with these or any other medical conditions should discuss the impact of massage therapy with their health practitioners.

On-site massage is offered by some companies to relieve stress in the workplace. Massage therapists, equipped with special chairs, deliver 15-minute back rubs right through your clothing. These short massage breaks are similar to those offered at malls, fitness shops and at least one major airport. They're not as thorough as a full Swedish massage, but "a little massage is better than none at all," says Edwards.

Sports massage is designed to loosen you up and invigorate you before an athletic event and speed recovery from exertion after a hard workout, such as a strenuous hike or a day of cross-country skiing.

CONTEMPORARY WESTERN MASSAGE: TARGETING PAIN

Practitioners of contemporary Western massage use a variety of techniques—myofascial release, myotherapy and neuromuscular therapy—to rub, pull and poke away the pain, says Edwards. In myotherapy and neuromuscular therapy, the therapist applies deep, sustained pressure on sensitive spots, called trigger points, within muscles. (Myo means "muscle.") Therapy is aimed at pain's source, whether caused by muscular adhesions ("sticky" muscles) or distortions in the fascia (tough bands connecting organs, muscles, tendons and other body tissues). Your therapist will use her fingers, palms and even her forearms and elbows to release tension from the fascia and restore the body's balance.

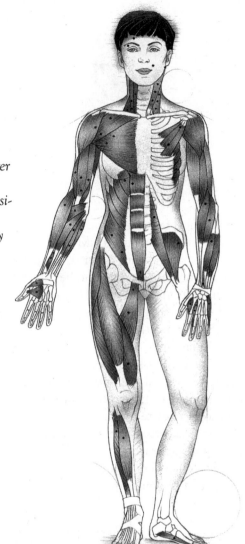

Trigger Points

Myotherapy and neuromuscular therapy (jointly referred to as trigger point therapy) focus on relieving pain in trigger points—tender, sensitive spots found in tight bands of muscle, as shown here. The theory is that trigger points are not only painful themselves but can also radiate pain to other parts of the body.

BODYWORK: A PHILOSOPHY OF BALANCE

Some other forms of massage, which are included under the broad term of bodywork, can help strike a healthy balance between the way your body is structured and the way you move. Practitioners will work to assist you in freeing restrictions, both physical and mental.

Rolfing: Keeping Gravity at Bay

Standing self-consciously in your bra and panties, you face a lithe, powerfully built man with piercing eyes. You take a deep breath and pull in your abs, as if to swallow the flab that's become your belly and thighs. He scrutinizes every inch of you. And then he says, "Your left shoulder is higher than your right. Your feet toe out. Turn sideways."

You turn. He points.

"You divert from the vertical here," he says. "Your pelvis is forward. Your shoulders are back. I'm going to try to lengthen your body to make you as tall and straight as possible. Stand still another minute . . . umm-hmm . . . and now we'll get started."

You're about to be Rolfed.

Rolfing was developed by Ida Rolf, Ph.D., a biochemist who was a research scientist at the Rockefeller Institute during World War I. Her interest in complementary healing—including other modalities such as homeopathy, yoga, osteopathy, chiropractic and the Alexander Technique—combined with her physical problems and those of her acquaintances led her to develop what she called Structural Integration (popularly known as Rolfing, for short).

"The ultimate goal of Rolfing is to bring the body into an ideal alignment with gravity so that gravity is assisting the body as opposed to wearing it down," says David Frome, physical therapist and Rolfing practitioner in Montclair, New Jersey. Rolfing doesn't focus on specific physical problems, he says. "Rather, Rolfing balances your structure to bring everything into alignment and allow healing to occur."

Dr. Rolf began teaching Structural Integration to chiropractors and osteopaths throughout the United States, Canada and Great Britain in the 1950s and 1960s. In 1972, Dr. Rolf and her followers established the Rolf Institute in Boulder, Colorado.

The process of being Rolfed involves ten hour-long sessions, says Frome. "Ten sessions allows us to work through the whole system of connective tissue (fascia). Each of the first seven sessions focuses on a different area. During the last three sessions, we reinforce what we've done. We concentrate on the outer layer of fascia during initial sessions, working progressively deeper as we go along," he explains.

Rolfing was once thought to be a painful therapy, but according to Frome, it's not any longer. "In the last 20 years, we've learned that Rolfers can accomplish their goals with a much lighter touch."

During a Rolfing session, you lie in various positions on a massage table. The Rolfer will use her hands, elbows or forearms to apply pressure of varying intensity. Along with the manual pressure, the Rolfer may ask you to move in specific ways. You'll feel as though you're being steamrollered smooth with deep, slow kneading motions and deep digging motions.

As the Rolfer works, she'll carefully watch the area under treatment. "When I work," says Frome, "I watch how you're breathing and how the tissue is responding, to continually check the impact of what I'm doing as I work."

Many Rolfers, like other bodyworkers, believe that the body stores its emotional history and experiences—from accidents such as falling out of a tree as a child to emotional upheavals that occur during abuse—in the tissues. "We contend that the process of Rolfing can release those emotional charges," says Frome.

How do those releases manifest themselves?

"Sometimes it will happen in the office during a session," says Frome. "But often a client will go home and have an epiphany of some kind. Or she'll express the release in her dreams. Once Rolfed, you may feel differently about yourself: more grounded, more in charge of your world. It's a very, very powerful therapy," he says.

Polarity Therapy: An Energizing Episode

Polarity therapy is based on the idea that the body has electromagnetic energy patterns, which must be in balance.

Its creator, Randolf Stone, was a chiropractor, osteopath and naturopath born at the turn of the century. Fascinated by the healing practices of other cultures, Dr. Stone's studies included Chinese medicine, herbology, reflexology, Indian Ayurvedic medicine, Middle Eastern spiritualism and Egyptian esoteric teachings.

As a result, his polarity therapy is a blend of Eastern and Western techniques that concentrate on unblocking the flow of energy through the body, says Ruth Kaciak, a bodyworker certified in polarity therapy and other bodywork modalities who works at the Open Center, a wellness facility in New York City.

During a polarity therapy session, the therapist will use a variety of motions (gently applied) aimed at balancing the body's energy. At various times during your session, she may hold you, rock you or use her hands lightly, or deeply, on your body.

In a typical session with a certified polarity therapist, a slight, wiry woman leads you up the stairs to a door marked "Wellness Room." Inside, incense burns. Candles glow. Tinkling, starry music emanates, it seems, from everywhere.

You are asked to remove your shoes and jewelry and to lie, fully clothed, on your back on a well-padded massage table. The therapist positions herself at the foot of the table. Gently, very gently, she pulls on your left leg and holds it for a moment or two.

"I feel an energy blockage in your hip," she comments, gently pulling some more. "Let's free that up."

Deft hands firmly press on points over your hipbone. It feels wonderful. An hour or so later, you've been gently stretched and pulled and occasionally kneaded all over your body. You leave feeling ten pounds lighter, ten years younger and energized enough to sprint across town.

Craniosacral Therapy: Massage for Your Head

Developed in the 1970s by John E. Upledger, D.O., craniosacral therapy is a gentle, hands-on method used to evaluate and enhance the craniosacral system—the membranes and fluid that surround the brain and spinal cord—to aid the body's natural healing processes. Dr. Upledger says that this therapy is effective for a wide range of conditions, including whiplash, migraines, eye problems, jaw pain and lower-back pain.

Describing craniosacral balancing as a gentle, noninvasive nervous-system and fascial-balancing technique, Kaciak explains that "craniosacral therapy works with structural alignment, energy and emotions."

Practitioners use a very light touch—generally about the weight of a nickel—to test for restrictions that block the flow of the cerebrospinal fluid.

You lie on the table as the healer places the palms of her hands very softly under the base of your skull. As you relax yourself into her hands, you feel warmth building and turning to comfortable heat, as if her hands had become tiny electric blankets. You are soothed, deeply soothed.

"Craniosacral balancing encourages the person undergoing therapy to capitalize on her own healing energy potential and not depend on the therapist's energy," says Kaciak. "Individuals may experience the energy during a session as warmth or a tingling sense of well-being."

The Trager Approach: Inner Peace in 90 Minutes

The method of hands-on healing known as the Trager Approach was developed by Milton Trager, M.D., an amateur boxer who became a doctor, using his hands to heal instead of fight. In 1980, he co-founded the Trager Institute to train Trager practitioners. Trager practitioners work with you to relax each of your body's muscle groups. Specific techniques vary from practitioner to practitioner, but, in general, a practitioner will work with an area until it has completely relaxed.

Lying down, you're urged by a low, gentle voice to "just let go," as warm, capable hands gently, firmly rock your head from side to side . . . from side to side . . . from side to side.

For the next 90 minutes, this gentle rocking will be repeated, in near-infinite variations, on your arms, your shoulders, your feet and your legs. The ever-so-gentle pulling, cradling and rocking that you'll receive all over your body may induce you to discover an inner peace so overwhelming that it may last for the rest of the day, or for the rest of the week or longer.

"Your body can be encouraged to remember what we did here today hours or days later," says certified massage and Trager therapist Bonita Cassel-Beckwith, who practices in the suburbs of Philadelphia. "When you want to regain this feeling of deep relaxation that you have reached, simply ask your neck, or any other part of you, how it felt during your Trager session. The body has a memory and will respond if you listen for its answer.

"At first, it's natural for someone to resist slightly," she says. "My job is to get you—and your muscles—to completely relax. A Trager practitioner is sensitive to every nuance of your muscles and knows how to coax them into relaxing or letting go."

A key part of the Trager Approach is what practitioners call Mentastics, mentally directed movements that suggest to the mind feelings of lightness, freedom and pleasure, says Cassel-Beckwith. "Mentastics enable those who've had a Trager session to continue feeling inner peace days, weeks and months later. The exercises help the body remember the relaxation that it discovered during the sessions."

CHOOSING A PRO

Unless you have an unlimited bodywork budget and oodles of time, it's unlikely that you'll be able to sample all of the healing riches that bodywork has to offer. But Kaciak has some wise advice.

"It's really not the technique that's important—it's the therapist and her level of skill and personal development," says Kaciak. "Bodywork is the craft and healing is the art; it transcends the technique that you use.

"Great therapists know how to help you tap into your own creative healing potential," says Kaciak. "Choose one who's skilled in several different bodywork techniques, then let her determine which of them—alone or in combination—is best for your needs." This is determined by careful listening to your body and mind and monitoring the response.

"A truly gifted practitioner, well-trained in several techniques, is like a chef with a huge spice rack at her disposal. She can blend appropriate bodywork styles together to provide optimum natural healing that's designed especially for you," says Kaciak.

SELF-MASSAGE FOR WHAT AILS YOU *NOW*

Practitioners agree that for optimum benefit—to relieve stress and ease stiff, sore muscle—nothing beats regular, professional massage. But with a little practice, you can give yourself an effective massage and treat yourself when time and money are short, according to Susen Edwards, licensed massage therapist, co-owner and instructor at the Somerset School of Massage in New Jersey and author of *The Healing Power of Self-Massage.*

"When you need to relax right now, self-massage is as close as your fingertips," says Edwards. She offers these special head and scalp and neck and shoulder massages for instant relaxation, whether you're stuck in traffic or facing a stress-provoking meeting.

Head and Scalp Massage

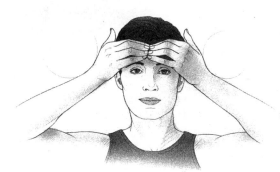

Place the pads of your four fingertips together at the center of your forehead. Very gently, smooth along the "worry" lines of your forehead from the center out to the temples. Repeat six times.

Next, using pressure no harder than the touch you'd use on your eyeball, make tiny circles on your temples, between the corner of your eye and your scalp. Repeat six times.

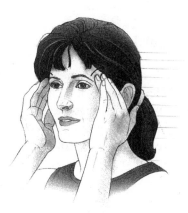

(continued)

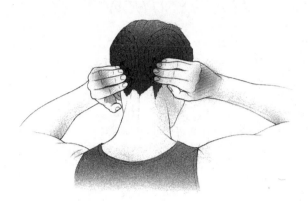

Then, using slightly firmer pressure with all of your fingers, massage your scalp with circular motions. Starting at the nape of your neck, work your fingers around until you have massaged each part of your scalp. As you massage, imagine that your scalp is loosening under your touch.

Finally, with your hand in a loose fist close to the scalp, grab a handful of hair and give it a little tug. Work until you've covered each section of the scalp.

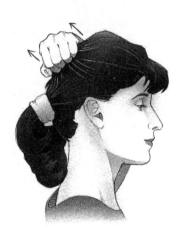

A Quick Fix for Chair Jockeys

This massage is great for when you've been seated for too long at your desk, in your car or on a plane, says Edwards.

"When you're stuck in a seated position for a while, you may begin to feel achy in your upper back, neck and shoulders. This massage will alleviate the problem pronto," she says. If you can't do this neck and shoulder massage comfortably, stop.

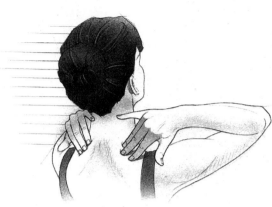

Neck and Shoulder Massage

Stand and tilt your head back slightly. Reach back, as shown, and use the pads of three fingertips, curved under a bit, to massage the muscles over your shoulder blades for about ten seconds. If you can't do this comfortably, stop.

Whole-Body Self-Massage

Try these other easy self-massage techniques for whatever ails you, suggested by Joan Johnson, licensed massage therapist at Ojo Caliente Mineral Springs in Ojo Caliente, New Mexico, and author of *The Healing Art of Sports Massage*. Or combine them with the head and shoulder massages, shown previously, for an all-purpose, 20-minute self-massage routine that you can do anytime, anywhere.

Hand Massage

Use the thumb of one hand to massage the palm of the opposite hand. Interlock fingers, as shown, and apply firm but gentle pressure to aching hands. Then switch hands.

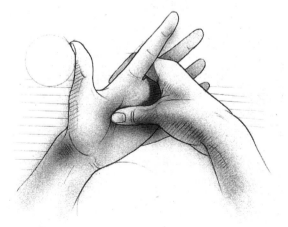

Foot Massage

Using lengthwise or circular motions, massage the bottom of your foot with both thumbs, concentrating on the arch area. Then use the fingers from both hands and, next, both palms to massage the bottom of your foot. Repeat on the opposite foot.

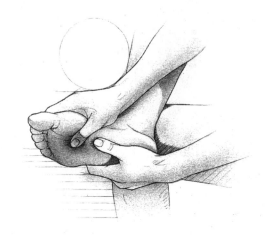

Calf Massage

Positioning your lower leg at a 45-degree angle to the floor, use your thumbs and/or fingers of both hands to squeeze, stroke, shake and knead the calf muscle. Repeat on the opposite leg.

Shin Massage

Reaching forward from a seated position, press both thumbs into the muscle running along the front of your lower leg. Begin near the ankle and stroke upward toward the knee. Repeat on the opposite leg.

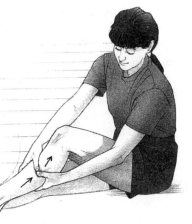

Quadriceps Massage

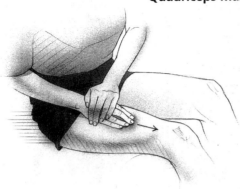

While seated with your right leg extended, cup the middle three fingers of one hand and bend the middle finger slightly. Using your opposite hand to help guide your cupped hand, firmly press and stroke your thigh toward the knee. Repeat on the opposite leg.

From a seated position, use both thumbs and fingers of both hands to shake, squeeze and knead at the back of your thigh. Then, divide the thigh muscle into longitudinal sections and, using your fingers and thumbs, stroke lengthwise toward your knee, working your way across, section by section. Finally, press your

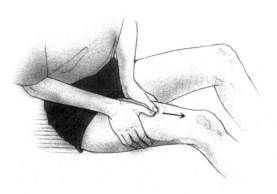

thumbs into the top of your thigh, as shown, and push your thumbs downward toward the knee. Repeat on the opposite leg.

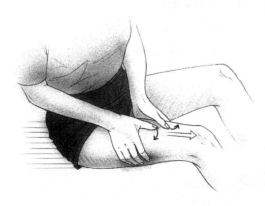

While remaining seated, continue to massage the quadriceps, alternating first one thumb and then the other. Press each thumb into the thigh in circular motions, working downward toward the knee. Repeat on the opposite leg.

Hamstring Massage

While seated against a wall, extend your left leg and bend your right leg at the knee with your foot flat on the floor. Use one or both of your hands to shake, squeeze and knead the muscle under the thigh, called the hamstring. Work the entire length of the muscle. Repeat on the opposite leg.

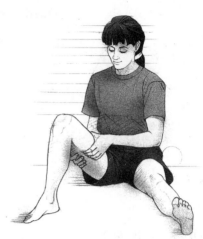

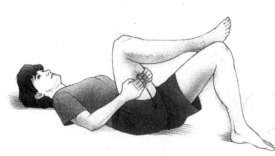

Lying on the floor, bend one leg and rest your foot on the bent knee of the opposite leg. Aligning your fingertips, as shown, press the fingertips of both hands into the hamstring muscle and press toward the buttocks. Keep the backs of the fingers of one hand touching the backs of the fingers of the opposite hand. Repeat on the opposite leg.

Buttocks Massage

Lying on the floor, bend one leg and bring your knee close to your chest. Use the fingertips of the outside hand to press firmly against the buttock, or "sit bone." Working in lengthwise sections, from the hip inward, press across the muscle, section by section.

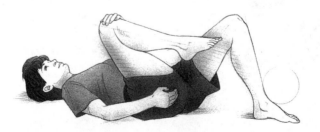

Lower-Back Massage

Lie flat on the floor with your knees bent and feet flat on the floor. Place a tennis ball under the area of your back that you want to massage. Pressing as much of your body weight against the ball as is comfortable, move your body against the ball, back and forth or in circular motions.

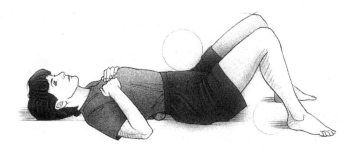

Biceps Massage

With the thumb of one hand, press the biceps muscle of the opposite arm, using long strokes from your elbow up toward your armpit, as indicated.

With the thumb and fingers of one hand, grip the biceps muscle of the opposite arm. Pressing your thumb lightly into the middle of the arm, where the biceps meet, rock the muscle back and forth. Repeat on the opposite arm.

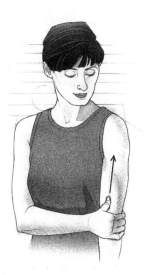

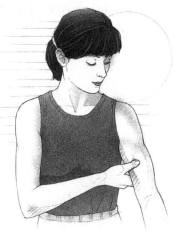

Triceps Massage

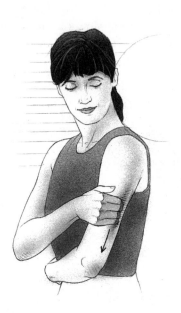

Bend one arm in front of you at a 90-degree angle. With the fingertips of the opposite hand, press the triceps muscles, located on the outside of your arm between your armpit and your elbow. Gentle press downward toward your elbow while slowly straightening your arm. Use lighter pressure near your elbow, where the triceps muscles join the triceps tendons. Repeat on the opposite arm.

Forearm Massage

Press your thumb into your lower forearm, with your palm held upward, as shown, and stroke the muscle. Then, turn the palm down and repeat. Repeat on the opposite arm.

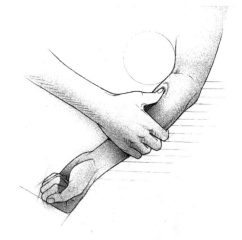

MEDITATION
A Menu of Calming Rituals

First thing tomorrow morning, before you rise, spend a few moments in bed doing something that will make you feel terrific: Meditate.

It's easy. Anyone can do it. Just breathe normally and tune in to the simple miracle of your respiration. Concentrate on the air as it fills your lungs. Note its release as you slowly exhale. Experience your body right now, this very instant, from head to toe. Feel how your body urges itself awake. Feel the sheets around your body. Feel the pillow under your head. Breathe out into the world around you with loving-kindness.

When you open your eyes, allow your eyes to be soft. Note the environment around you. Breathe into awareness as you see the morning light dance across your bedroom walls. Smell the morning air. Hear the morning sounds: the birds, the buzz of traffic or your children bounding down the stairs. Savor fully this moment in time in rich detail.

Now, go make breakfast.

Congratulations. You've just taken the first step toward practicing an ancient healing technique that's said to provide women with a litany of life-affirming benefits.

MEDITATION DEMYSTIFIED

Simply put, meditation is a form of contemplation that's thousands of years old and rooted in the traditions of the world's great religions. In fact, practically all religious groups practice meditation in one form or another.

Of the religions that use meditation, perhaps Buddhism, practiced widely in eastern and central Asia, is the best known. To Buddhists, the practice of meditation is essential for the cultivation of wisdom and compassion and for understanding reality.

Buddhists believe that our ordinary consciousness is both limited and limiting, says Jon Kabat-Zinn, Ph.D., in his book *Wherever You Go, There*

You Are: Mindfulness Meditation in Everyday Living. Dr. Kabat-Zinn is the founder and director of the Stress Reduction Clinic at the University of Massachusetts Medical Center in Worcester and associate professor of medicine in the school's Division of Preventive and Behavioral Medicine.

Meditation makes it possible to live life to the "full spectrum of our conscious and unconscious possibilities," writes Dr. Kabat-Zinn.

Prayer: Good for What Ails You

Meditation certainly has benefits for the woman who's meditating, but what about prayers? And, to take this question to the next step, can you be helped if someone else prays for you? Dale A. Matthews, M.D., prays for his patients. He also prescribes drugs for them and recommends surgery, when necessary. In a word, he does whatever it takes to help them get well, he explains. And he is certainly convinced that prayer is one of those things.

"Prayer works," says Dr. Matthews, associate professor of medicine at Georgetown University School of Medicine in Washington, D.C., and senior research fellow at the National Institute for Healthcare Research in Rockville, Maryland. Dr. Matthews has reviewed more than 200 studies linking religious commitment and health, cited in his book *The Faith Factor.*

Dr. Matthews says that he isn't the only physician who believes in the healing power of prayer—with good reason. He cites studies suggesting that people who pray are less likely to get sick, are more likely to recover from surgery and illness and are better able to cope with their illnesses than people who don't pray. Some evidence indicates that sick people who are prayed for also fare significantly better than those who aren't. In fact, some physicians report that people who are prayed for often do better even if they don't know they're being prayed for.

Prayer seems to have a positive effect on emotional and physical problems alike, says Larry Dossey, M.D., who reviewed 130 studies examining the efficacy of prayer for his book *Healing Words: The Power of Prayer and the Practice of Medicine.* He's also author of *Prayer Is Good Medicine.*

Written off by mainstream medicine for decades, prayer got a second look when researchers at the University of California, San Francisco, School of Medicine published a watershed study. To put prayer

AN ANTIDOTE FOR WOMEN'S SPECIAL STRESSES

Meditation can help you attain peace of mind. And it can also ease physical complaints such as premenstrual syndrome (PMS), tension headaches and other common health problems affecting women.

"Women's hectic role-switching can wreak havoc with their lives and

to the scientific test, they divided 393 men and women hospitalized for heart trouble into two groups. All the men and women got medical care. In addition, half were prayed for by volunteers outside the hospital. None of the men or women knew whether they were in the group being prayed for or not. Nonetheless, the men and women whose medical care was supplemented with prayer needed fewer drugs and spent less time on ventilators. They also fared better overall than their counterparts who received medical care but nothing more.

All types of prayer appear to work, says Jeffrey S. Levin, Ph.D., associate professor of family and community medicine at Eastern Virginia Medical School in Norfolk. Even the prayers of agnostics, who don't invoke a deity, get results.

"Some people offer a very directed prayer to a Father God asking that someone be healed," says Dr. Levin. "Others send their love or feel empathy for the person who is ill."

Empathy, in fact, is the key element in prayer, say Dr. Levin and Dr. Dossey.

"There has to be caring," says Dr. Dossey. "The desire for recovery has to be genuine, authentic and deeply felt. It has to come from a feeling of love and compassion."

As for why prayer gets results, researchers offer various natural and supernatural explanations but admit that they simply don't know for sure.

"Just because we don't understand the mechanism doesn't mean that it doesn't work," Dr. Levin adds. "After all, there was a time we didn't know why aspirin worked."

Prayer shouldn't replace conventional treatment, says Dr. Matthews, who is studying the effects of prayer on rheumatoid arthritis. But a growing body of evidence suggests that prayer should supplement it, he adds.

with their health," says Patricia Carrington, Ph.D., associate clinical professor of psychiatry at the Robert Wood Johnson Medical School of the University of Medicine and Dentistry of New Jersey in Piscataway and author of *Freedom in Meditation*.

"Office-efficient women from 9:00 to 5:00 often become homemakers, wives or mothers—sometimes simultaneously—at 5:01 sharp," continues Dr. Carrington.

"Meditation gives women a psychological buffer so that life's hectic pace doesn't knock them out," she explains. "It allows you to turn inward and be kind to yourself for a change. Practicing meditation is like taking a vacation once or twice a day. When you nurture yourself, you accrue a tremendous spin-off of benefits."

Take PMS, for example. Your body's response to high stress levels can worsen symptoms of PMS because stress can cause the muscle tension associated with PMS complaints such as fatigue, soreness and aching.

"When you meditate regularly, you dramatically reduce your body's response to stress, and that can ease the discomfort associated with PMS," Dr. Carrington explains. But she cautions that you not make the mistake of thinking that you can meditate PMS away in a session or two. You will probably need to meditate regularly for several months before your body responds positively.

Meditation can also improve irritable bowel syndrome, ulcers, high blood pressure and insomnia, among other stress-related conditions, says Dr. Carrington. "Eighty percent of the people who use meditation to relieve insomnia are successful," she adds.

Other physicians concur with Dr. Carrington. "Meditation can help prevent or treat stress-related complaints such as anxiety, headaches and bone, muscle and joint problems," says Adriane Fugh-Berman, M.D., former head of field investigations for the Office of Alternative Medicine at the National Institutes of Health in Bethesda, Maryland. "Meditation also provides women with an inner sense of clarity and calm, and that in itself may help ward off certain illnesses."

According to one study, meditation may even relieve the discomfort of fibromyalgia, a condition that causes fatigue and intensely painful "trigger points." When 77 men and women with fibromyalgia followed a ten-week stress-reduction program using meditation, all reported that their symptoms improved. And half described their improvements as "moderate to marked."

Finally, meditation frees women from tenacious preoccupation with the past and future and allows them to fully experience life's precious moments, says Daeja Napier, founder of the Insight Meditation Center and lay dharma teacher of insight meditation in suburban Boston.

"Many women tend to live in a state of perpetual motion and expectation that prevents them from appreciating the gifts that each moment gives us," says Napier. "We live life in a state of insufficiency, waiting for a mother to love us, for a father to be kind to us, for the perfect job or home, for Prince Charming to come along or to become a perfect person. It's a mythology that keeps us from being whole.

"Meditation is a humble process that gently returns us to the now of our lives and allows us to wake up and re-evaluate the way that we live our lives," says Napier. "We realize that the only thing missing is mindfulness, and that's what we practice."

MINDFULNESS: BEING PRESENT BRINGS PEACE

Mindfulness means fully experiencing what happens in the here and now. Mindfulness meditation is the art of focusing our minds on what's happening in and around us at this very moment.

Practitioners are taught to concentrate on their breathing and its passage through the body as they dismiss any distracting thoughts. Though it sounds simple, mindfulness takes practice, and the longer you practice, the easier the process becomes, according to Napier. "Breathing is the vehicle of transition from our conventional, anxiety-ridden, goal-oriented experience of stressful living into a natural state of functional calm and tranquillity."

Unlike other forms of meditation, mindfulness (also called insight) meditation works simply by focusing on your breathing, without using added words, images or sounds, says Napier. "Mindfulness teaches you to work with, rather than against, change in order to establish mental and physical calm."

Settle into awareness. Those who teach meditation say that it's helpful to begin the day with the kind of awareness exercise described at the beginning of this chapter, even before you get out of bed, says Napier. Use sights, sounds and senses to tune in to your body. Then, you're ready to begin meditating.

Find a meditation corner. "Set aside a special place that you can go to each day—a place where you are comfortable and where you're least likely to be interrupted as you meditate," says Napier. "Mark it with something simple like a cushion and a flower. A corner of your bedroom is often a good place to meditate."

Get comfy. Assume your most comfortable seated position, either on the floor with your back supported or in a chair. If you like, lean against a wall, using a cushion for added support.

Just breathe. At first, concentrate on the physical act of breathing, without trying to control or change your normal breathing pattern.

Dismiss distractions. If you get distracted by passing thoughts (and you will, especially in the beginning), avoid delving into them. Tell yourself that you'll deal with them later. Return to concentrating on breathing.

JOURNEY MEDITATION: TAKE A PEACEFUL MIND TRIP

Journey meditation combines imagery and visualization to achieve a meditative state. This form of meditation appeals to women who find peace by picturing themselves in a peaceful place, says Eileen F. Oster, registered occupational therapist and meditation instructor from Bayside, New York, and author of *The Healing Mind: Your Guide to the Power of Meditation, Prayer and Reflection.*

GettingStarted

Meditation

More and more doctors are prescribing meditation as a way to lower blood pressure, improve exercise performance in people with angina, help people with asthma breathe easier, relieve insomnia and generally relax the everyday stresses of life. It's easy to learn on your own. If you prefer formal instruction, here's how to pursue guidance.

Number of practitioners in the United States: Unknown.

Qualifications to look for: Psychologists with a Ph.D. and registered occupational therapists (O.T.R.) often use meditation and can offer you guidance in learning to meditate. Some clinical social workers (C.S.W.) can teach meditation as well. Otherwise, accreditations and standards for meditation training don't exist.

Professional associations: None.

To find a practitioner: To locate a psychologist trained in meditation, contact the Association for Transpersonal Psychology, P.O. Box 3049, Stanford, CA 94309. For a schedule of insight meditation retreats, contact the Spirit Rock Center, P.O. Box 909, Woodacre, CA 94973. To locate a journey meditation or movement meditation practitioner, contact Eileen F. Oster, O.T.R., P.O. Box 136, Woodmere, NY 11598.

Approximate cost: Psychologists or clinical social workers who teach meditation charge $100 to $200 per session—comparable to their normal session fees.

Here's how to begin.

Sit up straight. Get into a comfortable position. Either sit on the floor with your back against a wall, or sit in a chair with your feet on the ground and your hands resting on your knees or thighs. Have a pad and pencil nearby. Write down the worries, concerns or problems that you're afraid will distract you from meditation, and promise yourself that you'll deal with them when you're done.

Take a few cleansing breaths. Breathe in slowly and deeply for five counts, then exhale slowly for five counts.

Find a peaceful place. Close your eyes and concentrate on a soothing, tranquil place where you feel safe and calm. As distractions flutter through your mind, remind yourself that you'll deal with them when you are finished meditating.

A quiet beach is an ideal mental destination for many women, says Oster. Picture yourself resting on the sand. Feel the sun on your skin, hear the water lapping the shore, listen for the sounds of seagulls or see the ships gliding out to sea. You can use the same routine for any beautiful, serene place that calms you, says Oster.

Do it twice a day. You don't need to spends hours meditating, says Oster. "Most women will benefit from a 5- to 15-minute meditation practiced several days a week. A good rule of thumb for practicing journey meditation is to do it in the morning and then again later in the day. A peaceful meditative journey as you wake can improve the whole tone of your day," she adds.

Journey meditation is also an excellent antidote for afternoon slump, according to Oster. "If you can't take a nap at 3:00 P.M. when your energy suddenly ebbs, try taking a short journey break. In as little as ten minutes, you'll find that you've recharged your battery."

VIBRATIONAL MEDITATION: MAKING A JOYFUL NOISE

Also called sounding meditation, this technique uses the repetition of a word or sound as its focal point. Vibrational meditation appeals to women who find that making noise is a path to inner quiet, says Oster.

"We're taught to be nice and quiet as little girls—ladies aren't loud. Releasing sound and noise helps us release stress," says Oster. So it's especially beneficial to women.

Here's how to begin.

Get on your feet. Stand with your feet shoulder-width apart, your knees slightly bent and your hips centered, as though you're about to squat. Or, if you wish, sit or lie down. Keep your body loose and comfortable with your arms at your sides or on your hips. Begin by taking a few cleansing breaths.

Pick a word, any word. Choose a word that alternates vowels and consonants—like "serenity." The word that you select doesn't necessarily have to be a spiritual one, adds Oster. It just has to feel good when you say it.

Repeat after yourself. Repeat the word, chant the word, focus on nothing but saying the word over and over again. "Let the sound of the word vibrate through your body. Let the word resonate up from your abdomen and let it go to your hands, your feet. Let your muscles move as you chant the word," says Oster.

"Women have a tendency to clench their muscles when they're tense," she observes. "It's important to roll the sound through your body so that you can clear out the tightness in your muscles. Doing so promotes the meditative state of relaxation that feels like a natural high."

MOVEMENT MEDITATION: WALK, DANCE AND SHAKE OFF TENSION

Like the Eastern discipline of yoga, movement meditation combines breathing and gentle, flowing movements to create a meditative state. It appeals to women who tend to achieve a meditative state of mind by moving their bodies, says Oster.

"Movement meditation allows a woman to draw in *qi* energy from the Earth, which many healers—such as acupuncturists, acupressurists and some massage therapists—regard as the essential life force," says Oster. Qi, pronounced *chee* in Chinese and *kee* in Japanese, is energy that moves along meridians, or paths, throughout the body. It is an essential concept in Traditional Chinese Medicine and other Eastern healing techniques.

"Movement meditation is excellent to do first thing in the morning and can also be a prelude to prayer or another form of meditation," says Oster.

Here's how Oster recommends you practice movement meditation.

Center and concentrate. Take several deep, cleansing breaths. Then, move into a relaxed, squatting stance with your knees slightly bent and your hips and pelvis loose. Center yourself by visualizing your feet connected to the soil. Visualize the center of the Earth, from which we draw female energy, says Oster. Concentrate upon and honor the Earth.

Focus your awareness. Gently move your body in an undulating, snakelike swaying motion. See yourself as a flower opening up or as an animal moving through the brush. Dance, if you like.

If it pleases you, use sound or music to focus your attention on the movement and on the vibration. Allow yourself to get lost in the sense of movement and the beauty of your body as it moves. Feel the areas of your body that are tight and let the movement loosen them up.

MUSIC THERAPY
Orchestrating Good Health

Have a tension headache? You might try listening to a couple of Chopin nocturnes. Can't sleep? Some Sinatra may help. Got the blues? Then the blues, followed by some cool jazz and a bit of Bach, may be just the remedy.

For centuries, philosophers and poets have celebrated the healing power of music. Now, researchers are jumping on the bandwagon.

Increasingly, studies are finding that music offers wide-ranging therapeutic benefits. A serenade, it seems, can not only help alleviate stress, insomnia and depression but it can also improve concentration and memory, boost immunity and ease pain—even labor pain.

You may not be aware of it, but music appears to trigger a variety of physical changes, altering skin temperature, brain-wave patterns and levels of stress hormones in the bloodstream. Music also changes your breathing rate, heart rate and blood pressure.

"What we're realizing is that music and sound can be used as a tool for healing and well-being," says Don Campbell, a classically trained musician who is founder of the Institute for Music, Health and Education in Minneapolis and author of *The Mozart Effect* and *Music: Physician for Times to Come*.

Some hospitals already pipe music into rooms to help people relax and manage pain. But you don't have to be bedridden to enjoy the benefit of your favorite Bach or Beatles.

NOTEWORTHY RESULTS

The heroine of Jane Campion's film *The Piano* relies on music to lift her spirits, overcome loneliness and fear, and express joy and longing. She is, it happens, a gifted pianist. But talent isn't required, says Barbara J. Crowe, a registered music therapist and director and professor of music therapy at Arizona State University in Tempe.

In fact, most of the research into music's therapeutic effects has looked at a cross section of ordinary women. And the studies have shown that music brings many rewards.

One study used music in combination with imagery and breathing techniques to ease the pain of childbirth. A group of expectant mothers listened to music during labor. Each heard music for ten minutes, then went without for five, listened for the next ten, and so forth. When the music came on, the women breathed rhythmically and deeply or envisioned calming images, using techniques they'd practiced in advance.

"Every woman had fewer pain responses while listening to music," says study coordinator Suzanne Hanser, Ed.D., chairperson of the music therapy department at Berklee College of Music in Boston. The music, it seems, helped by both distracting and relaxing the women, she says.

Research suggests that stress can raise the risk of heart disease, weaken immunity, contribute to depression and anxiety and interfere with sleep, concentration and recall. By taking the edge off stress, music may stall these harmful effects—and might even reverse them.

Researchers at Stanford University studying depressed older adults found that those who used relaxation techniques while listening to music felt less depressed than those who didn't learn the techniques.

A University of Illinois study concluded that office workers who listened to music while performing moderately complex tasks were more relaxed, satisfied and productive than colleagues who toiled in silence.

You'll get even more than stress reduction from a close encounter with specific kinds of music, research shows. In a study at the University of California at Irvine, psychologists found that students who heard ten minutes of a Mozart piano sonata scored higher on a test of spatial intelligence than those who sat in silence or listened to instructions. But the researchers found no improvement in mental skills among students who listened to a hypnotic composition by Philip Glass or a highly rhythmic dance piece. It's possible that a complex musical composition, like a Mozart piano sonata, stimulates neural pathways that are important in certain essential mental skills, the researchers speculate.

A MUSIC THERAPY SESSION

Of course, music affects us emotionally and mentally as well as physiologically. It can move us to tears—of joy or of sorrow. Consequently, it's a powerful tool in psychotherapy.

"People have such a strong response to music," says Crowe. "Music therapy can be part of comprehensive treatment of depression or anxiety," she says. For treatment of these and other emotional disorders, music therapists may team up with therapists who specialize in other creative arts as well as psychologists and psychiatrists.

In an initial session with a music therapist, the two of you might discuss your goals and your musical preferences and abilities. What would follow would depend on what you hoped to accomplish. A therapist might ask you to try lyric analysis, for example. The two of you would discuss the lyrics to a song to explore your feelings, experiences and beliefs.

The results can be dramatic. Dr. Hanser recalls one woman who'd sat through a number of group therapy sessions without saying much, then burst into tears one day while the group listened to the Simon and Garfunkel ballad, "Bridge Over Troubled Water."

"She began to talk about her loneliness, of not having a bridge or a goal or something on the other side," says Dr. Hanser. "For her, the metaphor was so powerful that it led to tremendous insight."

PLAYING TO YOUR HEART'S CONTENT

A therapist might also encourage you to make music—to improvise vocally or with instruments in the therapy room. The idea isn't to play beautiful sonatas, but to play what you feel. If you're depressed because you

Getting**Started**

Music Therapy

Music therapy is a practice that is growing in the United States, with registered and certified music therapists paving the way. Here's who to consult, should you wish to give music therapy a try.

Number of practitioners in the United States: Approximately 6,000.

Qualifications to look for: Registered Music Therapist (R.M.T.) or a Certified Music Therapist (C.M.T.). Both require at least an undergraduate degree in music therapy from an approved program, completion of a clinical internship and board certification.

Professional associations: National Association for Music Therapy, 8455 Colesville Road, Suite 930, Silver Spring, MD 20910; American Association for Music Therapy, 1 Station Plaza, Ossining, NY 10562.

To find a practitioner: Contact the professional associations listed above.

Approximate cost: $35 to $50 per session.

habitually repress your anger, you may end up yelling and wailing or banging away on the lowest octaves on the piano. Not splendid music—but the expression of feeling is all for the better.

"Music therapy can really help people who aren't able to articulate all the things they're feeling and experiencing," says Dr. Hanser.

Once issues and feelings are out in the open, you and the therapist might explore these feelings further, and explore different ways of working with them, Crowe says. You might write a song together or do more improvisational music-making. The idea is to experience the feelings and different ways of dealing with them, rather than simply talk about them.

The woman who responded so strongly to "Bridge Over Troubled Water" went on to explore her feelings and options with more improvisational playing, Dr. Hanser adds.

"We created this bridge with the music we made," she explains. "The melody was about what it would feel like if she got to the other side, where hope is. While we were playing and chanting and singing, she didn't need to know or identify precisely what was on the other side—what her goal was. But by playing, she could sense that there was an option other than what she'd experienced in the past. She could feel there was hope, and actually express it by making sound that was hopeful. The fact that she could really experience this optimism gave her the confidence that eventually enabled her to articulate what she wanted and what she could do to get it."

GOING SOLO

With a few pointers, you can learn to use music to relax. You can also use it to be more productive, to feel better, to get to sleep or—if you put on that lively samba music—to get going during a workout.

The key, Campbell says, is selecting appropriate music.

If you're looking for some gentle strains to help you get to sleep, a slow, quiet Sinatra piece is more likely to get you there than Guns N' Roses. But maybe not. The same piece of music can have very different effects on different listeners, says Crowe.

"I'm leery when people claim that one type of music always has that type of effect," Crowe says. "Human interaction with sound is so complex; to prescribe like that is to misunderstand the complexity."

To find the right music, then, you have to experiment. Here's what the experts suggest.

Start with what you like. This advice may seem obvious, but music you don't like can make you feel more stressed out or irritated, says Crowe.

Put it to the test. Before you begin listening to a selection, check your pulse and note your breathing rate, says Campbell. Note whether your muscles are tense or relaxed and evaluate your mood. Are your thoughts louder than your feelings? Then listen to the music for 20 minutes, allowing your body to respond. Lie down, loosen up, dance, hum, clap—do whatever the music moves you to do and let the music release the stress from your body. Then check your pulse, breathing, muscle tension and mood again. In a notebook, jot down the name of the selection, and your feelings. Once you've made a few entries, use the information to help you use music to relax and change your mood.

Work with your mood, not against it. If you're sad and play happy music, it can make you feel worse, because it can seem an impossible standard to reach, says Crowe. "You need to make the change gradually," she explains. "So start with a piece matching your mood, then gradually change the music. If you start with the music that's a little sad, then begin to change the music, you can change your mood, too."

Ditto if you're trying to calm down and go to sleep. Start with music that matches your energy level and gradually shift to music that's slower and more subdued, Dr. Hanser says.

Tune in. Listen to sounds and feel vibrations in your own body, says Campbell.

Try humming. If you find yourself easily distracted or very stressed, says Campbell, try humming. "When you hum," Campbell says, "you're massaging your body from the inside out."

NATUROPATHY
Mix-and-Match Healing

In one room a woman with lower-back pain soaks contentedly in a whirlpool bath. In the next a doctor gives a neck massage to a woman with recurring migraines. Down the hall a grandmother complaining of chronic fatigue lies on a table, with a row of slender acupuncture needles in her back. Meanwhile, in the Chinese apothecary, a doctor concocts an aromatic herbal remedy for a woman with endometriosis.

At the naturopathic clinic at Bastyr University in Seattle, an array of natural therapies comes under one roof. It's the naturopathic way. Naturopathy, also called naturopathic medicine, incorporates a wide range of alternative treatments—Ayurvedic medicine (a traditional form of Indian healing), botanical medicine, exercise therapy, homeopathy, hydrotherapy, manipulation, massage, meditation, nutritional therapy and Traditional Chinese Medicine. Doctors of naturopathy mix and match different treatments, customizing therapy for each individual woman and her particular health condition.

Suffering from premenstrual syndrome? After taking you through a detailed interview and exam, a doctor of naturopathy (N.D.) may prescribe a high-fiber, whole-foods diet along with nutritional supplements, herbs and hydrotherapy. To prevent other health problems, she also might recommend meditation plus an exercise regimen.

The way naturopaths see it, their job is to teach you how to *stay* healthy. Should you fall, they're there to bolster your body's defenses with the best that natural medicine has to offer.

"The conventional medical approach is basically: Kill disease, kill disease, kill disease," explains Joseph Pizzorno, Jr., N.D., founding president of Bastyr University of Naturopathic Medicine.

"The natural medicine approach is to help the person live healthier. While we may use therapies that have a direct impact on disease, we're much more interested in utilizing therapies that help support the body's natural healing processes, rather than those that take over the healing process of the body."

COMPLEMENTS CONVENTIONAL MEDICINE

Naturopathy is an eclectic mix of therapies that traces its origins back more than a century to a time when conventional doctors doused their patients with heavy metals and were as apt to bleed them to death as save them. Gentler naturopathic alternatives like homeopathy and hydrotherapy won plenty of converts but lost them to conventional medicine when research led to improved surgical treatments and drug therapy.

Now, after decades on the sidelines, naturopathy is once more gaining ground. Bastyr's enrollment, for example, rose from 30 students in 1978, its first year, to 1,000 in 1996, nearly 20 years later. In 1994, Bastyr beat out Harvard and Columbia University, in New York City, for a hefty federal grant to study AIDS treatment. Not long after, the nation's third accredited school of naturopathic medicine, the Southwest College of Naturopathic Medicine, opened its doors in Scottsdale, Arizona. And in 1995, King County council officials in Washington voted to establish a government-subsidized naturopathic clinic in the greater Seattle area.

Dr. Pizzorno credits the growth of naturopathy to several factors. "To an extent, conventional medicine has reached the limits of what it can do by simply treating disease. Secondly, there's this growing awareness that you have to treat your body properly if you want to stay healthy, and people are looking for doctors who can teach them how. And finally, natural medicine makes a lot of sense."

Naturopaths don't reject conventional medicine out of hand. For acute health problems such as pneumonia and life-threatening illness such as cancer, conventional medicine is still your best bet, says Dr. Pizzorno. N.D.'s, who use blood, urine and other standard medical tests in diagnosis, will refer patients with such problems to M.D.'s. But naturopathic medicine is the ticket for chronic or less severe conditions that aren't life-threatening, he says.

Unfortunately, there aren't any scientific studies comparing naturopathy with conventional care. Even the best of researchers would be hard-pressed to design such a study: Naturopathy includes so many therapies, that controlling all the variables would be virtually impossible.

But studies have taken a look at individual therapies (like acupuncture, for example) for specific health problems. Results have been favorable. Sometimes they even got better results than conventional medical treatments, according to Dr. Pizzorno. Many herbal therapies have been extensively researched in Europe, he notes.

"I went to an M.D. first," says Ruth, a 26-year-old undergoing treatment at the Bastyr clinic. Diagnosed with Bell's palsy, a neurological disorder that causes partial facial paralysis, Ruth took her M.D.'s advice and took prednisone, a powerful steroid used to reduce inflammation. But her symptoms got worse.

"It got to the point that my vision and speech were affected. I really couldn't live a normal life," she says, looking quite comfortable, despite the acupuncture needles jutting out above her eyebrows and wrists. "Acupuncture helped right away. I wish I had tried it from the start."

Naturopathic Prescriptions for Good Health

The following is a roundup of advice culled from leading naturopaths—simple changes that they say can help any woman stay healthier, the naturopathic way.

Joseph Pizzorno, Jr., N.D., founding president of Bastyr University of Naturopathic Medicine in Seattle:

- Eat a high-fiber diet, focused on whole grains, beans, fruits and vegetables.
- Avoid refined foods, such as pastries and snack foods.
- Exercise at least four times a week for half an hour at a time.
- Do something to reduce stress every day—meditate, listen to relaxation audiotapes or take a nap, for example.

Mark Nolting, N.D., licensed acupuncturist and associate professor and chairman of the Department of Acupuncture and Oriental Medicine at Bastyr University:

- Take a class in traditional Chinese exercises and breathing techniques, such as qi gong (chi gung) or tai chi.
- Learn an Eastern self-healing technique, such as acupressure.
- Eat foods that are in season, in keeping with the tenets of Traditional Chinese Medicine.

Suzzanne Myer, R.D., assistant professor and director of dietetics at Bastyr University:

- Eat five to eight servings of fruits and vegetables daily.
- Include in your diet some green leafy vegetables, such as spinach, romaine lettuce or kale.
- Whenever possible, buy local, organically grown produce.

Alan Gaby, M.D., professor of therapeutic nutrition at Bastyr University:

- Eat more whole grains, nuts and seeds.
- Eat fewer refined foods, less sugar and less white flour.

MAKING THE MOST OF MANY OPTIONS

In naturopathic medical school, students study the basic sciences—anatomy, physiology, biochemistry, neurology, pathology and diagnostic techniques. In addition, they take courses in homeopathy, therapeutic nutrition, hydrotherapy, botanical medicine, spinal manipulation and other

- Drink adequate amounts of water—four to six glasses per day—preferably filtered, bottled water since chlorinated tap water is potentially harmful.

Douglas Lewis, N.D., faculty member of the physical medicine department at Bastyr University:

- To keep your muscles supple, stretch gently, especially after exercising and lifting weights.
- Learn yoga and practice a few yoga routines daily.
- Get incidental exercise—by parking your car far from your destination, for example, and taking the stairs instead of the elevator.

Mark Groven, N.D., physical medicine supervisor at Bastyr University Natural Health Clinic:

- When you shower, turn the water from warm to cold during the last 30 seconds. The change seems to improve circulation and stimulate the immune system.
- To strengthen your bones and avoid osteoporosis, take a class in weight training, or get a trainer to teach you the ropes.
- Buy supportive shoes. Look for a quality arch and a low to medium heel. Lace shoes are preferable. The more laces, the better.
- Adjust your work station. Look for a chair with arm rests and low-back support. Raise or lower your chair so that when you're seated, your thighs are horizontal and your feet are flat on the floor. If you work at a computer, adjust the monitor so that the screen is at eye level.
- Don't pile up your bed pillows. Sleeping on a high stack of pillows can cause neck and back pain. When you're lying down, your neck should form a straight line with the rest of your spine.

therapeutic modalities rarely taught in conventional medical schools.

One of the big advantages of the naturopathic approach, N.D.'s say, is that it offers so many options. To treat chronic muscle tension—a common cause of chronic pain—an N.D. might use spinal manipulation and massage, says Douglas Lewis, N.D., a faculty member of the physical medicine department at Bastyr University. But a naturopath might also prescribe hydrotherapy, at-home exercise routines and calcium and magnesium supplements. "The two minerals work as a wonderful muscle relaxer," he says.

After a woman that Dr. Lewis was treating injured her back and neck in a car accident, he recalls, the muscles surrounding the injured area tensed up, pinching nerves, cutting off circulation and causing pain that radiated out to her shoulder. He used manipulation and massage to ease the tension, prescribed supplements to relax the muscles and recommended at-home exercises. The combination of treatments worked better than any single natural remedy would have worked alone, he notes.

Natural remedies often work best in combination, as they support the body's own healing mechanisms and have a combined therapeutic effect, says Dr. Lewis. They tend to be gentler than prescription drugs and other conventional remedies, say practitioners.

"If I'm treating someone with, say, recurring sinusitis, I'll frequently recommend both dietary changes and herbal prescriptions," says Lisa Meserole, N.D., research consultant and faculty member in the botanical medicine department at Bastyr University.

It makes sense to combine food therapy with herbal remedies in cases like these, she says. Chronic recurrent sinusitis is often associated with a food or airborne allergy. According to Dr. Meserole, those with chronic sinusitis who normally consume a diet rich in dairy often improve when they eliminate dairy products. The residues in dairy foods seem to increase mucus production in susceptible individuals, she says. Combining dietary changes with the appropriate herbal tonics, she gets better results than she would if she prescribed either therapy singly.

"I'm not saying that herbs can't sometimes work alone," says Dr. Meserole, whose office bookshelves are stacked with botanical texts and jars containing plant samples. "But because they tend to be gentler and weaker than pharmaceutical drugs, herbs work better when combined with a holistic health program that is tailored to the individual."

THE GENTLER ROUTE

Depending on the state, some licensed N.D.'s can prescribe certain pharmaceutical drugs. But most prefer not to. They favor natural remedies, like herbs, precisely because the remedies are gentle and won't overwhelm the body's efforts at self-healing.

From the naturopathic perspective, symptoms are signs that the body is trying to heal itself. A rash, for instance, is a sign that the body is trying to protect itself from an irritant. Rather than override the body's attempts at healing—as when a person treats the rash by applying an anti-inflammatory cream—naturopathy aims to gently enhance the body's healing efforts.

A doctor of naturopathy might do this by prescribing a homeopathic remedy—in this case, an extremely dilute solution of a substance that would cause a rash in a healthy person. The theory behind homeopathy is that, by magnifying symptoms, the remedy will prompt the body to magnify its healing response. Again, the idea is to work with the body's healing efforts.

It seems to work.

"One woman that I treated had severe morning sickness, but her diet was fine, so I decided to prescribe a homeopathic remedy," recalls Pamela Snider, N.D., associate dean of the naturopathic medicine program at

Getting**Started**

Naturopathy

While naturopathic physicians aren't as numerous as osteopaths or chiropractors, their numbers are growing.

To find a naturopathic physician in your area, follow the guidelines listed below.

Number of practitioners in the United States: Approximately 400.

Qualifications to look for: Doctor of Naturopathy (N.D.) degree from an accredited naturopathic medical school—Bastyr University of Naturopathic Medicine in Seattle or the National College of Naturopathic Medicine in Portland, Oregon.

Professional associations: American Association of Naturopathic Physicians (AANP), 2366 East Lake Avenue, Suite 322, Seattle, WA 98102.

To find a practitioner: A directory of naturopaths is available for $5 from the AANP at the address listed above.

Approximate cost: $30 to $175 for an initial consultation. Follow-up visits usually cost less.

Bastyr University. The remedy—an extremely dilute solution of a substance that, in a nondiluted form, would have made a healthy woman queasy—did the trick. "Within two days, her morning sickness completely cleared up," says Dr. Snider.

SHARED PHILOSOPHY

Disparate as they are, all naturopathic treatments share this same philosophy: Help the body heal itself.

Sometimes a dietary and lifestyle change, possibly accompanied by an herbal tonic and a massage, are all the help that the body needs. Other times, a combination of vitamin and mineral therapy and hydrotherapy offers a sufficient boost.

"Some people need nutritional intervention, some need herbs, some need fasting and some need to be referred to an acupuncturist," says Dr. Snider. "We use the least-force approach, the one with the most ability to work with the body's inherent healing process."

AT-HOME FOLLOW UP

Naturopathic physicians offer a wide variety of therapies, but they ask their patients to do part of the job. Naturopathic "prescriptions" often include homework—exercises, dietary changes and stress-reduction programs that you have to follow through with at home.

To treat a woman with chronic migraines, for example, Dr. Lewis says that he may use massage and manipulation in the office and recommend both hydrotherapy and neck exercises for her to do at home.

For chronic constipation, Mark Groven, N.D., physical medicine supervisor at Bastyr University Natural Health Clinic, may recommend colon hydrotherapy—a type of enema that cleans your intestines—and herbal remedies, then suggest dietary changes and at-home exercise.

In addition to recommendations aimed at alleviating existing health problems, naturopathic physicians make recommendations aimed at preventing problems in the first place.

OSTEOPATHY
Manipulation Is Good Medicine

Many of Joyce Frye's patients don't realize she's not an M.D.—until she gets her hands on them.

Dr. Frye's staff calls her doctor. Her office is decked out with the usual medical equipment. Impressive-looking diplomas and licenses hang on the walls. "I suppose many of the people coming to see me for the first time don't know that I'm a D.O. rather than an M.D.—not that I make any attempt to hide it," says Dr. Frye, obstetrician/gynecologist and chairperson of the Gynecology Department at Presbyterian Medical Center as well as a clinical faculty member at Jefferson Medical College, both in Philadelphia.

Doctors of osteopathic medicine, D.O.'s, are fully qualified physicians. Like M.D.'s, they finish four years of medical school (at osteopathic medical colleges), complete residencies and take certifying exams. Like M.D.'s, they order x-rays, blood and other diagnostic tests, prescribe drugs and perform surgery. As a patient, you'd be hard-pressed to tell a D.O. from an M.D.

But there is a difference. D.O.'s have one tool at their disposal that most M.D.'s don't: hands-on osteopathic manipulation. Though all D.O.'s learn to manipulate bone, muscles and connective tissue, not all use manipulation after graduation. There was a time when osteopathic manipulation—something akin to chiropractic adjustment—wasn't as popular among D.O.'s. The demand, however, for alternatives to conventional medicine has reawakened interest in manipulation. By including it in a comprehensive treatment regimen, D.O.'s say manipulation is an effective complement to more mainstream therapies.

D.O.'s use manipulation to both diagnose and treat. Studies show that it can relieve back and neck pain and menstrual cramps. There's some evidence that manipulative techniques, alone or in combination with other therapies, can ease labor pain and delivery, relieve respiratory problems, soothe migraines and lower blood pressure. Osteopaths also use it to help relieve a wide array of other health problems, including premenstrual syndrome, pelvic pain, digestive trouble, ulcers, temporomandibular disorder, colds, sinus infections, carpal tunnel syndrome and fibromyalgia.

"There's a whole flock of benefits," says Robert C. Ward, D.O., professor of biomechanics and family medicine at Michigan State University College of Osteopathic Medicine in East Lansing.

Manipulation is a real boon to women during pregnancy. "During pregnancy, they can't take a lot of medication," explains Dr. Frye, who uses manipulation to treat expectant moms with sciatica, migraines, labor pain, joint pain and carpal tunnel syndrome. Before manipulating a new patient, she makes sure that the patient understands what manipulation and osteopathy are all about, she adds.

HISTORY AND PHILOSOPHY

Osteopathic medicine differs from conventional care in philosophy as well as practice. It was the inspiration of a nineteenth-century M.D. named Andrew Taylor Still. Disillusioned by traditional practice after two of his children died of spinal meningitis (despite state-of-the-art care), Dr. Still concluded that conventional medicine was missing something. The problem, he reasoned, was that it failed to recognize that health is as dependent on the soundness of the body's muscle and skeletal systems as it is on the body's vital organs.

Dr. Still went on to pioneer various manipulative techniques to correct musculoskeletal problems. And, on the heels of an unsuccessful attempt to convince mainstream medical schools to change their curricula, he

Getting**Started**

Osteopathic Medicine

In some regions, osteopathic physicians are nearly as common as M.D.'s. To find an osteopathic physician in your area, follow these guidelines.

Number of practitioners in the United States: Approximately 40,000.

Qualifications to look for: Doctor of Osteopathy (D.O.) degree.

Professional associations: American Osteopathic Association, 142 East Ontario Street, Chicago, IL 60611.

To find a practitioner: Contact the American Osteopathic Association (above) or the American Academy of Osteopathy, P.O. Box 750, Newark, OH 43050.

Approximate cost: $55 to $95 per session.

opened the first osteopathic medical school in 1892. There are now 19 schools of osteopathy—from the Greek "osteo" or bone, and "pathy" meaning disease—in the United States alone. M.D.'s still outnumber D.O.'s—only 6 percent of physicians are osteopaths—but the popularity and ranks of osteopaths are growing.

HANDS-ON EXPERIENCE

At the Philadelphia College of Osteopathic Medicine, the nation's largest school of osteopathy, a group of first-year students is learning how to manipulate muscles, connective tissue, joints and bones.

While one student lies facedown on an examination table, her partner presses on her back, just above her sacroiliac joint (the joint between the tailbone and hipbone), then bends her leg at the knee and rocks the leg back and forth. With this technique, an osteopath can test the sacroiliac joint's range of motion. The results can be particularly helpful in diagnosing the source of low-back pain, since limited flexibility of the joint is often the culprit, says Alex Nicholas, D.O., who leads the class.

Using a variety of techniques, a D.O. can detect not only abnormalities in range of motion but also uncover structural irregularities and changes in tissue texture and tenderness, which are additional diagnostic clues.

Dr. Nicholas asks his students how they would treat a patient who has limited sacroiliac joint mobility. Two students demonstrate. While one lies on her side on the examination table, her partner presses her upper leg down toward the floor, while rotating her pelvis out toward the wall, guiding the joint through the full range of motion.

In addition to improving mobility, Dr. Nicholas says, manipulation eases muscle tension and helps correct structural misalignments caused by injury, stress, poor posture or lack of exercise.

The osteopathic manipulative techniques that D.O.'s use are usually gentle and well-tolerated. A number of them resemble techniques that chiropractors use. But osteopathic manipulation has a different focus.

"Chiropractic concentrates more on the alignment of the bones," says William R. Loomis, D.O., an osteopathic physician in Spokane, Washington, and former president of the American Association of Orthopedic Medicine. "Osteopaths think that's important, but they think the soft tissues and connective tissues around the bones are extremely important."

Osteopathy focuses on the holistic concepts that emphasize the interplay among the body's many systems. The musculoskeletal system—all of it—gets as much attention as the cardiorespiratory system, the digestive system and all the rest.

"The idea is to have the musculoskeletal system working as efficiently as it can, thereby reducing the body's energy requirements, which in turn will reduce the workload on the heart and lungs," says Edward Isaacs, M.D., a Richmond, Virginia, neurologist and one of a small but growing number of medical doctors who are learning osteopathic manipulative techniques and incorporating these into their practices.

Improvements in musculoskeletal health can have all sorts of beneficial effects, practitioners say. Correcting pelvic misalignments, for example, can help alleviate severe menstrual cramps.

"The uterus doesn't just float in the abdomen; it's suspended by ligaments connecting it to the pelvic bones," explains John McPartland, D.O., an osteopathic physician in private practice in Middlebury, Vermont. "And if the pelvic bones are out of alignment, that puts pressure on the ligaments, which puts pressure on the uterus."

Since migraine headaches often start as tension headaches, Dr. McPartland says, relieving muscle tension can offer relief to browbeaten migraine sufferers.

For those with asthma, techniques that restore flexibility and strength to the chest muscles can make breathing easier. Why? If the diaphragm is more flexible, the patient can breathe more deeply, explains Dr. Ward.

For heart disease patients, the same techniques can help alleviate fluid-retention problems, since the motion of the diaphragm helps pump blood and lymphatic fluid through the body, Dr. Isaacs says.

DOMINO EFFECT

Manipulation seems to improve both circulation and nervous-system health in more subtle ways as well, easing other symptoms.

Among other things, it improves circulation by easing muscle tension. When muscles tense, they constrict both blood vessels and lymphatic channels, special vessels that channel excess fluid from tissues into the bloodstream. This limits the flow of blood and lymphatic fluid to surrounding tissues.

Because inadequate blood supply causes pain, manipulation helps relieve the pain by improving blood circulation, says Charles Steiner, D.O., adjunct professor of biomedical engineering at Rutgers University in New Brunswick, New Jersey. And because lymph helps clear dead cells and invading germs from the body, manipulation improves the body's ability to fight infection by enabling lymph to flow more freely, says Dr. Ward.

Animal studies suggest that manipulation may offer a variety of other benefits because it also has something of a calming effect on the autonomic nervous system, which governs involuntary functions like digestion, circulation and respiration. And various autonomic nerve pathways link the heart, intestines, stomach and other vital organs with the spine and brain.

Manipulating the section of the neck or back where the nerves to a particular organ join the spine seems to calm both the nerves and the organ they control, says Dr. Loomis. Consequently, manipulating the spot just beneath the shoulder blades, where the nerves controlling the dilation of blood vessels join the spine, seems to relax the nerves, thereby relaxing the muscles of the blood vessel walls and lowering blood pressure.

THE SCIENTIFIC EVIDENCE

To date, the best documented benefit of osteopathic manipulation is relief from neck and back pain.

A few scientific studies have found that manipulation helps take the edge off labor pain, speed labor and ease menstrual cramps as well. In a small-scale study, researchers at the University of Osteopathic Medicine in Des Moines, Iowa, found that manipulation performed within 12 hours of the start of menstruation relieved cramps and accompanying back pain for the duration of that period.

Other studies have found that manipulation can also help lower high blood pressure, alleviate breathing problems and decrease frequency of heart rhythm abnormalities. But studies examining manipulation's success in treating specific health problems are few and far between, says Philip Greenman, D.O., associate dean and professor in the Department of Osteopathic Manipulative Medicine at Michigan State University College of Osteopathic Medicine in East Lansing. And with good reason. Osteopathy has long taken a holistic view—focusing on overall health promotion rather than treatment of specific diseases and viewing manipulation as one element of a multi-therapy approach to care.

"It's this difference in philosophy that separates osteopathic medicine from mainstream orthodox medicine, and it's in this context that the profession uses manipulation," says Dr. Greenman. "Manipulation is not viewed as something good for a specific disease but as something good for promoting overall health. And most scientific studies look at the effects on this or that particular disease."

IF YOU GO

If you decide to see a D.O., remember that manipulation is just one of the tools that she'll use to diagnose and treat. In coordination with medical treatment, she may recommend changes in diet and exercise habits, prescribe at-home stretching and strengthening exercises and offer advice on dealing with stress.

She may also prescribe drugs or recommend surgery. By including manipulation in treatment, though, your D.O. may be able to lower the dose of medication that you're taking.

Unfortunately, manipulation seems to work better for some people than for others. Try three to five treatments before deciding whether it's helping you, suggests Dr. Loomis.

If it is, the frequency with which you'll need to schedule sessions will depend on what's ailing you. Some conditions clear up after just a couple of treatments. Others require follow-up sessions every month or two.

REFLEXOLOGY
Relaxation for Body and Mind

One of the fastest growing offshoots in the complementary health field, reflexology uses nothing more than strategically placed finger pressure, usually on the hands or feet, to reduce stress and stress-related health problems.

Under stress, humans instinctively practice reflexology, says Bill Flocco, reflexologist and director of the American Academy of Reflexology in Burbank, California. Mothers wring their hands the first time their teenagers drive the family car. And many of us find ourselves rubbing our feet at the end of a long, hard day at work or pulling on our ears as we ponder a sticky problem.

The technique, reflexologists say, relieves tension, improves circulation and enhances nerve function. While some practitioners work solely with the feet and hands, others include the ears as well.

Reflexologists see the feet and hands as a mirror of the body. Certain areas on each foot and hand, they say, are linked to all body parts. The right foot corresponds to the right side of the body and the left foot corresponds to the left side of the body. Theoretically, the big toe relates to the head, including the brain; the sole of the foot relates to all parts of the body, including organs and glands; and the heel area relates to the pelvic area, including the bladder, reproductive organs and sciatic nerve. By working the appropriate areas of the feet or hands, practitioners say that you stimulate a reflex response that affects the corresponding areas of the body.

And that, Flocco says, is why Academy Award winners so often pull their earlobes before accepting their Oscars and launching into their acceptance speeches. The earlobe corresponds to the head and brain, he says. Pulling it helps clear the mind. Similarly, during court trials, defendants wring their hands on the stand because the palm supposedly represents the diaphragm, spine and internal organs and stimulating that area can relieve abdominal tension. Ditto for the sole of each foot, which allegedly explains why we instinctively rub our feet after grueling days at the grindstone.

Reflexology Zones

Reflexologists believe that your body is divided into energy zones and that every tendon, ligament, organ, muscle, bone and brain cell falls within these zones. Each area on the soles of your feet corresponds with parts of your body, so gentle pressure applied to these spots, shown here, can relieve pain and stress. Because of individual differences, some practitioners suggest that you work the broader areas as well. (Some practitioners use different versions of this diagram.)

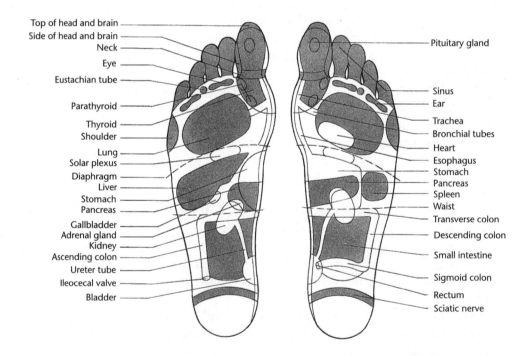

Top of head and brain
Side of head and brain
Neck
Eye
Eustachian tube
Parathyroid
Thyroid
Shoulder
Lung
Solar plexus
Diaphragm
Liver
Stomach
Pancreas
Gallbladder
Adrenal gland
Kidney
Ascending colon
Ureter tube
Ileocecal valve
Bladder

Pituitary gland
Sinus
Ear
Trachea
Bronchial tubes
Heart
Esophagus
Stomach
Pancreas
Spleen
Waist
Transverse colon
Descending colon
Small intestine
Sigmoid colon
Rectum
Sciatic nerve

GAINING GROUND

Reflexology as we know it today was developed in the mid-1930s by Eunice Ingham, a physical therapist in Rochester, New York.

The Office of Alternative Medicine for the National Institutes of Health hasn't researched reflexology. However, research that has been conducted has found reflexology to be effective against premenstrual syndrome (PMS). Researchers at the American Academy of Reflexology and the California Graduate Institute in Los Angeles randomly assigned 35 women with PMS to two groups. One group had 30 minutes of ear, foot and hand reflexology once a week for eight weeks. The other group had sham reflexology sessions—too little or too much pressure on inappropriate spots on the feet, hands and ears. While women in the first group had 46 percent fewer symptoms, women in the control group reported 19 percent fewer symptoms. Beyond that, little has been done in the way of scientific research.

Nonetheless, reflexology is thriving. "Experience tells us that it works," says Flocco, co-author of the PMS study.

The International Institute of Reflexology, a training organization for reflexology in St. Petersburg, Florida, estimates that it has trained more than 70,000 practitioners worldwide. Massage therapists, physical therapists, medical doctors, chiropractors, allopathic physicians, naturopaths, podiatrists and nurses now use or recommend reflexology for stress-related health problems such as back, shoulder and neck pain, headaches, chronic indigestion, headaches, overeating and anxiety as well as many other health problems.

"Reflexology is a very effective treatment to reduce stress," says Ray C. Wunderlich, Jr., M.D., a St. Petersburg physician who refers stressed-out men and women to reflexologists.

And Marian Small, R.N., naturopathic physician and clinical instructor of acupuncture at Bastyr University in Seattle, uses ear reflexology on women suffering pain of all sorts.

Practitioners and clients like the fact that reflexology is noninvasive—it doesn't require taking drugs or invading the body with foreign matter or materials, thus causing no side effects—and may lend itself to self-treatment. You can learn basic reflexology routines at a weekend workshop at a school of reflexology or from a book, notes Dwight Byers, president of the International Institute of Reflexology and author of *Better Health with Foot Reflexology.*

A TYPICAL SESSION

Reflexologists don't claim to treat specific illnesses. In a given session, they'll work the entire length and width of each foot or hand. But they will give extra attention to whatever part of each foot or hand corresponds to the body part that's causing you trouble.

A typical reflexology session lasts 30 to 60 minutes and clients remain clothed, though barefoot, throughout. Long-term problems may require several sessions, says Laura Norman, reflexologist in New York City and author of *Feet First: A Guide to Foot Reflexology*. And clients whose lifestyles are habitually stressful usually do best with weekly sessions, she adds.

If you're curious about how reflexology is applied, consider the following scenario: Teaching a weekend reflexology class in midtown Manhattan, Flocco demonstrates proper technique on Amelia, a student with a not-so-leisurely job for New York City's subway system.

He starts by asking her a few questions. Does she have any health problems? She says that she thinks she's pulled something and has some pain near her stomach. Does she see a doctor regularly? Eat properly? Exercise? She says that lately she hasn't been eating well. So Flocco suggests a few dietary changes, then asks her to take off her shoes and socks and hop up on a padded reflexology table that is similar to a massage table.

Flocco checks her ears, feet and hands for tender spots and discolorations. According to theory, such irregularities can be warning signs that corresponding body parts aren't working right. Flocco notes a discolored area in the upper groove of Amelia's ear and tender spots on her palm and the sole of her foot—all areas that correspond to the stomach.

After gently rubbing Amelia's ear for awhile, he starts pressing firmly with his thumbs and fingers. He covers the entire ear but gives the discolored spot extra attention. Then it's on to the other ear, the hands and, finally, the feet. When Flocco has finished, Amelia says that the pain near her stomach has faded. Extremely relaxed, she dozes off on the table.

S-O-O-O RELAXING

No wonder she fell asleep: First and foremost, practitioners attribute reflexology's successes to its stress-reducing effect.

"The primary benefit of reflexology is relieving stress and tension, which is the cause of over 75 percent of our health ills," says Byers, who is also the nephew of Eunice Ingham, founder of modern reflexology. Doctors implicate stress as a culprit in a multitude of health problems—from migraines and muscle spasms to back, shoulder and neck aches, to compulsive eating, high blood pressure, depression, anxiety and sluggish immunity.

According to Flocco, stress also interferes with the function of the nervous system, leading to a buildup of substances that irritate the nerve endings.

Reflexology may work in the same way that acupuncture and acupressure do, prompting the body to produce the neurochemicals responsible for producing feelings of well-being, relieving pain and reducing inflammation throughout the body, says Bruce Pomeranz, M.D., Ph.D., neurophysiologist and professor at the University of Toronto School of Medicine and one of the world's foremost acupuncture researchers.

Instead of inserting needles into strategic points on the body, reflexologists apply pressure to points on the feet, ears and hands. So pressing a reflexology point on the ear could well relieve pain by stimulating nerves which then trigger the release of painkilling neurochemicals in the brain, just as acupuncture does, says Dr. Pomeranz.

Reflexology, practitioners say, is not a substitute for medical treatment but a supplement to medical care. "We don't diagnose," says Norman. "So it's always a good idea to get a diagnosis from your doctor before consulting

Getting**Started**

Reflexology

Reflexologists study the science and art of relieving common areas of pain and stress that can accumulate over time. Practitioners believe that working on certain spots can help your body return to its natural balance and give it a chance to heal.

Number of practitioners in the United States: Approximately 10,000.

Qualifications to look for: Experts suggest that you look for certification from the American Reflexology Certification Board, an independent testing service, but there is no one standard training program for reflexology. Practitioners learn reflexology at reflexology institutes, community colleges, adult education programs and other schools—so the quality and extent of training varies widely.

Professional associations: American Reflexology Certification Board, P.O. Box 620607, Littleton, CO 80162; International Institute of Reflexology, P.O. Box 12642, St. Petersburg, FL 33733.

To find a practitioner: Contact one of the associations listed above.

Approximate cost: $35 to $100 per session, depending on where you live.

a reflexologist." Norman believes that most illnesses are brought on or aggravated by stress. So if your doctor diagnoses a stress-related problem, she advises heading for a qualified reflexologist.

Dr. Wunderlich says that he often refers patients to reflexologists for relief from neck and muscle pain, poor digestion, tension headaches, fibromyalgia and PMS.

And Dr. Small recommends it for aches, pains and PMS as well.

REFLEXOLOGY SELF-TAUGHT

If you're interested, you can learn the basics of reflexology in a special weekend workshop, through an adult education program, or a community college. For a short-hand version, try the standard techniques that follow. These techniques won't qualify you as a full-fledged reflexologist. But you'll get the basic idea.

Finger Walk

Using the edge of your index finger, take small "bites" of your foot. This is done by bending your finger joint closest to the nail and imagining that your finger is taking tiny bites of your foot. Place your thumb on the other side of your foot for leverage. Each area should be worked four or five times before moving on to work the adjoining area.

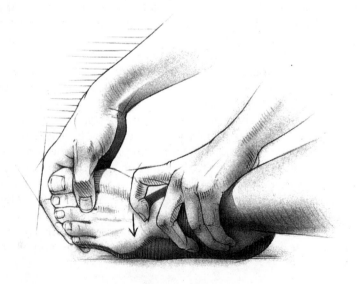

Thumb Walk

Using the outside edge or tip of your thumb, slowly and gently "walk" it along the area that you want to work. This is done by bending the thumb joint closest to your thumbnail. Each time that you bend and unbend this joint to move it forward, imagine that the thumb is taking tiny bites of your foot. Placing your fingers around your foot so that they are directly underneath your thumb will help you apply more even pressure to the areas. The pressure should be gentle but steady. Work each area at least four or five times before moving on to the next area.

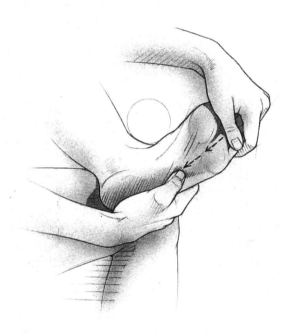

THERAPEUTIC TOUCH

Smooth Out Your Energy Field

When Janet Ziegler's 14-year-old son Daniel broke his collarbone in a cycling accident, the doctor who set the break predicted that the bone would take at least two months to heal.

In the interim, Ziegler decided to treat her son with Therapeutic Touch, a healing technique based on the laying on of hands. A registered nurse trained in the technique, Ziegler gave Daniel a five-minute session three or four times a day.

Two and a half weeks later, Ziegler recalls, she looked out her kitchen window and saw Daniel swinging by his hands from the neighbor's porch railing.

"I said, 'Get down! You have a broken collarbone. You'll hurt yourself!'" says Ziegler. "And he said, 'No, Mom, it's better.' So I took him back to the doctor, who took an x-ray, which showed that the bone was completely healed."

According to Ziegler and others who practice Therapeutic Touch, the therapy enhances the body's ability to heal itself. Research indicates that this healing method helps anxiety, speeds wound healing, induces feelings of relaxation and decreases the perceptions of headache pain. Therapeutic Touch isn't a replacement for conventional treatment, they note, but it is an effective adjunct—that is, a natural way to enhance and speed recovery.

Therapeutic Touch is so effective that every woman should learn it and use it on her family, her friends and herself, says Ziegler, a clinical nurse specialist in Allison Park, Pennsylvania, and coordinator for Nurse-Healers Professional Associates, a professional organization for practitioners of Therapeutic Touch. "I treat women in my office when they have cramps or premenstrual syndrome, and in five minutes, they feel so much better. I use it at work and at home. I really don't know how I would have raised my kids without it."

GROWING RECOGNITION

Developed in the early 1970s by Dolores Krieger, R.N., Ph.D., a New York University nursing professor, and Dora Kunz, a self-taught healer, Therapeutic Touch was at first written off by the medical establishment. Though still controversial, the technique has been gaining credibility ever since. It's now part of the curriculum at more than 100 universities nationwide.

"For some individuals, Therapeutic Touch can be a very important part of the overall healing process," says Jeremy Geffen, M.D., an oncologist in Vero Beach, Florida, who treats cancer with conventional treatments such as chemotherapy and radiation but encourages his patients to supplement those treatments with alternative therapies like Therapeutic Touch.

HEALING WITH ENERGY

Therapeutic Touch is something of a misnomer. A practitioner doesn't need to actually touch the person that she's treating. Usually, she touches

Getting**Started**

Therapeutic Touch

Therapeutic Touch is one of several hands-on healing techniques. Those who practice it believe that it helps the body to heal itself. While not as widely practiced as therapeutic massage, you can find a practitioner by following these guidelines.

Number of practitioners in the United States: Nurse-Healers Professional Associates has 1,500 members, but thousands of other practitioners use Therapeutic Touch.

Qualifications to look for: No certification exists for Therapeutic Touch. Look for a practitioner who has completed a training course approved by Nurse-Healers Professional Associates.

Professional associations: Nurse-Healers Professional Associates, 1121 Locust Street, Philadelphia, PA 19107.

To find a practitioner: Contact the Nurse-Healers Professional Associates at the address listed above, or ask the administrator of a hospital, nursing home or hospice whether any staff members do Therapeutic Touch.

Approximate cost: Cost varies widely. Also, some hospitals and institutions offer Therapeutic Touch as an integral part of health care, at no additional charge.

the "energy field" surrounding the person or, if she's working on herself, the field surrounding her own body. According to the theory underlying Therapeutic Touch, each of us is surrounded by a human energy field, like an all-body halo. These fields extend out several inches from the skin surface, practitioners say.

When we're healthy, Dr. Krieger explains, our fields are symmetrical or balanced and energy flows evenly through them. But physical and emotional problems—everything from broken bones to depression—cause asymmetries or imbalances in the fields. Therapeutic Touch aims to balance them out, she says.

Reiki Practice: Aid to Healing?

Reiki is the Japanese word for "universal life energy," and reiki therapists believe they can tap into this energy and use it to enhance healing.

Both reiki (pronounced ray-key) and Therapeutic Touch work with energy, although they are separate practices based on different theories. According to reiki theory, practitioners can channel universal healing energy to balance and enhance the flow of vital energy through their own and others' bodies. A harmonious balance of energy in the body aids healing, explains licensed massage therapist Thomas Claire, a reiki master who practices in New York City and author of Bodywork: What Type of Massage to Get—And How to Make the Most of It.

Reiki practitioners generally touch their clients, albeit very gently. Usually, the person lies on a massage table, fully dressed. (There's no need to undress because the energy permeates clothing, Claire says.)

During a typical 60- to 90-minute healing session, practitioners place their hands, palms down, over your major organs and glands and over various spots that are believed to be centers of subtle energy, called chakras. If the practitioner is treating herself, she holds her hands over the same spots. A practitioner usually holds her hands over each spot for 3 to 5 minutes. During that time, reiki theory has it, the person undergoing treatment draws in whatever energy she needs from the universe through the medium of the practitioner.

Reiki differs from Therapeutic Touch in yet another way, notes Claire. You can't learn to tap or use the energy simply by mastering the hand positions and wanting to heal. You have to go through an initiation—a ritual—in which a reiki master attunes you so that you can become a channel for the healing energy.

"You're not healing the person yourself when you do Therapeutic Touch; you're reordering her energy field so that her body can efficiently heal itself," says Ziegler.

If you visited a practitioner of Therapeutic Touch, she would begin the session by getting a sense of imbalances in your energy field. Holding her hands two to six inches above you, she'd begin at your head and work down to your feet. Some practitioners say that a balanced energy field feels like a barely perceptible but steady breeze; but different individuals sense it differently. Imbalances, on the other hand, may feel more tingly or slightly cooler than other areas, and areas with deficient energy may feel empty or

There are three degrees of reiki, each requiring an attunement, explains Joyce J. Morris, a reiki master teacher in Encino, California, and author of *Reiki—Hands That Heal*. After four attunements, says Morris, you're at the first degree of reiki and can transmit healing energy by touching anything alive. To achieve the second degree, you learn sacred symbols, how to send healing energy over a distance and how to amplify the energy of the first degree and treat mental, emotional and addictive problems. After the third and final initiation, you become a reiki master, trained to do reiki attunements.

Reiki is based on ancient Tibetan healing techniques that were rediscovered in the mid-1800s when Mikao Usui, a professor at a Christian seminary in Kyoto, reportedly discovered the keys to the practice in ancient Sanskrit texts. Practitioners say that he discovered the way in which to use them for reiki healing during a mystical experience atop a sacred Japanese mountain.

The secrecy surrounding reiki invites skepticism, acknowledges Claire, who says that he was skeptical himself, initially. But even die-hard skeptics say that they feel something happening during the treatment. People report feeling tingling, heat and spinning sensations and seeing colors. In one study, students who were learning first-degree reiki had higher blood levels of hemoglobin (the oxygen-carrying component of blood) than before the training, suggesting that some kind of beneficial change occurred.

Though you don't have to get initiated to benefit from reiki treatment, the attunement will enhance the treatment, Claire says. Once you're attuned, you can apply the technique to your friends, family and yourself—a real benefit, since reiki masters suggest that you give yourself a treatment every day for optimum results.

congested. A practitioner "balances" the energy field with her hands, using various techniques, as the occasion demands.

No one knows exactly why Therapeutic Touch gets results. Since the practitioner doesn't necessarily touch the client, results can't be attributed to the physiological and psychological effects of physical touch, which science recognizes. Practitioners offer various explanations, based on electromagnetic and quantum physics and psychology. At this point, though, it's not clear which explanations, if any, are correct.

MASTERING THE BASICS

Many practitioners of Therapeutic Touch are doctors, nurses, psychotherapists or other health professionals. But with training, anyone can learn the technique, says Dr. Krieger, author of six books about Therapeutic Touch, including *The Therapeutic Touch Inner Workbook*.

"I've taught the technique to well over 43,000 health professionals in addition to many laypeople," Dr. Krieger says. "And my students have probably taught as many," she adds.

If you want to learn Therapeutic Touch, your best bet is to take classes with a practitioner. "Getting feedback from a teacher or mentor really helps," says Ziegler. Eight to 12 hours of training will cover the essentials.

If you're unable to train with a practitioner, you can still learn the rudiments of Therapeutic Touch.

Let's suppose that you want to treat a friend who's been having muscle aches or headaches. First, find a quiet place in which to work and ask your friend to sit on a stool. Treating someone who's seated in a backless chair gives you access to her entire energy field, says Ziegler. Since the energy field permeates clothing, there's no need to undress for a session, she says. (If your friend has to lie in bed, that's okay, too.)

Once your friend is in position, follow these steps.

Center yourself. This is the most important part, says Dorothy Woods Smith, R.N., Ph.D., associate professor of nursing and instructor of Therapeutic Touch at the University of Southern Maine in Portland. "To center yourself, tune out what's around you. Quiet your mind so that you can become acutely aware and focused throughout the process."

Assess. Become attuned to the energy field around the body of your subject. Holding your hands two to six inches above her, start at her head and continue to work downward to her feet. Smooth your hands over the area above her face, then the sides and back of her head and finally her shoulders. In your mind, compare what you feel on the right side with what you feel on the left; compare sensations in front with those in back. Continue working downward, over her torso, pelvis and both legs. Look for and note signs of imbalance, says Dr. Smith. These may feel like differences in warmth and coolness or as a tingling. The person you're treating won't feel the imbalance.

Even out perceived areas of buildup or deficiency in the energy field. Move your hands downward and outward from the top of each uneven area using a flowing motion, says Dr. Smith. "The strokes should be rhythmic."

Evaluate. To complete the session, reassess your friend's energy field to make sure that you've balanced it out, says Dr. Krieger.

TOUCHING TIPS

Following a similar procedure, you can also do Therapeutic Touch on yourself. Sit in a backless chair and repeat the above process. You should be able to cover your entire field, though it may be a little more difficult to cover the area between the back of your shoulders and waist, according to Dr. Krieger.

Whether you're using Therapeutic Touch on friends, family or yourself, you can do it a couple times a day. But as a beginner, you should limit each

Getting**Started**

Reiki Therapy

Reiki practitioners balance and enhance the flow of energy in your body by touching your body in certain ways while you're fully clothed. Here's how to find a practitioner near you.

Number of practitioners in the United States: Thousands of reiki therapists practice in this country, and 1,000 reiki masters practice worldwide.

Qualifications to look for: Look for a practitioner who is a reiki master (that is, one who has complete all three levels of reiki initiation) or one who has been initiated by a reiki master.

To find a practitioner: Contact The Reiki Alliance, P.O. Box 41, Cataldo, ID 83810-1041.

Approximate cost: $30 to $100 per one-hour session.

session to five minutes. Otherwise, you'll overload the person you're treating, or yourself, with energy, Ziegler says. That can cause irritability, a sympathetic nervous response, she explains.

You should be particularly careful not to overdo it with the very young, the very old or pregnant women since they can get overloaded easily, Ziegler adds.

Of course, you and any family member can see a professional if there's one in your area. The professional might ask you to come about once a week for a session lasting 20 to 30 minutes, she says.

TRADITIONAL CHINESE MEDICINE
Still Valid after 2,500 Years

Enter the waiting room of a Traditional Chinese Medicine practitioner and you've left the world of the medically familiar behind. The air may be strangely scented with unfamiliar herbs. Jars may be stuffed with gnarled roots, shells, dried plants and blackened wormlike creatures, even sea horses, and placed right next to modern, colorfully wrapped patent medicines with labels printed in Chinese. The walls may be hung with delicately inked rice-paper panels in oriental motifs. Here, even the Muzak sounds exotic.

Clearly, this is like no doctor's waiting room that you've ever been in. You have taken a great leap of faith, suspending for the moment your life-long reliance on modern Western medicine.

Take a deep breath. Relax. You're about to participate in a healing art that's been around for more than 2,500 years, one that is used today by an estimated one-quarter of the world's population.

What prompts women to give Traditional Chinese Medicine a try? Usually, some kind of chronic pain, says Barbara Bernie, licensed acupuncturist and president of the American Foundation of Traditional Chinese Medicine (TCM) in San Francisco. "Although we don't have statistics on how many people visit TCM practitioners, experience tells me that many people first try acupuncture, one of TCM's therapeutic treatments, for chronic pain that hasn't responded to traditional Western medicine.

Tsung O. Cheng, M.D., professor of medicine and a cardiologist at George Washington University School of Medicine in Washington, D.C., agrees. "TCM offers excellent pain relief." Dr. Cheng several years ago saw an acupuncturist for lower-back pain with satisfactory results.

A TOTAL HEALING SYSTEM

But Traditional Chinese Medicine is much more than the practice of acupuncture. It is a medical system, combining acupuncture with the use of medicinal herbs, massage and dietary therapy. Practitioners also often recommend exercise, breathing disciplines and meditation in the form of qi gong (chi gung) and tai ji (more commonly known as tai chi) as part of an ongoing, holistic wellness program.

And when it comes to women's health concerns, practitioners say that TCM can't be beat.

"I think that women's reproductive and endocrinological problems are well-addressed by Traditional Chinese Medicine," says Martha Howard, M.D., co-director of Wellness Associates, a Chicago-based family medical practice. "I treat menstrual irregularities, premenstrual syndrome, ovarian cysts and symptoms of menopause very successfully with TCM." Dr.

Chinese Herbs: Not to Be Used Casually

An ancient book, the *Shen Nung Pen Ts'ao Ching*, ranked the 365 herbs that, 2,500 years ago, formed the backbone of herbal medicine in China.

Though the work was revised over the centuries that followed, authorities say that the herbal wisdom it contains is "as popular and useful today as when it was written."

"The observations that the ancient Chinese sages made about medicinal herbs were very wise, and they stand the test of time," says Zoe Brenner, a licensed acupuncturist and Traditional Chinese Medicine (TCM) practitioner in Bethesda, Maryland.

"In Chinese medicine, hundreds of medicinal herbs are used in thousands of combinations," says Christina Stemmler, M.D., a Houston physician who integrates TCM and acupuncture with Western medicine and previously headed the American Academy of Medical Acupuncture. While some Chinese herbs, like astragalus and ma huang, sound distinctly exotic, others are as familiar as licorice and cinnamon.

But treating with Chinese herbs is a healing art that takes years of study to practice effectively, notes Brenner. "Chinese herbs are rarely used singly or to treat single symptoms. That's because *your* headache is caused by a variety of imbalances within *your* system; the herbs that I prescribe to treat it are selected and blended just for you. Your friend's headache may spring from totally different causes, and the

Howard says that TCM is just one of a variety of complementary therapies that she prescribes, including good nutrition, exercise, proper rest, vitamin supplements, stress reduction, herbs, acupuncture and others.

"Premenstrual syndrome is easily treated with acupuncture and Chinese herbs," says Christina Stemmler, M.D., a Houston physician who integrates TCM and acupuncture with Western medicine and previously headed the American Academy of Medical Acupuncture. "I believe that a TCM approach can ease hot flashes in the majority of women who are so treated."

Traditional Chinese Medicine can also provide effective pain relief during labor and childbirth, according to Dr. Howard.

---

herbs that cure your headache may only make your friend's feel worse," she says.

Brenner contends that endorsements given to some Chinese herbs as cure-alls are misplaced.

"Folk remedies refer to dang gui (also known as dong quai) as a panacea for women's reproductive problems. Though this herb can be highly effective, it should be compounded for your particular condition, probably in combination with other herbs," says Brenner. "Taking it on your own could worsen your symptoms."

Another Chinese herb that's been misused, says Brenner, is ma huang. "Ma huang has been touted as a 'safe and natural' weight-loss aid, but in reality, it's like taking herbal speed—amphetamines," she cautions. "It's similar to the decongestant pseudoephedrine, and while it can cut your appetite, over time, it can make you tired and deplete your energy. I've known its misuse to lead to strokes and heart attacks."

According to Brenner, "There's a popular misconception that says, 'If it's natural, it can't hurt you.' But many natural medicinal herbs, in fact, are toxic. In the right hands, they can heal, but use them incorrectly and you're asking for trouble."

So what does modern wisdom say about the ancient practice of Chinese herbal medicine? "It's a highly effective healing art, but one that should be left to qualified, experienced TCM practitioners," concludes Brenner.

WISDOM FROM THE WORLD'S OLDEST MEDICAL BOOK

Traditional Chinese Medicine emanates from a culture that is vastly different from our own. So if you decide to consult a TCM practitioner, be prepared to hear some very strange terminology. You'll learn about yin and yang, about the five elements of nature, about your body's meridians and about the status of your qi, or vital energy. These are health attributes that don't show up on Western diagnostic tools such as x-rays and CAT scans.

Not to worry, says Andrew Weil, M.D., professor of herbalism and director of the Program of Integrative Medicine at the University of Arizona College of Medicine, near Tucson, and best-selling author of *Spontaneous Healing* and *Health and Healing*. "Just because we cannot detect, perceive or measure forces and factors that Chinese doctors say are important in

Qi Gong: China's Extraordinary Healing Art

Part meditation, part movement and part breathing, qi gong (pronounced CHEE-goong) is an ancient Chinese system of healing exercise credited with some very powerful health benefits.

Qi gong's gentle breathing and meditation exercises help to circulate your energy and get your body back into its proper alignment, says Martha Howard, M.D., co-director of Wellness Associates, a Chicago-based family medical practice. Dr. Howard teaches qi gong as part of her Traditional Chinese Medicine practice. "Qi gong is a meditative form of healing art," she says. "Practicing it can both relax you and enhance your energy level."

A flurry of research projects have linked qi gong with lowering blood pressure, increasing the body's ability to use oxygen efficiently, boosting the immune system, slowing the aging process and increasing levels of serotonin and endorphins—brain chemicals that help soothe and calm.

"If you can't find a class in qi gong, tai ji (commonly known as tai chi) offers similar benefits," says Ching-Tse Lee, Ph.D., a qi gong master, chairman of the psychology department at Brooklyn College and director of the Tao and Zen Research Center in New York City. "It's especially good for stress reduction and can help you learn to meditate."

managing illness does not automatically mean they do not exist," Dr. Weil explains in his book *Health and Healing*.

Though some of the TCM concepts seem decidedly exotic to Westerners, the fact is that they have withstood the test of time, says David Molony, Ph.D., licensed acupuncturist and executive director of the American Association of Acupuncture and Oriental Medicine, who practices in the northern suburbs of Philadelphia. And, he notes, "according to the Chinese, who've had nearly 3,000 years of experience to back up their science, conventional medicine, which is only a couple of hundred years old at best, has yet to be proven."

In other words, while Westerners think of TCM and other nonmainstream medical practices as new, experimental alternatives, to practitioners and their satisfied patients, modern Western medicine is the real "alternative" medical system.

Nearly 2,500 years ago, *The Yellow Emperor's Classic of Internal Medicine* was written as discussions between Huang Ti, the legendary first emperor of China and the pioneer of Chinese medical science, and six Chinese scholars. A summary of ancient medical practices, the world's oldest medical book reveals the principles of Traditional Chinese Medicine. These principles, which were originally based on observations of nature, still guide modern TCM practitioners today.

"Traditional Chinese Medicine is all about nature's balancing act," says Martin L. Rossman, M.D., physician, certified acupuncturist and clinical associate in the Department of Medicine at the University of California at San Francisco. "The ancients suggested that we take a cue from nature's seasonal activity, and that still makes sense today."

Winter is the season when nature rests, for example, says Dr. Rossman. Animals hibernate to conserve their energy. Plants go dormant. Trees lose their leaves. And what do humans do (at least, in Western cultures)?

"They party!" says Dr. Rossman. "Starting around the holidays, at a time of year when nature dictates that we slow down, we shop till we drop, work way past the natural sunset and run ourselves ragged with holiday activities. It's no wonder that by January and February, many people, especially women, are exhausted, and inevitably more vulnerable to colds and flu bugs."

USER-FRIENDLY TCM

To prepare you for what to expect if you consult a Traditional Chinese Medicine practitioner, here's a brief run-down of the basic concepts behind this ancient healing art.

About Yin and Yang

"Yin and yang signify two opposite yet complementary forces, which create movement in all aspects of our lives," explains Dr. Rossman. "Yang is the desire to become something and yin is the desire to return to nothing," says Dr. Rossman. TCM holds that balance and harmony between these, with shifting balances to suit the season and situation, are essential to good health.

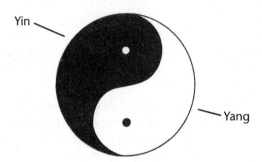

The Chinese character for yin translates to the shady side of a hill and can be thought to represent darkness; the character for yang is the sunny side, representing light. They represent opposite but complementary qualities in every aspect of one's life. Traditional Chinese Medicine strives to achieve balance and harmony of these qualities for good health.

These are some of the traditional yin and yang associations, cited by Dr. Rossman.

Yin	Yang
Moon	Sun
Rest	Activity
Earth	Heaven
Flat	Round
Space	Time
Cold	Hot
Inhibition	Excitement
Right	Left
Water	Fire

The Five Natural Elements

In Traditional Chinese Medicine, the interaction of five natural elements plays a role in determining your health. When there is an imbalance in the natural harmony of these elements, health problems can ensue.

An ancient Chinese medical text, the *Shang Shu*, describes the interaction of the five elements as follows: "The five elements are water, fire, wood, metal and earth. Water moistens downward; fire flares upward; wood can be bent and straightened; metal can be molded and can harden; and earth permits sowing, growing and reaping. That which soaks and descends (water) is salty, that which blazes upward (fire) is bitter, that which can be bent and straightened (wood) is sour, that which can be molded and become hard (metal) is pungent and that which permits sowing and reaping (earth) is sweet."

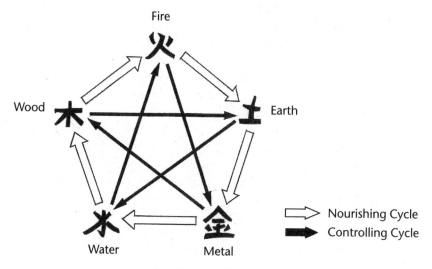

Five Natural Elements

The five elements are an essential principal of Traditional Chinese Medicine. The elements—water, fire, wood, metal and earth—symbolize and link five different qualities and states of natural phenomena. In addition, the elements correspond to different colors, seasons and internal organs.

The theory behind this system may sound esoteric, almost beyond our Western understanding. But from an Eastern perspective, it's all quite logical. According to Dr. Stemmler, "The five elements arose from the ancients' observations of nature, and today we know that these observations translate into many of our current concepts of physics. Each element is associated with certain energies that affect specific organs, emotions and spiritual states."

"Chinese medicine has effective and valid ways of treating a variety of health problems," says Elaine Stern, licensed acupuncturist and TCM practitioner in private practice and at the Pacific Institute in New York City.

Qi, the Essential Life Force

To the Chinese, qi (also written as chi and pronounced "chee") is the river of energy that courses through our bodies and gives us life.

"Think of qi as the force that organizes a bunch of chemicals into a living, breathing human being," says Dr. Rossman. "Qi doesn't just sit around in a puddle; it flows through the body through special channels that we call meridians, much like the blood flows through arteries and veins."

Dr. Rossman says that it's especially easy to explain the concept of qi to women that he treats. "I tell them that qi is whatever took a microscopic cell and caused it to grow into your beautiful baby."

TCM practitioners use Chinese herbs, acupuncture, moxibustion and massage—treatments designed to restore the balance and healthful flow of qi throughout the body. They also emphasize prevention first and encourage their patients to follow an appropriate diet, sleep well and live life in alignment. TCM is a second line of defense after living a balanced life.

A VISIT TO A TCM PRACTITIONER

Your first Traditional Chinese Medicine visit is likely to be quite different from the doctor visits that you're used to.

You know the drill. You don a too-small gown and perch on a paper-covered table in a drafty room that smells of industrial-strength antiseptic. There you wait, far longer than you'd like, surrounded by fearfully modern medical equipment. The waiting, however, is not without purpose: It gives you plenty of time to consider just how that equipment may be used—on you.

"A Western medicine exam is typically a hurried process," says Dr. Howard. Think back to your last physical, when, very likely, you were rushed through as if on an assembly line.

In contrast, you're likely to feel a good deal less hurried and a whole lot more nurtured during a visit to a TCM practitioner. First of all, TCM uses completely different methods of diagnosis than does Western medicine. The practitioner will do nothing more invasive than examine your tongue and take your pulse. In TCM, diagnosis can be summed up in five words:

- Asking
- Looking
- Hearing
- Smelling
- Touching (palpation)

A Medical History Like No Other

Before she does anything else, the TCM practitioner will interview you (unlike a Western doctor, who may question you while you're up on the examining table). But be prepared to answer a lot more questions than you're used to being asked—some more personal and graphic than those that your family doctor usually asks.

You may feel like your Western doctor seems rushed—"just the facts, ma'am"—prompting you to pass over problems that you think are important.

In contrast, a TCM practitioner will want to know everything about you in infinite detail—details that she will take very seriously. You'll be asked about your lifestyle, your eating and sleeping patterns and about your monthly cycle, even about the color and content of your menstrual flow and how it changes during your period. You'll be asked if temperature affects you and whether you generally feel hotter rather than colder or vice versa.

Your diet and habits will be carefully questioned; so will your food preferences. Do you eat foods hot, cold, spicy or bland? Crave sweets? Salty foods? Do you drink coffee? How often? Do you smoke? Drink? And do you chew your food thoroughly? For how long? How do you deal with your emotions? What is the quality of your relationships? What is your stress level?

Finally, your output is at least as interesting as your input: Your TCM practitioner will also want to discuss the color, consistency and frequency of your bowel movements and urine flow.

Looking and Learning

If you think that your TCM practitioner seems to be looking very closely at you during the course of your exam, you're absolutely right.

Though a good practitioner of Traditional Chinese Medicine is far too subtle to stare obviously, she will be carefully observing many things during the course of her examination of you.

In *The Yellow Emperor's Classic of Internal Medicine*, it is said that "one should observe minute and trifling things as if they were normal size . . ." and that "those who are experts in examining patients judge their appearances. . . ." Your practitioner will carefully examine your face, studying your eyes, nose, ears, teeth and gums, throat, arms, legs and skin.

After she's checked you out physically, your practitioner will consider your spirit and emotions and your demeanor, because not just your body but also your mind and spirit will speak about your overall vitality and health patterns.

Revealing Sounds and Scents

How you sound has a lot to do with how you feel. So as you answer her questions, your practitioner will listen to the sound of your voice, your breathing and any coughs—even to the way your stomach gurgles.

To a classically trained TCM practitioner, a woman's body scent (if unperfumed) may provide valuable clinical information. Body odors, which an experienced TCM nose differentiates as rancid, burned, sweet, rank and putrid, indicate various imbalances within the body's system. Similarly, bad breath or foul-smelling excreta signal specific imbalances.

Stick Out Your Tongue and Say Nothing

A thorough examination of your tongue is another essential diagnostic tool used by practitioners of Traditonal Chinese Medicine.

Practitioners say that tongue diagnosis is remarkably reliable, especially in complicated conditions, since the tongue nearly always reflects your body's basic pattern of balance.

"The tongue is a place where the TCM practitioner can see what the inside of your body looks like," says Dr. Molony. "Interpreted correctly, the tongue accurately depicts the state of your health because it represents, in microcosm, your body and how it functions."

The practitioner will note your tongue's color, shape and how, or whether, it's coated. A thin white coating is said to be a normal sign that the stomach is digesting food properly. A thick coating may indicate imbalance. The moistness of your tongue is also a factor in your diagnosis.

What your practitioner learns from examining your tongue gives her additional information about a range of factors that are influencing your health.

Tongue Diagnosis

Different areas of the tongue are said to reflect the state of the internal organs. Traditional Chinese Medicine practitioners use the tongue's color—pale, pale red (normal), red, deep red, purple and blue—the shape of the tongue and its coating and moisture to diagnose the state of your well-being. The zones, shown here, cover many areas of the body in addition to the specific zone named. For example, the lung and heart zones cover the organs and body functions above the diaphragm, such as the esophagus or respiration.

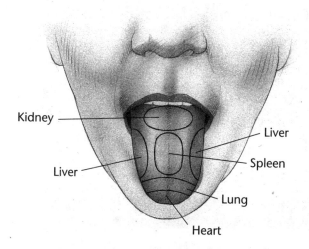

Kidney

Liver

Liver

Spleen

Lung

Heart

A Different Take on Pulse-Taking

For a Western doctor, taking the pulse is simply a matter of noting the rate, rhythm and regularity of your heart rate at a peripheral artery, like your wrists. As such, taking a pulse doesn't take much time and can be learned with ease.

But when a well-trained TCM practitioner takes your pulse, years of training are on display. Pulse-taking is an essential TCM diagnostic tool, one that requires not only refined sensitivity but also a high degree of concentration on the part of the practitioner. Pulse-taking is considered a fine art and is said to be a difficult skill to acquire.

In Traditional Chinese Medicine, pulse-taking relies on fingertip palpations of 12 separate pulses, 6 on each wrist. When taking your pulse, the practitioner will regulate her breathing pattern to yours to enable her to tune in to your pulse sounds.

The first three fingers of the hand are used at three levels of the wrists' radial artery, the same one used for Western pulse-taking. The best TCM practitioners will be able to note 28 different pulse variations on frequency, rhythm and density.

Each pulse is believed to correlate with the activity of a different organ. Combined with your medical history and other parts of the exam, the subtle qualities of each pulse and how they fit into your pattern of health leads your practitioner to your diagnosis and the best method of treatment for you.

IS TRADITIONAL CHINESE MEDICINE RIGHT FOR YOU?

"The advantages of Traditional Chinese Medicine fit nicely with the disadvantages of Western medicine," says Glenn S. Rothfeld, M.D., clinical instructor in the Department of Community Health at Tufts University School of Medicine in Boston and a practitioner in Arlington, Massachusetts. "It's a classic yin/yang relationship."

TCM excels when you have diverse symptoms that don't form a coherent picture, says Dr. Rothfeld. "Western medicine will have you going

Getting**Started**

Traditional Chinese Medicine

Informally referred to as TCM, Traditional Chinese Medicine combines acupuncture with Chinese herbs and massage. To find a practitioner in your area, follow these guidelines.

Number of practitioners in the United States: In the thousands.

Qualifications to look for: Certification by the National Commission for Certification for Acupuncture and Oriental Medicine (NCCA). Practitioners may also be licensed acupuncturists (L.Ac.), trained physicians (M.D.'s or D.O.'s) or doctors of oriental medicine (D.O.M.).

Professional associations: American Association of Oriental Medicine, 433 Front Street, Catasauqua, PA 18032.

To find a practitioner: Contact the NCCA, P.O. Box 97075, Washington, D.C. 20090-7075.

Approximate cost: $75 to $150 for an initial visit, including a complete evaluation and medical history. Follow-up sessions cost from $25 to $100.

to specialists who treat your symptoms independently. For example, you might see an ear, nose and throat specialist for your sinus problems and a gastroenterologist for your stomach problems. A TCM practitioner would see all those symptoms as part of an overall pattern and would treat you accordingly." In fact, he adds, stomach disorders are especially well-suited to TCM.

"When you see a gastroenterologist for your stomach problems, you may endure a lot of uncomfortable tests before the doctor diagnoses you with, say, irritable bowel syndrome and leaves it at that, because there isn't much that Western medicine has in its bag of tricks that works," says Dr. Roth-feld. "But TCM offers ways of treating the various symptoms that are called irritable bowel syndrome."

"Western medicine has some tremendous assets," says Dr. Stemmler. "It's far superior when it comes to surgical procedures. It excels at treating life-threatening diseases affecting the cardiovascular system as well as various serious illnesses affecting vital organs in the body." But, continues Dr. Stemmler, "such illnesses occur rarely or often later in someone's lifetime. Most daily ailments affecting the very young to the middle-aged are less serious and do not require a full trauma team at your bedside or the use of potentially dangerous drugs and expensive and uncomfortable procedures. TCM can serve this large sector of the general population well. There is definitely a well-defined place and time for each approach: Eastern or Western. Knowing when to use one, the other or both simultaneously is going to be the challenge of the new generation of dually trained physicians."

VEGETARIAN DIETS
No Meat, Plenty of Benefits

Ruth Heidrich is arguably one of the world's healthiest women. A marathoner and Ironman triathlete, she competes in an average of 50 races annually. And she's broken at least one world fitness record.

She wasn't always so healthy.

"I used to *think* that I was one of the world's healthiest people—I had given up red meat, and I was running," says Heidrich, who has a Ph.D. in health management, nutrition and exercise. "But then, at age 47, I found out that I had breast cancer."

While recuperating from cancer surgery, Dr. Heidrich met John McDougall, M.D., tireless advocate of meatless eating and author of *The McDougall Program* and *The New McDougall Cookbook*, and she soon became a strict vegetarian, eating no animal food whatsoever. And that, she says, made all the difference. She set her sights on the triathlon shortly after and hasn't stopped moving since.

"The cancer never recurred and I've never felt this good in my life," says Dr. Heidrich.

On a typical day, she cycles, swims or runs for two to three hours, writes and lectures on the merits of the meatless life. She has published two books, *A Race for Life: From Cancer to Ironman* and *A Race for Life Cookbook*. "It's the healthiest way to eat," she says.

THE BENEFITS KICK IN IMMEDIATELY

The vegetarian way may well be the healthiest way for everyone to eat. By far, the best documented health benefit of vegetarianism is a reduced risk of heart disease, the number one cause of death among women. Numerous studies find that vegetarians run a lower risk of heart disease than meat-eaters do.

A number of factors seem to come into play: First, women who eat a vegetarian diet are less likely to be overweight. They have lower blood cholesterol levels because their diets tend to be lower in total fat, saturated fat and dietary cholesterol. And vegetarians eat more fiber, which has been shown to lower cholesterol levels.

Research also suggests that the plant protein on which vegetarians rely—found in soybeans and other legumes—has an edge over the animal protein that nonvegetarians eat, at least as far as heart protection goes. Why? Animal protein is high in lysine, an amino acid that speeds up cholesterol production in the body. Soybeans, on the other hand, are low in lysine and high in arginine and glycine, two different amino acids that don't have this effect.

Vegetarians also tend to have lower blood pressures than meat-eaters do. In one study, 500 men and women who enrolled in an intensive program—a low-fat vegetarian diet, moderate exercise and stress reduction—saw their blood cholesterol levels drop an average of 11 percent in just 12 days. That wasn't all. Their blood pressures sank 6 percent, and their weight fell an average of 2.2 pounds.

Getting**Started**

Vegetarianism

If you decide to try a vegetarian diet and you're pregnant or nursing or have a chronic health condition such as diabetes, it's a good idea to consult a dietitian or other health professional trained in nutritional counseling, to ensure that you're getting all the nutrients that you need. Here's how to find a qualified nutritionist near you.

Number of practitioners in the United States: Approximately 69,000 registered dietitians and nutritionists.

Qualifications to look for: Registered Dietitian (R.D.). Some states require dietitians and nutritionists to be licensed. Also, M.D.'s, D.O.'s and Ph.D.'s in nutrition are qualified to give nutritional advice. Those with master's degrees in nutrition may also be qualified, depending on your state's licensing requirements.

Professional associations: American Dietetic Association, 216 West Jackson Boulevard, Chicago, IL 60606-6995.

To find a practitioner: Contact the Vegetarian Resource Group of the American Dietetic Association at the address listed above.

Approximate cost: $50 to $100 per hour for an initial consultation and $25 to $50 for shorter follow-up sessions, depending on where you live.

Even if you've been eating meat for 40 years, a switch to vegetarianism can do your heart good, says Erica Frank, M.D., assistant professor of family and preventive medicine at Emory University School of Medicine in Atlanta. In one study, a team of researchers at the University of California in San Francisco put men and women with heart disease on a very low fat vegetarian diet and an exercise and stress-reduction program. The regimen actually slowed or decreased the progression of the disease.

The benefits don't stop there. Some studies suggest that a vegetarian diet may offer protection against some cancers. An Asian study found that the Chinese, who eat an average of one ounce of meat per day and no dairy products, have a breast cancer death rate of 8.75 per 100,000 women (compared to 43.9 for American women) and 23.4 deaths per 100,000 people for lung cancer (compared to 80.4 for Americans). Research makes a strong case for protection against lung cancer. Some evidence shows that vegetarianism may protect against colon and breast cancer, too.

Again, a number of factors seem to play a part. Vegetarian diets are usually rich in fruits and vegetables, which in turn are rich in antioxidants—nutrients that protect cells from damage wrought by cancer-causing substances. Plus, vegetarian fare tends to be low in fat, and some research hints at a dangerous link between high fat intake and some cancers. Finally, there's the high fiber content of vegetarian meals. Fiber seems to reduce the risk of colon cancer, scientists speculate, by diluting potentially harmful bile acids in the digestive tract.

A vegetarian diet can also be kind to your bones. Research finds that vegetarians may run a lower risk of osteoporosis than carnivores. Why? They're less likely to overdo it on protein, says Randall White, M.D., adjunct assistant professor of human and natural ecology at Emory University. Excess protein prompts the body to excrete calcium, an important bone-building mineral, he explains.

Finally, vegetarianism may help ease the symptoms of rheumatoid arthritis. In a few Scandinavian studies, people with arthritis who switched to vegetarian diets after brief fasts reported less pain, stiffness, joint tenderness and swelling than those eating meat.

Women who adopt a vegetarian diet seem to benefit whether they're lacto-ovo vegetarians—who eat eggs and dairy but no other animal food—or vegans (pronounced vay-gun or vee-gun)—who eat no animal products whatsoever. A lacto-ovo vegetarian diet can be just as healthy as a vegan one, as long as it includes only moderate amounts of eggs and dairy and not too much fat, says Reed Mangels, R.D., Ph.D., nutrition adviser to the Vegetarian Resource Group based in Baltimore.

"At virtually any age, if you decide to go on a lacto-ovo vegetarian or vegan diet, it will improve your health," Dr. Frank concludes.

BUSY WOMEN *CAN* GO MEATLESS

Estimates put the total number of adult American vegetarians—vegans plus lacto-ovo vegetarians—at roughly 12.4 million. According to one poll, nearly 70 percent of the total are women. Surprised? Dr. Mangels isn't.

"I think more women are vegetarians largely because they're usually the health care gatekeepers in families," she says. "In general, we tend to know more about food than our spouses, and we seem to be more health conscious."

Whether you take the vegan or lacto-ovo route, the vegetarian way is easier than ever, says Dr. Mangels. Responding to demand, food manufacturers offer all sorts of vegetarian fare. Many vegetarian foods are based on soybeans, a versatile legume that serves as a nutritious alternative to meat

A Typical Vegan Diet—Totally Vegetarian

A vegan diet contains no animal food whatsoever—no meat, no eggs, no dairy, no yogurt, no ice cream. This one-day menu, outlined by Reed Mangels, R.D., Ph.D., nutrition adviser to the Vegetarian Resource Group based in Baltimore, and adapted from the group's *Vegetarian Journal Reports*, gives some idea of what to expect should you decide to adopt a vegan diet.

Breakfast
Eggless banana pancakes. (Combine 2 mashed bananas with ½ cup each of rolled oats, cornmeal and whole-wheat flour. Add 1 tablespoon baking powder and 1½ cups water. Mix thoroughly. Pour batter into oiled skillet and cook over low heat until done. Makes 3 servings.)
1 cup orange juice
1 cup fortified soy milk

Lunch
2 bean tacos with ½ cup shredded lettuce and sliced tomatoes
1 medium apple

Dinner
1 cup vegetarian chili
1 slice cornbread
½ cup steamed broccoli
½ cup steamed cauliflower
½ cup pineapple chunks

Snack
½ cup soy ice cream

and dairy products. Today, most supermarkets carry not only soy milk and tofu (soybean curd) but also veggie burgers and meatless breakfast links (sometimes called soysage), soy lunchmeats, soy hot dogs, soy cheese and soy ice cream as well as egg substitutes and a wide selection of frozen vegetarian entrées.

"There are great resources out there—a huge supply of supermarket foods that simply didn't exist when I became a vegetarian years ago," marvels Jennie Collura, president of the North American Vegetarian Society in Dolgeville, New York.

Contrary to popular belief, it's easy to get the protein that you need from a vegetarian diet. In fact, the American Dietetic Association finds that vegetarians usually meet or exceed requirements for protein.

It is true, however, that only animal protein—found in meat, dairy, eggs and the like—contains a good ratio of the amino acids that your body needs to produce hormones and enzymes and build muscle. Individually, neither legumes nor grains nor seeds contain an ideal ratio of the necessary amino acids in sufficient quantity. Combine them, though, and they'll give you everything that you need. And you don't have to combine them in the same meal. Eating legumes and grains or nuts and legumes over the course of a day or two will do the trick, says Dr. White.

Here's how to get started.

Stock up on beans and peas. Look to staples such as chili, bean burritos, baked beans and split pea soup for the "meat" in your diet, says Dr. Mangels. The American Dietetic Association suggests that women who are vegetarians aim for two to three servings a day of high-protein legumes, namely beans, lentils, soy food and peas.

Serve soy. Make at least one of your servings of legumes a soy food, like tofu or soy milk, suggests Mark Messina, Ph.D., nutritionist in Port Townsend, Washington, author of *The Simple Soybean and Your Health* and co-author of *The Vegetarian Way*. Studies suggest that soy may offer added protection against heart disease and some types of cancer and may help alleviate menopausal symptoms, he explains.

Load up on grains, fruits and vegetables. Whether you elect a vegan diet or include eggs and dairy, try to eat at least six servings of grain products, four or more servings of vegetables and at least three servings of fruit daily, nutritionists advise.

Think variety. Every food brings its unique combination of nutrients to the table, say nutrition researchers. When choosing produce, be a colorful shopper—pick up dark leafy greens for bone-building calcium and the B vitamin folate, deep yellow fruits and vegetables for beta-carotene and related disease-fighting substances, and citrus fruits or other produce, like oranges, green peppers and strawberries, for vitamin C.

Keep track of milk and eggs. If you're a lacto-ovo vegetarian, nutritionists say, you can serve yourself up to three servings of dairy products, like skim milk and nonfat yogurt, each day and up to four whole eggs weekly. (All the fat and cholesterol in eggs are in the yolks, so use mostly whites). If you're a vegan, give yourself extra servings of breads, cereals, vegetables and fruits instead of those eggs and dairy.

NUTRIENTS TO WATCH OUT FOR

Women vegetarians need to take a few extra steps to make sure that they're getting all the nutrients they need, says Barbara Deskins, R.D., Ph.D., associate professor of clinical dietetics and nutrition at the University of Pittsburgh. If you swear off meat, follow this advice.

'C' that you get iron. Red meat is a particularly good source of heme iron, the most easily absorbed form. Spinach, beans and other plant food contain smaller amounts of iron, all in the form of nonheme iron, which is less easily absorbed. But research shows that vitamin C helps your body absorb nonheme iron. So if you don't eat meat, nutritionists recommend that you boost your absorption of nonheme iron by eating iron-rich plant food like soybeans, lentils or other dried beans, or dark leafy vegetables such as spinach or kale, as well as foods high in vitamin C, like peppers, tomatoes and citrus fruits.

Serve yourself some cereal. Ready-to-eat cereal is usually fortified with both iron and vitamin C. "So an easy way to get the iron that you need is to eat fortified cereal every day," says Dr. Deskins.

Keep tabs on iron intake. Before menopause, women need 15 milligrams of iron daily. So keep track of your intake, says Dr. Deskins. If tallying up your daily iron intake is inconvenient, ask your doctor whether you should take a multivitamin/mineral supplement with iron. Once you're past menopause, though, your iron needs and odds of developing a deficiency drop considerably, so you really don't have to keep tabs then, she says. But you'll want to consult your doctor to decide if you should continue taking a multivitamin.

Watch that zinc. You'll find zinc in both plant food, like cooked beans, and animal food, like roast beef and pork chops. Like iron, however, the zinc in plant food isn't nearly as plentiful or well-absorbed as the zinc in animal food. So you'll either have to keep a tally of the zinc that you get from the food you eat (something few of us have the time to do) or take a multivitamin/mineral supplement, says Dr. Deskins. Look for a supplement offering between 50 and 100 percent of the Recommended Dietary Allowance (RDA), which is 12 milligrams, for zinc.

FOR VEGANS ONLY

If you go the vegan route and steer clear of dairy and eggs, you'll have to keep track of a couple more nutrients.

Bank on tofu, orange juice and soy milk for calcium. A cup of skim milk (one of the richest sources of dietary calcium available) supplies 302 milligrams of calcium. In comparison, a 3½-ounce serving of broccoli (one of the richest plant sources of calcium) contains 205 milligrams of calcium. So on a vegan diet, it's harder for women to consume the amount of calcium considered optimal for good health (1,000 milligrams a day for most women ages 25 to 50; 1,200 to 1,500 milligrams a day if you're pregnant or nursing; and 1,500 milligrams a day if you're past menopause).

Dr. Mangels recommends that vegans consume at least three servings of calcium-rich nondairy foods daily. Calcium-fortified tofu, calcium-fortified orange juice and calcium-fortified soy milk are particularly good sources. (Read labels for actual amounts.) In addition to broccoli, kale, collard and mustard greens can supply useful amounts of additional calcium. If you're worried that you may not be getting enough calcium from the food that you eat, consider a supplement, advises Dr. Mangels.

In the long run, though, you can probably keep your bones strong and healthy with less calcium than the average omnivore—a person who eats both plants and animals. Why? Because you're less likely to eat excess protein, which prompts your body to excrete calcium, explains Dr. Frank.

Look to fortified soy milk for vitamin D. As it turns out, fortified dairy products or fortified cereal are also reliable sources of vitamin D, needed for fracture-resistant bones. Your skin will synthesize this vitamin when exposed to the sun. (Full-strength sunscreen, however, prevents this synthesis.) Unless you live in a sunny locale and spend at least 15 to 30 minutes outside every day, you'll need a reliable food source, Dr. Mangels says. Or choose a multivitamin/mineral supplement.

Look for nutritional yeast with B_{12}. Found almost exclusively in animal products, B_{12} is a key player in your body. It plays a role in the production of blood and DNA and helps keep your nervous system running well. You can find B_{12} in fortified soy milk and cereals and a special cheesy-tasting yeast called Red Star Nutritional Yeast T6635. Use the yeast the way that you would Parmesan cheese, says Dr. Mangels. Two teaspoons a day should get you the RDA for vitamin B_{12}—two micrograms a day, for women.

"A lot of fermented soy food, like tempeh and miso (a soybean paste used for soup), are touted as having B_{12}, but they're not reliable sources," Dr. Mangels cautions. If you're not good at keeping tabs, take a multivitamin that gives you the RDA for B_{12}.

Pregnant? Pay attention. A well-planned lacto-ovo or vegan diet is fine during pregnancy, says Charles Mahan, M.D., professor of obstetrics and gynecology at the University of South Florida in Tampa. Just make sure that you talk to your obstetrician about what you're eating. If you're a vegan, have a registered dietitian analyze your diet and make sure that it includes everything you and your baby need, he says.

While you're pregnant and nursing, you'll need more protein, calcium and B vitamins (folate, riboflavin, thiamine and niacin), says Dr. Deskins. "Adding another glass of low-fat milk or calcium-fortified soy milk would be a good idea because that adds calcium, protein and thiamine," she says. "In addition, you might have another half-cup of legumes since most are excellent sources of folate (a B vitamin essential for normal fetal growth), or have another serving of vegetables or fruits (also rich in folate)."

A Typical Vegetarian Menu

As long as you don't go overboard on eggs and dairy products, a vegetarian diet with milk and eggs—known as a lacto-ovo vegetarian diet—can be as nutritious as a vegan diet, says Reed Mangels, R.D., Ph.D., nutrition adviser to the Vegetarian Resource Group based in Baltimore. To get started, try this one-day menu.

Breakfast
1 ounce wheat, corn or bran flakes with ¼ cup raisins
1 cup skim milk

Lunch
Whole-wheat pita pocket bread stuffed with 1 cup mixture of raw
    Swiss chard, sliced tomatoes, shredded lettuce, sliced avocado
    and 2 diced hard-boiled eggs, dressed with mustard
1 cup vegetable soup
1 medium orange

Dinner
1 cup cooked pasta with ½ cup chick-peas and ½ cup tomato sauce,
    sprinkled with 1 ounce shredded low-fat mozzarella cheese
1 slice whole-wheat bread or a whole-wheat roll (spread with mar-
    garine, fruit jelly or fruit butter, if desired)
½ cup mixed steamed broccoli and carrots
1 medium pear

Snack
2 oatmeal cookies

AN EASY TRANSITION

If you'd like to try a vegetarian diet, here's some advice on making a smooth transition.

Jump in—or pace yourself. If you're the type who likes to make big changes all in one fell swoop, you can switch to a vegetarian diet overnight, says Dr. Frank. But if you like gradual transitions, take it slow.

Go slow. If you're used to eating a lot of refined foods, such as white bread, lunchmeat and chips, take it slow, suggests Dr. Deskins. Unlike most vegetarian fare, refined foods are low in fiber. Abruptly increasing your fiber intake may cause intestinal gas and bloating. By slowly increasing your consumption of high-fiber whole grains, legumes, seeds and nuts, you're less likely to feel uncomfortable, she says.

Start with a couple of meatless days each week. If you're accustomed to planning your menus around meat, get used to two meatless meals a week, then move to three and beyond, suggests Suzanne Havala, R.D., registered dietitian in Charlotte, North Carolina, and nutrition adviser to the Vegetarian Resource Group.

Make your favorite foods—without meat. Stumped for meatless meal ideas? "Make a list of meatless dishes that you already eat, like baked beans or pasta with tomato sauce, and make those more often," Havala suggests. Other popular options include vegetarian chili, meatless lasagna and pizza with mushrooms, onions and peppers instead of sausage or pepperoni.

Substitute. To diversify, start substituting vegetarian versions for other favorites. Trade veggie burgers for beef patties, soy franks for hot dogs, bean burritos for the beefy variety, "soysage" for sausage, and pasta with tomato and basil sauce for linguine bolognese, Dr. Mangels suggests.

Prepare dishes without fat. A vegetarian diet isn't automatically low in fat or cholesterol. Look for low-fat and nonfat cheese, tofu and tempeh and fat-free mayonnaise and other spreads. Don't fry your food—bake, broil and steam instead, says Dr. Mangels.

Go easy on nuts. Nuts, seeds and nut butters are good sources of protein, but they're also high in fat, so eat them in moderation, Dr. Deskins says. Use no more than two tablespoons of peanut butter on your sandwich. Eating nuts? Call it quits after a quarter-cup.

Avoid junk food. Loading up on baked goods, chips and sweet treats will pack on extra fat and calories, canceling some of the benefits of a vegetarian diet. So limit junk food, says Dr. Mangels.

VISION TRAINING
"Eye-Robics" for Tired Eyes

You might have eyes like a hawk, and the only glasses you need are the ones you pour your orange juice into every morning. But visit an optometrist's office who performs vision training (sometimes called vision therapy), and you may discover that your eyes aren't as picture perfect as you thought.

Glance into the cheiroscope, which resembles a microscope with two lenses instead of one. Through the lenses, you see a picture of an elephant you're supposed to trace.

No problem, right? Surprise: As you peer through the binocular lenses, which force each eye to work on its own, you keep losing sight of the elephant's outline. In fact, even the pencil point with which you're trying to draw seems to disappear.

That's because in order for your drawing to line up with the picture, *both* eyes have to do their thing. But optometrists who practice vision therapy say that often, one eye "shuts down" without you ever knowing it—mainly because the brain sees the information it's receiving as conflicting—and your other eye takes over, resulting in eyestrain and headaches, says Glen Steele, O.D., chief of pediatrics and vision therapy service at Southern College of Optometry in Memphis.

Correcting problems like that—known as suppression—is what vision therapy is all about.

"We're changing the way people go about trying to see," says Dr. Steele. "Not only that but also how they use the information that comes in. If your brain can't use the information, it shuts down."

TRAIN YOUR EYES TO SEE BETTER

Although optometrists often work with children who have problems like crossed eyes or wandering or lazy eye, adults have other, sometimes more subtle, issues to deal with. Optometrists report that a common adult problem is convergence insufficiency, in which the eyes either can't align themselves properly or are unable to sustain that alignment. The result, they say, is often blurry close-up vision or occasional double vision that many people write off as tired eyes.

So how do optometrists remedy these problems? Some use vision therapy, also called visual training, or a series of prescribed visual tasks to help you relearn effective seeing skills, says Stephen Miller, O.D., director of the Clinical Care Center of the American Optometric Association in St. Louis.

You do these tasks for an hour or two a week in the optometrist's office along with some additional eye exercises at home for anywhere from three to nine months—depending on your condition—under the guidance of an optometrist who's skilled in vision therapy.

"It's not a remedy for people who've been wearing glasses all their lives," says Dr. Miller. "But it helps with eye focusing and coordination. A 30-year-old woman may be able to see okay to drive to work in the morning, for example. But any extra stress on the eyes during the day may cause eyestrain, discomfort and blurred vision. Vision training can enhance eye coordination and focusing skills to a point where the eyes work more comfortably and efficiently."

A COMPUTER-AGE PROBLEM

Back in the days when we were hunters and gatherers, survival depended on being able to spot game at great distances. But in this computer age, almost all of our tasks are within 15 inches of our faces, says Arthur Seiderman, O.D., director of the Vision Development Center in Norristown, Pennsylvania, and author of *20/20 Is Not Enough: The New World of Vision.*

On top of that, gazing into a computer screen all day is extra-hard on the eyes, says Dr. Seiderman. And it's something that women especially have to worry about, he says. "Your eyes can compensate for vision problems up to a point. But lots of women who've rejoined the work force after taking a few years off to raise their little ones discover that they've lost the ability to compensate for visual problems. In fact, it's hard to imagine anyone putting in four to six hours on the computer who *doesn't* have a visual problem."

The fact that your eyeglass prescription gets stronger and stronger as you get older has a lot to do with environmental demands, says Mark Greenberg, O.D., chairman of the sports vision section of the American Optometric Association in Pearl River, New York. Working at a computer causes the eye's focusing muscles to lock in, which means they can't relax.

So you need stronger and stronger corrective lenses.

"Wearing stronger glasses corrects the symptom and not the problem," says Dr. Greenberg. "What you need to do, and what visual training can help you with, is learn to relax those focusing muscles."

The effect of all that close-up work on your eyes could go unnoticed, Dr. Seiderman notes. "It causes subtle focusing problems that might keep you from being able to concentrate on reading. I'm sure nine out of ten people realize that they're fatigued but don't connect the problem to their eyes."

HOW TRAINING CAN HELP

Many vision skills are actually developed as you grow, in the same way you learn to stand, walk and run, says Dr. Miller. Not everyone's eyes have the same focusing and eye coordination abilities.

To a certain extent, how well you see is determined by genetics. After all, if both your parents were nearsighted, you have a much greater chance of needing glasses yourself, says Dr. Steele. But vision therapy can help you to see better with or without glasses and reduce eyestrain and fatigue, especially in men and women who work at computers.

"The eye muscles are like any other muscles in the body in that they can be enhanced and strengthened," says Dr. Greenberg.

The kind of training you get in vision therapy varies, depending on what's wrong with your eyes, says Dr. Seiderman. But the real focus is on getting both eyes to work as a team. That means doing routines in which each eye works alone in order to equalize their skills, doing routines that work the two eyes at the same time but separately to eliminate the problem of the brain rejecting the messages of one eye, and doing routines in which both eyes work together, he says.

In one session, for example, you might follow moving targets with one or both eyes. Or you might look through an instrument with each eye seeing a different picture to help you relearn to use the eyes together again. By using different power lenses that force the eye to change focus, the eye develops new and more efficient means of focusing or refocusing, says Dr. Miller.

FOCUSING ON SELF-HELP

Although vision training should be done under the direction of an optometrist, you may wish to use the following general vision therapy eye exercises at home.

Do a pencil push-up. A good exercise for dealing with eye coordination (convergence) problems, where the eyes have a hard time working together to look at close objects, is the pencil push-up, notes Dr. Miller. Hold a pencil vertically at arm's length directly in front of your face and slightly below eye level. Gradually bring the pencil closer and closer to your nose.

At some point, you should see two pencils, says Dr. Miller. If the "double vision" doesn't occur until the pencil is almost to the nose, you probably don't have a convergence problem. But some people may see double at five or six inches from their nose. "If that's the case, relax your eyes by looking at something across the room, then look back at the tip of the pencil, which should still be near your nose, and try to be able to see just one. Then move it out to arm's length and bring it in again," he says. Repeat this for about 10 to 15 minutes.

"Over several days or weeks, you should be able to gradually bring the

Getting**Started**

Vision Training

Vision training, also known as vision therapy, should be done under the direction of a licensed optometrist. But not all optometrists provide vision-training services. The following information will help guide you in your search.

Number of practitioners in the United States: Approximately 2,500.

Qualifications to look for: Consult a Doctor of Optometry (O.D.). Although not required, optometrists practicing vision training may be members of the College of Optometrists in Vision Development (COVD). Members considered fellows in this organization must have more than 200 hours of postdoctoral continuing education in vision training, pass a qualifying exam and continue to earn 30 additional hours of education per year. Some optometrists have vision-training technicians in their offices to assist them in providing services.

Professional associations: College of Optometrists in Vision Development (COVD), P.O. Box 285, Chula Vista, CA 91912.

To find a practitioner: Contact either COVD or the Optometric Extension Program Foundation (OEP), 1912 East Carnegie Avenue, Suite 3-L, Santa Ana, CA 92705.

Approximate cost: $40 to $160 per hour, depending on where you live, what type of training you are receiving (group therapy or one-on-one) and the length of the session.

pencil closer each time until it's almost to your nose before you see two," he says.

Practice with an ice cream stick. You can use an ice cream stick (like a Popsicle stick) to work on improving peripheral vision, which is the vision that goes out to each side, notes Dr. Greenberg. "Take an ice cream stick and draw a little letter on it. Move your left arm out as far as you can to the side while still being able to read the letter on the stick without turning your head," he says. Then switch the stick to your right hand and try to hold it as far to the side as you can while still reading the letter. Alternate right and left, for about four minutes total. Practice a couple of times a week, and you should eventually see an improvement in your peripheral vision, says Dr. Greenberg.

Take a thumbnail view of TV. To further stimulate peripheral vision, select an action-filled show like a sporting event on television, suggests Dr. Seiderman. Position your chair so that when your arm is extended, your thumb is 12 inches from the screen. Hold your arm straight out in front of you with your thumb up. Keep your eyes focused on your thumb while trying to be aware of the action on either side of it. Do this for two minutes. Repeat a couple of times a week.

Read the writing on the wall. Instead of staring nonstop into a computer screen, give your eyes a focusing break, suggests Dr. Greenberg. "Take two pieces of paper—one with written material held at a distance of 16 inches and one with newspaper headlines posted about 20 feet away," he says. Then, to help strengthen your focusing abilities, read the paper at a distance of 16 inches and then look over at the paper that is posted 20 feet away. Repeat this exercise, shifting your focus from near to far, for about three minutes using both eyes. Repeat at least once every hour or so while working at a computer screen. When you can do this easily, change the distance of the paper you hold in your hand from 16 inches to 13 inches, then 10 and then 7.

Nose in on the news. Another focusing exercise is to take a newspaper or magazine, hold it at normal reading distance and then gradually move it closer until the print blurs, notes Dr. Miller. Then look at something across the room and back at the newspaper again. Try to see the print clearly. Repeat for about five minutes, two or three times a day.

Stretch your eye muscles. Another convenient way to take a break from the computer is to stand and stare out the window toward something in the distance, notes Dr. Greenberg. Or, if your work station has no windows, look toward each of the four corners of a nearby wall, without moving your head. Do this clockwise first, then counterclockwise. "That really stretches the eyes," he says. "Do it with your eyes open and then closed, to get the feeling of a real stretch while really relaxing the eyes."

VITAMIN AND MINERAL THERAPY
Nutritional Weapons against Disease

As far back as Cleopatra's day, people realized that they could prevent and treat different health problems by eating certain foods. The ancient Egyptians, for instance, ate liver to ward off night blindness. Fifth-century Chinese sailors grew potted ginger aboard their ships and nibbled on the shoots to steer clear of scurvy, a disease marked by loose teeth and bleeding gums.

It wasn't until the early twentieth century, though, that researchers discovered special substances in foods that prevent and cure the likes of scurvy. That potentially fatal disease turned out to be the result of too little vitamin C, a nutrient plentiful in ginger shoots. And night blindness? A nasty consequence of insufficient vitamin A, a nutrient abundant in liver.

Over time, scientists put together everything they knew about the vitamins and minerals women, men and children need to ward off severe deficiency. In 1943, the Food and Nutrition Board of the National Academy of Sciences established a dietary standard known as the Recommended Dietary Allowances (RDAs).

WHY "AVERAGE" ISN'T GOOD ENOUGH

Glance at any cereal box—or just about any packaged food—and you'll notice that the vitamin and mineral contents are listed as percentages of Daily Values (DVs), not RDAs. Daily Values are essentially the recommended amounts needed by the general population, ages four and up, to ensure adequate nutrition. Daily Values are easier to use when referring to people in general, not individuals. They're less precise than the RDAs.

Take, for example, your need for calcium, a mineral essential for healthy bones. The Daily Value for calcium, for the population as a whole, is 1,000 milligrams a day. The RDA for women over the age of 25 is lower—800 milligrams of calcium a day. For pregnant or nursing women, it's considerably more—1,200 milligrams a day. So for women, the RDAs are more meaningful than Daily Values.

THE CASE FOR MORE

The RDAs serve as benchmarks—guides to assessing the nutritional value of foods in terms of what men, women and children need to avoid nutritional deficiency. As new information evolves, the board periodically revises their recommendations.

As a tool for combating nutritional deficiency, the RDAs are adequate, says Shari Lieberman, Ph.D., clinical nutritionist and certified nutrition specialist in New York City and co-author of *The Real Vitamin and Mineral Book*. "But a growing number of studies suggest that to stay truly healthy, we need doses of most vitamins and minerals that are higher than the RDAs. The RDAs won't ensure optimal health for women," she adds emphatically.

Like-minded nutritionists, physicians and researchers agree. The RDAs are high enough to prevent the kind of extreme deficiency that can lead, in a relatively short time, to diseases like scurvy.

But many of the allowances aren't high enough to prevent less pronounced deficiencies that can slowly and surreptitiously trigger the physiological changes that lead to cancer and degenerative disorders such as heart disease, they warn.

Doses that are higher than the RDA can help prevent and also help treat a wide range of common health problems, says Michael Janson, M.D., director of the Center for Preventive Medicine in Barnstable, Massachusetts, and author of *The Vitamin Revolution in Health Care*.

Evidence suggests that beyond-RDA doses of certain vitamins and minerals can prevent and treat fatigue, depression, diabetes, asthma, infections, allergies, osteoporosis and arthritis, Dr. Janson says. Minerals for which there is no RDA, like chromium, may help prevent or treat diabetes.

Evidence also suggests that, in addition to vitamins and minerals, other protective nutrients may help a number of health problems unique to women, such as premenstrual syndrome, menstrual cramps and menopausal symptoms, among others. For example, the Food and Nutrition Board has yet to establish RDAs for bioflavonoids—plant compounds found in fruits and vegetables—but studies show that bioflavonoids can help to cool menopausal hot flashes, guard against heart disease and prevent breast cancer, says Dr. Janson.

ANTIOXIDANTS TO THE RESCUE

The best documented benefits of vitamin and mineral therapy are reduced risks of heart disease and cancer. Numerous studies suggest that higher doses of carotenes (some of which your body converts into vitamin A), vitamins C and E, the mineral selenium and other assorted plant compounds can help protect you from both. Collectively, these protective nutrients are known as antioxidants.

Antioxidants come to the rescue by disarming toxic molecules called free radicals, Dr. Janson explains. Free radicals are the unstable by-products of all sorts of chemical reactions. Industrial manufacturing often produces free radical–generating molecules. So do normal physiological and metabolic processes that take place inside our bodies.

Like the proverbial bull in a china shop, unstable free radicals damage any cells that they come in contact with. Widespread damage can accelerate aging at the cellular level, promote the buildup of plaque that clogs the arteries to our hearts, damage cell membranes and DNA and lead to cancer.

At levels higher than the RDA, antioxidants seem to protect cells from free radical damage. For example, the RDA for women for vitamin C is 60 milligrams. For vitamin E, the RDA for women is 12 international units. And there is no RDA for beta-carotene. But consider: A study conducted in the United States suggests that beyond-the-RDA doses of vitamin E can protect women against heart disease. The Nurses Health Study, an ongoing study of 87,000 women, found that women who'd been taking 100 international units of vitamin E daily—eight times the RDA—were 34 percent less likely to have heart attacks than women who didn't take supplements.

As for the role of antioxidants in cancer protection, the evidence is equally promising.

- Several population studies have found that women who average 300 milligrams of vitamin C daily—five times the RDA—reduce their risk of breast cancer by 30 percent.
- In a Latin American study, women who consumed more than 300 milligrams of vitamin C daily ran a 31 percent lower risk of cervical cancer than women with intakes of less than 153 milligrams.
- In an Iowa study, women who averaged 66 international units of vitamin E daily had one-third the risk of colon cancer of women who averaged 36 international units.

Over-the-RDA doses of antioxidants have been shown to ease and prevent debilitating health problems, such as osteoarthritis, as well. A Boston University Medical Center study found that high vitamin C intake can slow the progression of osteoarthritis by helping prevent the loss of cartilage in joints. Moderate to high doses of vitamin C ranging from 141 to 2,319 milligrams also appear to reduce knee pain. But proceed with caution: Doses of vitamin C higher than 1,200 milligrams can cause diarrhea in some people.

Research suggests that antioxidants can also help treat adult-onset diabetes. If you have diabetes, your cells have trouble using glucose, the simple sugar that serves as your body's primary fuel. There are two types of diabetes. With Type I, which usually appears in childhood, your body produces little or no insulin, the hormone that ushers glucose from your bloodstream into your cells where it can be used. With Type II, which usually appears in adulthood, your body produces insulin, but your cells refuse to accept insulin or the accompanying glucose. Shut out of your cells, glucose builds up in your bloodstream. Glucose buildup can damage your blood vessels, nerves, kidneys and eyes, leading to kidney failure, loss of vision and other problems.

Vitamin E may help women with diabetes, however. In an Italian study, men and women with Type II diabetes who took 900 milligrams of vitamin E daily (112 times the RDA) were able to use glucose more efficiently. After four months of supplementation, tests showed that their cells were more receptive to insulin and allowed more glucose inside. Talk to your doctor before taking high amounts of Vitamin E.

Chromium, an essential mineral for which there's no RDA, also appears to improve glucose tolerance in women with diabetes and lower levels of artery-clogging cholesterol, says Dr. Lieberman. She recommends 200 to 400 micrograms of chromium daily if you have high cholesterol, and sometimes more if you have diabetes. It's a good idea, however, to first consult your doctor about this approach, if you'd like to explore it. If she consents to giving it a try, she may need to adjust any medication that you've been prescribed.

B VITAMINS GET HIGH MARKS

Ranking with antioxidants in the benefits department are folic acid and vitamin B_6. In a Canadian study, people who had high intake of vitamin B_6 or folic acid had lower risks of heart disease and heart attack. Studies suggest that a high daily dose of the B vitamin folic acid can also help prevent cervical dysplasia, abnormal changes in the cells in the opening to your uterus. These changes may lead to cervical cancer.

Folate seems to boost resistance to the human papillomavirus, the most common cause of cervical dysplasia. In a University of Alabama study, women with low levels of folate who were infected with the virus, which is sexually transmitted, were five times more likely to develop dysplasia than women who had plenty of folate in their bloodstream. The RDA for folic acid is 400 micrograms for expectant mothers (it helps prevent birth defects) and 180 micrograms for everyone else.

If you suffer from migraines, riboflavin—another B vitamin—may help, says Alan Gaby, M.D., professor of therapeutic nutrition at Bastyr University in Seattle and author of *Every Woman's Essential Guide to Preventing and Reversing Osteoporosis*. The RDA for riboflavin is 1.3 milligrams. In one study, migraine sufferers who took 400 milligrams of riboflavin a day experienced two-thirds fewer debilitating headaches.

BEYOND THE RDAs

Considering the evidence, Dr. Lieberman, Dr. Janson and others say that to get truly protective amounts of vitamins, minerals and other nutrients, you need to take supplements.

Getting even the generally accepted requirement of certain vitamins and minerals from food alone can be difficult, even for people who choose their foods carefully, says Dr. Janson. Consuming protective amounts is harder still.

To consume enough vitamin E to protect yourself from heart disease—400 international units, according to some studies—you'd have to finish off 40 cups of almonds, a rich source of vitamin E, Dr. Janson says. So supplements of vitamins and minerals in pill form are a convenient way to bridge the gap.

A STARTER PLAN FOR PREVENTION

That said, it's hard to say precisely how much higher than the RDA you should go. Some studies, for example, suggest that 100 international units of vitamin E will help keep heart attacks at bay. Others suggest that 800 international units is appropriate.

Why the discrepancy? In part, what's considered ideal for one woman isn't necessarily the ideal dose for another, says Dr. Gaby. Differences in genetic makeup, health status and lifestyle create different needs. Women with diabetes, for instance, seem to need more vitamin E to protect their hearts than do women who don't have diabetes, explains Dr. Lieberman.

The differences don't end there. Research suggests that if you take birth control pills, you'll need more folic acid than women who don't take the

Pill. And if you're pregnant, Dr. Gaby says, you'll need more vitamin B_6, along with up to 1,000 extra milligrams of calcium and up to 500 extra milligrams of magnesium. "Evidence suggests that those nutrients, in higher amounts, help prevent pregnancy-induced high blood pressure," he says. (If you have heart or kidney problems, check with your doctor before taking magnesium supplements.)

You also need to consider your environment. If you live in midtown Manhattan, you'll need more of vitamins E and C than women living in the country, says Dr. Lieberman. "Research shows that people who live in polluted environments need more antioxidants," she points out.

To design your basic vitamin and mineral regimen, follow these guidelines.

Take three-or-more-a-day multis. You can meet most of your needs easily and conveniently with a good multivitamin/mineral supplement, says Dr. Gaby. Look for a multi that gives you 10 to 20 times the RDA of the B vitamins, 500 to 1,000 milligrams of vitamin C, 200 to 400 international units of vitamin E and at least 500 milligrams of calcium and 300 milligrams of magnesium, he says.

Standard one-a-day multis are too small to give you everything that you need, says Dr. Gaby. You'll have to choose a multiple-dose multivitamin/mineral supplement—one that you take three to six times a day. You can find them in health food stores.

Supplement your supplement. Even the best multiple-dose multi won't give you everything that you need. Unless your doctor advises you otherwise, shoot for at least 600 to 1,200 milligrams of calcium and 300 to 600 milligrams of magnesium daily, Dr. Gaby says. If your multi gives you 600 milligrams of each, make up the difference with individual supplements plus calcium- and magnesium-rich foods such as leafy greens, yogurt and almonds. The RDA for women for magnesium is 280 milligrams—less than half that for calcium. But research suggests that unless otherwise indicated by your doctor, you're better off taking just as much magnesium as calcium, he explains.

Dr. Lieberman agrees. "Taking a lot of calcium every day without sufficient magnesium can induce a magnesium deficiency, which may raise your risk of osteoporosis and heart disease, too."

Consider natural supplements. Some evidence indicates that your body can more easily absorb and use naturally occurring vitamin E than synthetic vitamin E. Dr. Lieberman recommends natural brands primarily because they're less likely to contain artificial dyes and additives.

Check the expiration date on the bottle. Supplements lose their potency over time. Most supplements keep for three years unopened and for one year once they are opened. To keep vitamins and minerals from deteriorating, store supplements in a cool, dry, dark place, Dr. Lieberman says.

Take your supplements with food. Supplements are best absorbed and less likely to upset your stomach when taken with food, says Dr. Janson. He suggests that you take a third of your vitamins and minerals with breakfast, a third with lunch and a third with dinner.

Don't substitute pills for food. Advocates of vitamin and mineral therapy say that even if you take supplements, you need to pay attention to

Getting**Started**

Vitamin and Mineral Therapy

"Taking vitamins and minerals isn't a substitute for medical care," says Michael Janson, M.D., director of the Center for Preventive Medicine in Barnstable, Massachusetts, and author of *The Vitamin Revolution in Health Care*. "It should complement medical care. Before starting a supplement program, check with your doctor. Some medications can interfere with vitamin and mineral absorption. And some supplements can affect your need for certain drugs." Your doctor may need to advise you on what vitamins or minerals to take and in what quantities, and monitor you. Or your doctor may refer you to a nutritionist for that kind of advice.

But whether you get advice on supplements from your doctor or from a nutritionist, ask her to explain the rationale behind her recommendations, says Shari Lieberman, Ph.D., clinical nutritionist and certified nutrition specialist in New York City and co-author of *The Real Vitamin and Mineral Book*. "The person you see should be able to explain why they're recommending a particular dose and cite the research on which the doses are based."

Here's how to locate a professional qualified to give nutritional advice.

Number of practitioners in the United States: Unknown.

Qualifications to look for: Doctor of Medicine (M.D.), Doctor of Osteopathy (D.O.), Doctor of Naturopathy (N.D.) or Certified Nutrition Specialist (C.N.S.).

Professional associations: American Association of Naturopathic Physicians, 2366 Eastlake Avenue East, Suite 322, Seattle, WA 98102; American Holistic Medical Association, 4101 Lake Boone Trail, Suite 201, Raleigh, NC 27607; American Preventive Medical Association, 459 Walker Road, Great Falls, VA 22066.

To find a practitioner: Contact one of the professional associations listed above. They each charge a $5 fee for this information.

Approximate cost: $80 to $300 per session, depending on where you live.

your diet. They emphasize that you should include at least five servings of vegetables and fruits daily. Besides vitamins and minerals, nutritious food supplies other critical nutrients—protein, carbohydrates and essential fatty acids—best supplied by food, not pills.

A diet that includes fruits and vegetables also supplies hundreds of other plant compounds, known as phytochemicals, that researchers believe may be as crucial to health as the vitamins and minerals listed on your cereal box. (One family of protective nutrients, the carotenoids, includes 500 members.) While a handful of these protective nutrients are available in supplement form, others are still available only in plant foods like fruits, vegetables and grains. Also, new phytochemicals are discovered every year, so you'll be ahead of the game if you rely on plant compounds for these nutrients.

CUSTOMIZING YOUR SUPPLEMENT PROGRAM

Depending on your family medical history, your personal health status and your lifestyle, you may want to take extra amounts of certain vitamins or minerals, Dr. Lieberman says. Talk to a nutritionist or your doctor for advice on how vitamins and minerals best fit into your life.

Consider antioxidants. Dr. Janson recommends extra antioxidants for most women. He suggests 25,000 international units of mixed carotenoids and 2,000 milligrams of mixed bioflavonoids.

Don't go overboard. Excessively high doses of certain vitamins and minerals can be toxic. For example, doses of vitamin B_6 higher than 62 times the RDA of 1.6 milligrams can cause unstable gait and numb feet. Doses of vitamin A higher than 10,000 international units are not advised for pregnant women. Excessive amounts have caused birth defects.

Consult a professional. "I don't think people should run off and pop the latest pill they've read about," says Dr. Gaby. "Instead, consult a professional."

Not all doctors are convinced that all women need to take supplements or higher-than-RDA doses of vitamins and minerals. But the number of converts is growing. At one gathering of cardiologists, says Dr. Gaby, a good 70 percent of the doctors raised their hands when asked if they took vitamin E. At one time, he says, they would have laughed at the notion.

Not only are M.D.'s taking supplements, and particularly antioxidants, they're also recommending them for their patients, Dr. Lieberman says. "More than 90 percent of my clients are referred to me by physicians."

Know your medical history. Evidence suggests that vitamin or mineral therapy can benefit a growing list of health conditions. But determining the right dosage requires an accurate diagnosis and sometimes a blood test.

A case in point is iron, a mineral needed to form hemoglobin, the substance that helps your red blood cells transport oxygen from your lungs to the rest of your body. Women who have iron-deficiency anemia may need extra iron before menopause because we lose some when we menstruate. Women also need extra iron while they're pregnant, to nourish the developing fetus. After menopause, though, our iron needs drop, says Dr. Janson. In fact, several studies suggest that excess iron may contribute to heart disease before and after menopause.

The RDAs for iron take these changes into account and will meet most women's needs, says Dr. Janson. So you shouldn't take more than the RDA unless your doctor tells you to, he advises.

Folic acid is another example. In one study, 47 women with cervical dysplasia saw significant improvement after taking 10,000 micrograms a day for three months, notes Dr. Gaby. So he recommends up to 10,000 micrograms of folic acid a day if you have, or are at risk of, dysplasia. But high doses of folic acid can hide symptoms of a form of anemia that can lead to permanent nerve damage. So you shouldn't take doses higher than 400 micrograms without medical supervision.

If you have kidney stones, ask your doctor before taking extra vitamin C, since high doses of the vitamin can aggravate the condition, says Chris Meletis, doctor of naturopathy and clinic director, chief medical officer and medicinary director at the National College of Naturopathic Medicine in Portland, Oregon.

Also, in some people, high doses of vitamin C can cause diarrhea. If that happens to you, lower your dose, says Adriane Fugh-Berman, M.D., former head of field investigations for the Office of Alternative Medicine at the National Institutes of Health in Bethesda, Maryland. If you have diarrhea, it means that you're taking too much, she says.

Use caution with medications. With some medications there may be a limit on the amount of a vitamin or mineral you should take. For example, taking 100 international units or more of vitamin E thins the blood, says Dr. Fugh-Berman. So if you're taking blood-thinning drugs, you need to limit your intake of vitamin E. Also, people on blood thinners must be sure not to overdo it with too much vitamin K or any other fat-soluble vitamins.

Separate supplements and prescription drugs. Iron supplements will interact with certain prescription drugs in ways that may prevent their absorption. Iron supplements will keep your body from properly absorbing thyroid drugs, for instance, says Jacob Teitelbaum, M.D., clinician and researcher on the treatment of chronic fatigue syndrome at Anne Arundel Medical Center in Annapolis, Maryland, and author of *From Fatigued to Fantastic!* If you take your medications in the morning and at night, take iron supplements around lunchtime, he suggests.

YOGA
Fitness with a Twist

Started as a spiritual discipline 6,000 years ago in India, the practice of yoga has newly emerged as a powerful remedy for ailments ranging from menstrual cramps to rashes and from mood swings to varicose veins, making it a valuable healing tool for women.

And don't worry—you don't have to contort your body into awkward positions to practice yoga. In a typical yoga routine, you clear your mind, breathe deeply and gently ease yourself into different poses.

After an hour, you feel renewed—almost as if you've done an aerobic workout. The result is better posture, increased flexibility and a host of other benefits, without the sweat and jolting of your joints and bones.

"Anybody can do yoga," says Carrie Angus, M.D., medical director for the Center for Health and Healing at the Himalayan International Institute of Yoga Science and Philosophy in Honesdale, Pennsylvania. "A beginner doesn't need to put her foot behind her head or twist herself into a pretzel. So don't worry that it will be too demanding."

Yoga is more than just a physical experience, emphasizes Larry Payne, Ph.D., director of the Samata Yoga Center in Los Angeles and chairman of the International Association of Yoga Therapists. "It quiets the distractions of the mind, so it's very good for relieving stress and improving concentration."

Yoga is more popular now than ever, says Dr. Payne. In fact, he says, more people in the state of California are doing hatha yoga, based on poses and breathing techniques, than in the entire country of India.

"Yoga is the mind-body fitness for the 1990s," he says. "It was the original non–impact aerobics—the original mind-body workout."

FINDING YOUR INNER PEACE

The term *yoga* comes from the Sanskrit word meaning "to yoke"—joining the mind and body together, says Richard C. Miller, Ph.D., a yoga instructor and psychologist in San Rafael, California, co-founder of the

International Association of Yoga Therapists and founder of the Marin School of Yoga. "Some people interpret yoga as the union of different forces or energies," he says.

In India, the sage Patanjali compiled the following yoga sutras, or eight steps to spiritual enlightenment.

1. Physical practice of a wide range of yoga poses, or postures
2. Breath control
3. Focusing the senses (sight, sound, touch, taste and smell)
4. Concentration
5. Meditation
6. Cleansing disciplines like cleaning, washing and bathing
7. Moral practices like truth and nonviolence
8. Enlightenment (the culmination of all the steps)

Different branches of yoga may focus only on specific aspects, says Dr. Miller. For example, some kinds of yoga, such as Desikachar yoga, emphasize breathing, while others, such as Iyengar and Pattabhi Jois yoga, focus on physical poses.

The physical, spiritual and psychological aspects of yoga make it a useful therapy for health ailments, says Dr. Angus. Physically, yoga can build strength and improve flexibility because it stretches and strengthens the muscles, she says. It's good for the spine because it loosens the back and aids good posture, like correcting slumped, rounded shoulders. Correcting posture misalignment helps free the rib cage, allowing you to breathe more deeply. Dr. Angus says that this strengthens the body's ability to heal itself.

Yoga can also counteract negative emotions such as anger, anxiety and depression, says Dr. Angus.

"Doing yoga postures and concentrating on breathing is soothing and relaxing. And it gives you something else to focus on," says John Orr, an instructor of physical education at Duke University in Durham, North Carolina, and formerly an ordained Theravadin Buddhist monk who practiced in Thailand and India.

After people start doing yoga to relieve stress or physical problems, they gradually discover the deeper psychological benefits, says Orr. "In spending quiet time alone, you get to know yourself better. So yoga keeps you in touch with your physical, mental and spiritual self."

YOGA, FOR TOTAL HEALTH

"Tired of taking pills and tired of solutions that don't get to the root of the problem, more and more women are turning to yoga as a lasting solution," says Dr. Angus.

And practical, regular yoga can work wonders, says Lee Lipsenthal, M.D., medical director at the Preventive Medicine Research Institute in Sausalito, California. "It can lower risk of heart disease, high blood pressure and stroke."

To see what happens to a heart that's under stress, imagine this: You're sitting at your desk when suddenly you remember that tomorrow's deadline was bumped up to today. Inside, your adrenal gland releases adrenalin and other glucocorticoids—chemicals that increase blood flow to the skeletal muscle system, decrease blood to the internal organs and increase tone in the muscle of the blood vessel walls. The result: a higher likelihood that the artery will spasm and close, causing a heart attack.

The calm and well-being that yoga creates has been shown to counter that stress reaction, says Dr. Lipsenthal. "What we find is that with yoga, the heart disease begins to regress and blockages in the arteries shrink," he notes. "The goal is to get people to slow down, which in turn lowers their blood pressure and their heart rate."

And because of its emphasis on joint flexibility, yoga also has orthopedic benefits, says Dr. Lipsenthal. A joint is a place where two bones meet, bridged by muscles and tendons. "If the muscles are tight, the bones are more likely to rub together, but if they're loose, they have more freedom, less inflammation and less chance of injury."

SPECIAL BENEFITS FOR WOMEN

Because of yoga's effect on stress, it can help with conditions that have both psychological and physiological components, such as fibromyalgia (painful "trigger points" in the muscles), arthritis and migraine headaches, says Dr. Lipsenthal.

Women especially can benefit from yoga. It's claimed to ease the pain of premenstrual syndrome (PMS) as well as help ease the discomforts of pregnancy, childbirth and certain changes associated with menopause, such as hot flashes. Your doctor may be able to advise you on whether or not yoga can help, says Ramanand Patel, a senior instructor of Iyengar yoga at the Iyengar Yoga Institute in San Francisco.

"It is believed that breathing through your left nostril, for example, creates a cooling breath. This can be used to cool the system down and ease hot flashes," says Dr. Lipsenthal.

Also, evidence suggests that women who practice yoga are better off emotionally—less irritable and more congenial—than others. One study compared 12 women between the ages of 27 and 55 who did yoga postures, meditation and breathing exercises to 13 women who had no experience with relaxation exercises and who didn't do yoga exercises. The women who practiced yoga scored much better on self-tests designed to measure both positive emotions (such as euphoria) and negative emotions (such as excitability).

Although yoga has hundreds of poses, most routines contain about 20 different ones, with specific poses used to help specific ailments. Poses that emphasize sitting on the floor with your legs spread or lying on your back with your open legs up on the wall, can ease cramps and PMS, for example, says Dr. Angus.

Poses that focus on your pelvis help direct energy to the area and ease menstrual problems, she adds. Bloating, for example, is said to be caused by stagnation of bodily fluids in the pelvic cavity. When you stretch that area, you get fresh blood pumping to the underlying muscles and tissues.

Citing another example, Patel says that back bends help lift your spirits because they open the chest, while bending forward from a standing position can worsen depression because it causes the chest cavity to compress and restrict breathing.

Which routine of poses should you choose? It all depends on your physical problems, says Dr. Miller. "There would be a different one for women with back pain than for women with bladder problems," he says. "When teaching yoga, I always individualize the postures to each person in the class."

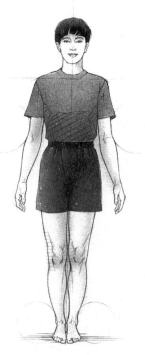

Mountain Pose

Stand with your feet close together so that the inner bones of your ankles touch and the edges of your big toes touch. Rock back on your heels and stretch the soles of your feet, then set your feet back down. Next, raise your heels to stretch your soles in the other direction.

Standing with your knees gently locked and your thighs lightly tightened, breathe normally. Keeping your back straight, tighten your buttocks and stomach muscles. Then lift your rib cage and arch your back slightly while pulling back your shoulders. Turn your upper arms out and reach down, with your palms facing the thighs, as shown. Hold your head up and face forward, with your neck straight. Hold the pose for 30 to 40 seconds, then relax. Repeat the pose once or twice.

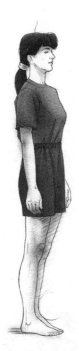

Note: If you ho
sure, consult ;
doing this pose.

To begin, stand in a position w...
your hands at your sides and your
feet together. Exhale.

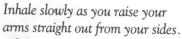

Inhale slowly as you raise your
arms straight out from your sides.

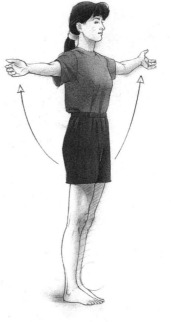

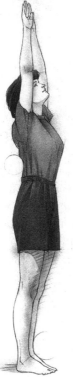

Continue raising your arms until
they meet, thumb to thumb, over
your head. Look up and gently
stretch.

(continued)

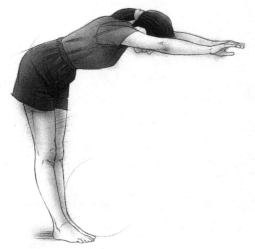

Begin to exhale as you bend forward from the hips. Continue
bending until you have
completely exhaled.

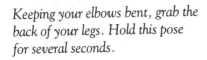

Keeping your elbows bent, grab the
back of your legs. Hold this pose
for several seconds.

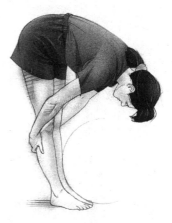

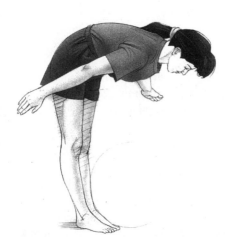

Inhale slowly as you let go of your
legs. Lift your body upright while
raising your arms to your sides and
over your head. Exhale and return
to the standing position. Repeat this
pose twice.

Windmill Pose

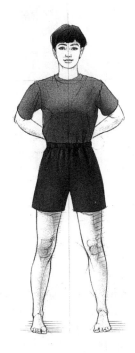

Note: If you have lower-back pain, use caution when doing this pose.

Start with your feet shoulder-width apart and your fingers spread on both sides of your spine to support your lower back. Your hands will stay there for the duration of the pose. Point your toes slightly inward.

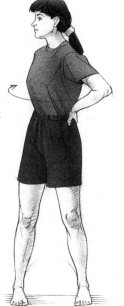

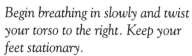

Begin breathing in slowly and twist your torso to the right. Keep your feet stationary.

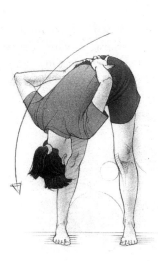

Bend forward at the waist while exhaling. Bring your forehead as close to your right knee as possible.

(continued)

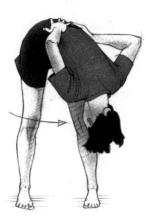

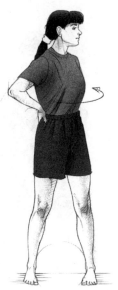

In one continuous motion, swing your head and torso slowly toward your left knee. Exhale completely by the time you reach this position.

Begin inhaling as you lift your torso and face left. Finish inhaling when you are in a standing position, as shown. Hold your breath and twist back to the right. Repeat the entire sequence six times, three times in each direction.

Corpse Pose

This pose requires little movement. You focus on the release of muscle tension. Lie on your back on a mat or the floor. Rest your arms at your sides with your palms facing up. Stretch your legs out straight with your feet in a relaxed position. (If you feel pain in your lower back as you do this pose, bend your legs by raising your knees and placing both feet flat on the floor and continue with the pose.) Hold this pose for 30 seconds to several minutes. Your eyes should be closed while you breathe deeply and concentrate on relaxing your muscles.

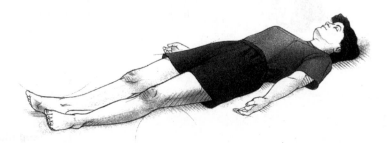

Head-to-Knee Pose

To begin, sit on the floor or a mat with your legs straight out in front of you with your feet together. Keep your torso, head and neck straight. Bend your left knee and slide your left foot toward your crotch, resting the sole of your foot as high on the inside of your right thigh as possible.

Lift your arms straight over your head as you take a deep breath, stretching as high as possible while you expand your chest. Bend forward as you begin to exhale, keeping your back straight and your head between your arms. Rest your hands on your right leg, making sure to keep the back of your right knee in contact with the ground. Relax, breathe normally and hold the position for five to ten seconds.

If you want to stretch farther, keep this same position and stretch forward from the base of your spine as you take a deep breath. When you exhale, try to bring your head as far as possible down to your right leg, then breathe normally and relax. Wait for five to ten seconds before you begin to inhale and lift your head, neck and back. As you straighten to the sitting position, keep your arms in line with your head. Breathe out and slowly lower your arms. Repeat the stretch with your left leg, then do this sequence two more times.

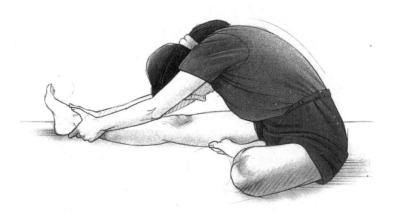

Spine Twist Pose

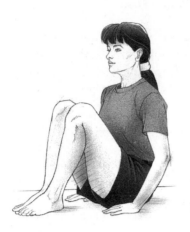

Note: If you have spinal disk problems, use extreme caution when attempting this pose, or skip it entirely.

Begin the spine twist by sitting on the floor or a mat with your knees drawn to your chest and your hands resting, palms down, on the floor on either side of your body.

With your left leg bent, as shown, lower your right leg to slide it under your left leg. Your right heel should be tucked in front of your left buttock. Your right knee should be touching the floor while you raise your left leg over it to place your left foot on the outside of your right knee.

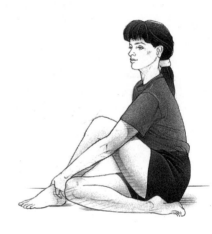

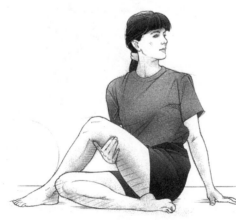

After straightening your spine and lifting your rib cage, twist to the left, as shown. Put your left hand behind your right foot and bring your right arm under your left leg to grab the back of your thigh. Turn your head and shoulders so that they are facing left.

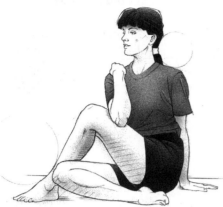

With your arm bent, place your right elbow on the outside of your left knee. Use your right elbow to rock your left knee back and forth a few times.

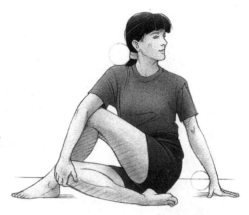

Pull your left leg as far to the right as you can and extend your right arm. Keep your right arm on the outside of your left leg and, depending on your level of flexibility, grab your right knee or left ankle.

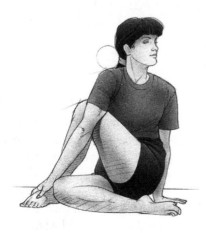

Be sure that your back is straight and your left hand is as close as possible to the base of your spine. Look forward and breathe in deeply. Slowly exhale as you gently twist your spine to the left. Turn your head also and look as far to the left as possible. Do not use your hands and arms to move your body farther. They should only be used for balance as you hold the pose and gently breathe for several seconds. Unwind, and repeat on the other side.

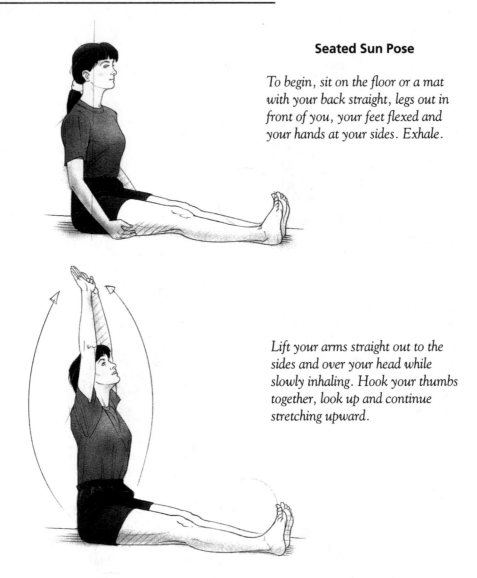

Seated Sun Pose

To begin, sit on the floor or a mat with your back straight, legs out in front of you, your feet flexed and your hands at your sides. Exhale.

Lift your arms straight out to the sides and over your head while slowly inhaling. Hook your thumbs together, look up and continue stretching upward.

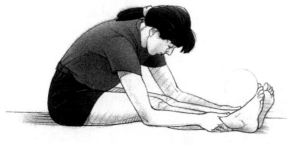

Exhale as you bend slowly forward from your hips, keeping your upper arms parallel to your jaw. With your elbows bent, grasp your ankles, as shown, and pull your torso toward your legs. (If you can't reach your ankles, grab your calves.) Hold for one or two seconds.

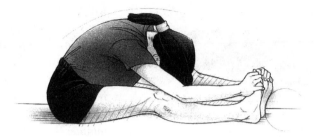

If you can, touch your toes, with your elbows bent, and hold for one to two seconds, keeping your thumbs on top of your big toes and your index fingers on the bottoms. Inhale slowly as you lift your chest back to the starting position. Start with your hands at your sides and then, as you inhale, lift your arms straight out and over your head again with your thumbs hooked together. Look up and stretch slowly, exhale and lower your arms. Repeat twice.

Baby Pose

Note: Do not do this pose if you have high blood pressure.

To begin, sit on the floor with your knees bent and your heels beneath your buttocks. Keeping the tops of your toes flat on the floor, let your arms hang freely at your sides.

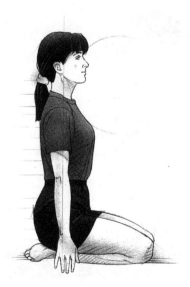

(continued)

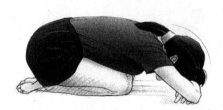

Slowly lean forward at the waist and rest your arms crossways on the floor in front of you. Rest your forehead on your forearms, as shown, keeping your neck straight and relaxed. Breathe normally and hold this position for up to five minutes.

Variation: If you have arthritis in your knees, vary this pose. Start by sitting in a chair with your hips pushed against the back of the chair and your feet flat on the floor and slightly apart. Then lean forward at the waist and let your head drop between your knees, keeping your neck straight and relaxed and letting your arms hang at your sides with your hands near your ankles.

Half-Boat Pose

Lie flat on your stomach with your arms out in front of you on the floor or a mat. Both your forehead and palms should be touching the floor. Keep your legs together, with your muscles completely relaxed.

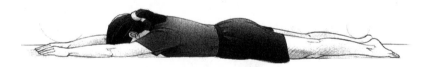

Slowly lift your arms, head and torso off the floor as you take a deep breath. Breathe evenly and keep your head between your arms at all times while you hold the pose for five seconds. Breathe out, lower your body back to the floor and relax. Repeat twice.

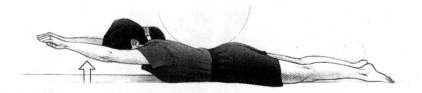

Return to the starting position and move your feet 12 to 18 inches apart, keeping your legs straight. Lift your legs and feet and keep your upper body and arms relaxed while you breathe in slowly. Hold the pose for five seconds while breathing evenly. Breathe out and slowly lower your legs back to the floor. Repeat this sequence twice.

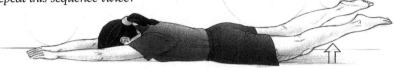

Cobra Pose

Lie facedown with your forehead and the tops of your toes touching the floor. Your palms should also be touching the floor with your hands placed on the ground next to your armpits.

Note: Avoid this pose if you are menstruating, have open wounds in the abdominal region or have undergone abdominal or pelvic surgery within the past several weeks.

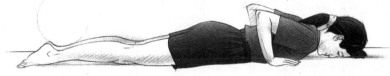

Look straight up as you inhale and lift your head slowly off the floor. Next, use your back muscles to lift your stomach and chest off the floor. As you rise, curl your spine and keep your hipbones on the floor at all times—don't try to push up with your arms. Close your mouth and jut your lower jaw forward to stretch your throat muscles. Keeping your elbows bent and your torso off the ground, as shown, hold the pose for several seconds. Then slowly lower your body back to the starting position, allowing your stomach to touch the ground first, followed by your chest and then forehead, while you exhale. Repeat twice.

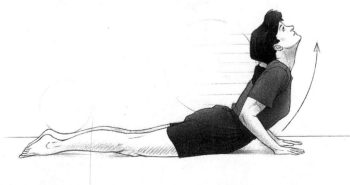

Butterfly Pose

Sitting on the floor or a mat, keep your back straight and draw the soles of your feet together and hold with both hands. Just like the wings of a butterfly, slowly raise and lower your knees several times.

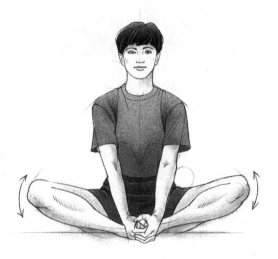

Gently stretch the muscles on the insides of your legs by slowly leaning forward from your hips. Hold this position for about two minutes while breathing normally and keeping your back straight. Each time you exhale, try to lean forward a little farther.

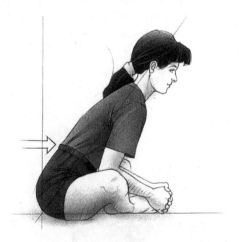

Menstral Cramp Pose

Lie on your back with your knees bent and your feet flat on the floor, spread apart. Hold your ankles firmly and arch your pelvis, as shown, as you inhale. Hold for a few seconds. Relax and lower your pelvis as you exhale. Repeat several times.

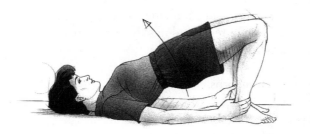

Premenstrual Syndrome Pose

Begin by lying facedown on the floor with your arms at your sides. Bring your feet up to your buttocks by bending your knees and grasp first one foot and then the other. (Flex your feet, if it makes them easier to reach.) Then lift your head, elevate your knees and then raise your trunk as far off the floor as possible as you inhale. While squeezing your buttocks, hold the pose for 10 to 15 seconds, imagining that your body looks like a gently curved bow.

To release the position, allow your chin to touch the floor first, then release your feet and slowly return to the original position. Repeat this pose five times.

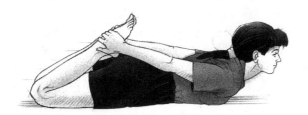

DEEP BREATHING: A REMEDY IN ITSELF

"Just relax and take a deep breath." Most of us have heard those words in times of maximum stress-ocity. But how often are you really making the most of each breath—drawing on oxygen supplies from deep in your diaphragm rather than in the shallow reaches of your chest?

One of the most important parts of yoga is how it teaches you to really breathe, notes Dr. Angus. "You learn to breathe with your diaphragm, which helps you relax and stimulates the part of the nervous system that calms us down," she notes. "And relaxing helps increase your immunity. It is incredibly healing."

Unfortunately, it's not as easy as you'd think. Most people breathe too fast, through their mouths, or not deeply enough, notes Dr. Miller. Instead, breathe through the nose, which filters and warms the air, and then let it out from your mouth. "You should use the whole rib cage as well as the abdomen and diaphragm," he says. "That kind of breathing helps distribute the body's vital energy throughout the body."

To get the most bang for your breath, take these tips from yoga experts.

Get down to basics. One neat way to learn how to breathe properly is to lie on your back on the floor with a book on your abdomen, notes Dr. Miller.

When you inhale, push up against the weight of the book and lift it. As you exhale, allow the book to drop down. The focus on raising and lowering the book will force you to breathe diaphragmatically. Try not to make the chest cavity expand, and put all the emphasis on the abdomen, Dr. Miller advises.

Try the hands-on method. Another way to make sure that you're taking abdominal breaths is to spread your fingers across your abdomen and stretch your thumbs toward your spine, says Dr. Miller. As you breathe, your abs should push out against your fingers and the back of your spine should expand as well.

Take your time. To work on making your breathing deeper and fuller, practice taking longer, slower breaths, suggests Dr. Miller. "Normal breathing is 8 to 12 breaths a minutes. I have people do between 4 and 8 breaths a minute," he says. "It's not unusual to be able to do just 2 in one minute."

By slowing down, the breath has time to enter all the spaces in the lung tissue so that the lungs have more air entering them, he notes.

Clear out the gunk. Learning to do a cleansing breath is a great way to clear out the body's toxins and breathe in more positive energy, says Dr. Angus.

"Lie on your back in the corpse pose (see page 316) and breathe so that your belly rises and falls," she says. As you exhale, she adds, "imagine breathing out from the top of your head and down your spine, then down to your legs and feet." When you inhale again, reverse the order so that you're breathing in through all those parts of your body—or at least imagine that you are.

Some people can exhale for nearly 20 seconds, while others can only do it for 6 seconds before they're gasping for breath, she says. Over time, your lungs increase their capacity and you can breathe out for longer and longer.

AN AT-HOME YOGA ROUTINE

Convinced that yoga is worth a try? Follow these directives from expert instructors.

Get an early start. You can do yoga at any time of the day, but Dr. Miller recommends doing it in the morning. "The effect lasts eight to ten hours, so you can enjoy it for the rest of the day."

Get comfortable. Using a mat, blanket, rug, cushion or chair, sit with your upper body erect but relaxed. Take a minute to check in mentally and put aside all the things that you've been thinking about.

Quiet your mind. Each yoga class begins and ends with a few minutes of quiet meditation to quiet your mind, Dr. Angus says. "It's about focusing the mind on one thing, like your breath or a word such as *peace* or *love*. In that stillness, you can have all kinds of revelations about what you need in life and what's true for you."

A quiet mind can help ease anxiety and depression. You come to realize that lots of things are uncontrollable and that you have to let go of what you can't control.

When clearing your mind for yoga, you should sit up either on the floor or in a chair, with your head, neck and trunk in a straight line, and take 10 to 15 deep breaths, says Dr. Angus.

Focus. Once your body starts to relax, focus on one sound or one object. "For example, think 'so' while you're breathing in and 'hum' as you breathe out. It takes patience, so if you can do it for one minute, you're doing great," says Dr. Angus. With practice, you will be able to focus your mind for longer and longer periods.

Don't make it difficult. Although classes usually run 60 to 90 minutes, a home yoga routine could be effective at 20 to 30 minutes, notes Dr. Miller.

After doing deep breathing for 2 to 3 minutes, do varying yoga poses, synchronized with deep breathing, for about 15 minutes. Repeat this three days a week.

Don't push yourself. In yoga, the philosophy of "no pain, no gain" just doesn't apply, says Dr. Miller. "Trying to do more than your body can handle is the way that people injure themselves," he says. "You should be listening to your body the whole time."

WANT MORE?

If you like what you experienced during the breathing exercise, you may want to try more yoga, maybe even a lot more. A class is usually the best

Getting**Started**

Yoga

If you'd like to learn yoga from an instructor, or your health care practitioner has recommended yoga for a specific health condition, here's how to locate instructors in your area.

Number of practitioners in the United States: Unknown.

Qualifications to look for: No national standards exist for yoga instruction. Training standards vary from school to school and range from intensive six-week courses to two-year programs. Most, however, average about 100 hours of training. Ask your instructor where she was trained and for how long.

Professional associations: American Yoga Association, 513 South Orange Avenue, Sarasota, FL 34236; International Association of Yoga Therapists, 20 Sunnyside Avenue, Suite A-243, Mill Valley CA 94941. Other sources: American Yoga College, P.O. Box 1746, Sedona, AZ 86339-1746; Himalayan International Institute of Yoga Science and Philosophy, R.R.1, Box 400, Honesdale, PA 18431.

To find a practitioner: Contact one of the professional associations listed above or consult a massage therapist or health care practitioner in your area. You can also check the Yellow Pages or the teacher's directory in the annual July/August issue of *Yoga Journal*.

Approximate cost: $25 per class, if you register for a series of classes at a yoga center. Some health clubs include yoga instruction with membership at no extra change.

way to go, says Dr. Miller. "A class provides a community that gives you a support system so that you'll want to practice at home when you don't go to class."

You can find yoga classes everywhere—at the local YMCA or at area fitness clubs, says Dr. Payne. It's a good idea to check out the class before you commit to it, says Dr. Payne. Here are some things to check for before making a commitment.

- A clean classroom
- Clear distinction between class levels
- A tone, or energy, from the instructor and exercises that fit your expectations
- A nonpressured environment where you won't be intimidated into doing postures with which you're not comfortable

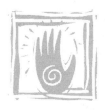

PART 3

PUT
NATURAL HEALING
TO WORK
FOR YOU

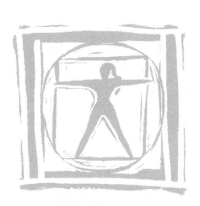

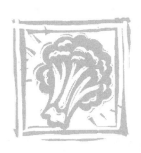

ALLERGIES

Make Peace with Hay Fever and Food Sensitivities

If you think of your body as a battleground on which a fight for your survival is constantly raging, then you're thinking just like your immune system does.

A network of specialized cells and the organs that produce them, your immune system maintains a continual search and destroy mission against alien organisms—viruses, bacteria, fungi and parasites. Its job, quite simply, is to get them before they get you.

WHEN YOUR INNER DEFENSE SYSTEM GOES HAYWIRE

Usually, the battle that your immune system wages against potentially harmful invaders is pretty efficient. But if you're one of many women with allergies, your immune system becomes just a little too efficient, and that's when trouble can ensue.

When your immune system takes aim against a harmless foreign substance like pollen, your body releases histamines and other chemicals that produce symptoms of an allergic response. Those symptoms can range from a little case of the sniffles to (less commonly) a full-blown, life-threatening, body-wide reaction called anaphylaxis, marked by breathing difficulties and a dangerous drop in blood pressure. Various foods, drugs, pollen, animal dander, dust mites, plants or insect stings can spark allergic reactions.

Environmental pollution, food additives and pesticides have combined to make people more allergically reactive than ever before, says Martha Howard, M.D., co-director of Wellness Associates, a Chicago-based family medical practice. "We treat more and more people with allergies these days. It's practically an epidemic."

Here's what alternative medicine has to offer for two of the most common types of allergy, hay fever and food allergies. (For details on relieving asthma, which is often—but not always—triggered by allergies, see page 490.)

HAY FEVER: LET NATURE CURE

It's not caused by hay, and you don't get a fever when you have it. So precisely what is hay fever, anyway?

Sometimes described as the most common and annoying allergy around, hay fever affects something like 40 million Americans, who suffer through it with sneezing, wheezing, runny noses and itchy, watery eyes. There are two varieties: Seasonal hay fever occurs only when certain allergens, such

---

How I Healed Myself **Naturally**

She Was Allergic—To Everything!

Mary Swander, a 46-year-old author, essayist, poet and university professor living in Kalona, Iowa, had food allergies of one sort or another for most of her life. Finally, she decided to do something about her problem.

"I consulted an allergist, but the doctor accidentally injected me with too much of one of the allergens that he was testing me for," says Swander. "I became chemically sensitive to practically everything." Swander was diagnosed with environmental illness, an autoimmune disorder in which the body erroneously produces antibodies, or immune substances, in reaction to substances that would normally be harmless.

Swander became violently allergic to just about everything that she ate, breathed or touched—most foods, pollutants, chemicals, cleaning supplies, smoke and odors. She was especially allergic to perfumes. "I was so sensitive that if my mail even traveled in the same bag as women's magazines loaded with perfumed cards, I'd have a bad reaction," says Swander. When she ventured outside her house, she had to wear a surgical mask to filter out fumes and odors.

Swander consulted a second allergist. He placed her on an elimination diet limited to foods that she'd rarely or never eaten before. For a while she lived on a diet that included caviar, lobster, frog's legs, rattlesnake, raccoon and bear steaks (her favorite). As Swander's doctor explained, her body hadn't produced antibodies to those unfamiliar foods—so she wouldn't have an allergic reaction.

as pollen, are airborne; perennial hay fever is a year-round allergy to things like animal dander and dust mites.

"Allergies to airborne irritants tend to run in families," says Lisa Meserole, doctor of naturopathy, research consultant and faculty member in the botanical medicine department at Bastyr University of Naturopathic Medicine in Seattle. "Women who have hay fever can be environmentally sensitive in other ways: They might have eczema or other skin problems, or their bodies might overreact to mosquito bites," she continues.

The medical approach to managing hay fever often calls for taking antihistamines—over-the-counter or prescription medications that relieve symptoms by blocking the release of histamines, the substances responsible

Swander followed the diet for three years, rarely eating the same food twice. "I pretty much worked my way through the entire animal and plant kingdoms," she says. "It got to the point where friends would drop by with a pheasant that they'd just hit with their car, asking me, 'Mary, is this something you can eat?' "

After three years, Swander consulted Nicholas Gonzales, M.D., an immunologist in private practice in New York City. "He put me on a very specific nutritional regimen that included vitamins, minerals and herbs to adjust my body's acid-base balance. And he put me on a detoxification program to clear my system of allergy triggers. It's quite strenuous and very involved, but it's working," she says.

As part of her treatment, Swander has been forced to simplify her life. She lives in a former schoolhouse among Amish farmers. She grows her own organic produce, and she raises her own organic turkeys on pesticide-free feed that is untreated with antibiotics.

"I'm much more functional now," says Swander. "I can travel, though I have to sleep in a room with windows that open and I have to air it out first. I bring all of my own organic food, water and pots and pans with me."

Though it sounds like a lot of trouble, Swander says that the effort is worthwhile: "I'm feeling better than I have in years." She has even written a book about her experience, *Out of This World: A Journey of Healing.*

for hay fever symptoms. Problem is, antihistamines can leave women tired.

Thankfully, natural medicine offers some highly effective alternatives that, combined with basic avoidance tactics, may eliminate (or at least lessen) your need for fatigue-provoking drugs. Here are the experts' tips.

Move or modify. "The classic recommendation for hay fever is to reduce your exposure as much as possible," says Dr. Meserole. "If you have a bad seasonal allergy—hay fever triggered by pollen, for example—and you can't actually move to another part of the country, then you have to eliminate pollen from the air that you breathe."

Dr. Meserole advises her patients to use air filters at home and in the office and to clean their home furnace vents regularly. (Conventional physicians often give the same advice.)

Boost your immune system. Supporting your general health helps your immune system fight off outside invaders, says Dr. Meserole. "So eat plenty of fruits and vegetables, be sure to exercise regularly and get enough sleep—and make sure to laugh heartily several times a day."

"When your immune system is stressed out due to a poor diet, lack of sleep or other problems, you can become apparently allergic to things that wouldn't normally cause you to react," says Dr. Meserole.

"And when you're really run down and exhausted, your adrenal glands and the hormones that they secrete—epinephrine and norepinephrine—are affected. White blood cells fail to migrate properly, histamine release is off-balance and as a result, your body mounts an ineffective and overreactive immune response to allergens," explains Dr. Howard.

Try an herbal helper. "I encourage doctors to use freeze-dried stinging nettles (*Urtica dioica*) for people who have hay fever," says Andrew Weil, M.D., professor of herbalism and director of the Program of Integrative Medicine at the University of Arizona College of Medicine, near Tucson, and best-selling author of *Spontaneous Healing* and *Health and Healing*. Speaking at a seminar at the Columbia University School of Medicine on herbal healing in New York City, Dr. Weil said, "The effects of stinging nettles are very dramatic for hay fever. It's a far better choice than antihistamines and is one of the most effective herbal remedies that I know of."

"Use freeze-dried nettles in capsules, tinctures or teas according to label directions," says Dr. Meserole. Try a small dose first since some people are sensitive to nettles. Nettles are available at health food stores.

Meditate hay fever into submission. Practicing meditation or yoga regularly can help turn hay fever around, says Dr. Meserole. "Both disciplines allow you to reach the ideal state of relaxation that makes it easier for your body to heal itself and ease allergic symptoms."

Take C and see. "High doses of vitamin C alone, between two and five grams a day (2,000 to 5,000 milligrams in divided doses), will reduce hay fever symptoms in some people because vitamin C at these levels has an antihistamine action," says Dr. Meserole. "Though I've also seen it not work, it's totally safe, cheap and readily available." (If you're prone to kidney stones, however, you shouldn't exceed 500 milligrams of vitamin C a day. Also, excess vitamin C above 1,200 milligrams a day may cause diarrhea in some people.)

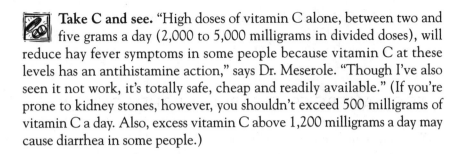

Homeopathy for Hay Fever

"Homeopathic remedies offer hope for people with hay fever," says Michael Carlston, M.D., assistant clinical professor at the University of California, San Francisco, School of Medicine.

The surest way to successfully treat hay fever with homeopathy is to consult a homeopath, says Dr. Carlston. During your first visit, which can last up to two hours, you will be closely questioned about your symptoms, lifestyle and your medical and psychological history. Your answers will enable the homeopath to precisely select a remedy for you from among more than 2,000 known homeopathic remedies.

"Success depends on exactly matching your symptoms to the right remedy," says Dr. Carlston. "Each homeopathic remedy is associated with the symptoms that it's said to cure. The closer the match between your symptoms and the remedy's symptom profile, the better your chances are for successful treatment."

You can also try self-treating with homeopathic remedies that you find in health food stores or some drugstores, says Dr. Carlston. Use homeopathic preparations specially blended for hay fever or try these remedies.

Allium cepa. If your hay fever is characterized by watery eyes, a burning mouth, hoarseness and a cough made worse in warm weather or a warm room, a dull headache, and eyes that are sensitive to light, Dr. Carlston suggests using Allium cepa—derived from the herbal family that includes garlic, shallots, leeks and onions—in concentrations of 6c or 12c. (Concentrations are expressed in c's and correspond to the potency of a homeopathic remedy.)

Arsenicum album. If your eyes and nasal passages are irritated and you experience a burning sensation with a lot of sneezing, or if you're fatigued and restless and your symptoms are worse when it's cold, use Arsenicum album—an extremely dilute form of arsenic—in concentrations of either 6c or 12c, suggests Dr. Carlston.

Euphrasia officianalis. This remedy is especially useful when the focus of the allergic reaction is the eyes—that is, if you experience watery eyes and blinking, says Dr. Carlston. Look for concentrations of 6c or 12c.

FOOD ALLERGIES: CLEARING UP THE CONFUSION

When it comes to dealing with food allergies, the solutions are more complicated—mainly because reactions to food are so confusing, says Melvyn Werbach, M.D., assistant clinical professor of psychiatry at the University of California, Los Angeles, and author of *Nutritional Influences on Illness* and *Healing with Food*.

Foods can cause two kinds of reactions in people who are sensitive. As with allergic reactions to airborne allergens like dust, one is a true allergic reaction to certain foods that causes specific symptoms like hives, watery eyes, sneezing, wheezing and sinus congestion.

Seafood, especially shellfish, is among the foods that most commonly trigger true allergic symptoms. Nuts are also villains, and some people have very severe reactions to them. (And peanuts, which are legumes, cause more allergy-related deaths than any food.) Wheat, corn, milk, soy and eggs have all been implicated as allergy-causers. And allergists have found that egg whites are even bigger troublemakers than the yolks.

The second kind of reaction—food sensitivity—isn't an allergy in the true sense of the word. That is, your body doesn't release histamine or other chemicals typically triggered by allergens. Food sensitivity causes a broad variety of less specific reactions.

"Severe food sensitivity can cause all kinds of problems, ranging from headaches and stomachaches to confusion and other vague complaints," says Dr. Werbach. Food sensitivity has been implicated in conditions as diverse as eczema, arthritis, colitis, ear infections, asthma and glaucoma.

According to Dr. Werbach, the science of food sensitivity is advancing, and doctors are increasingly aware of the problem.

"We now know that partially broken down proteins can get into the immune system through the intestines," explains Dr. Werbach. "This tendency, called gut permeability, or leaky gut syndrome, can sensitize people to foods like milk and wheat."

Doctors have also discovered that food sensitivities can come and go, says Dr. Werbach. Eating certain foods frequently can sensitize you to them, he adds. "I remember one woman, for example, who was sensitive to cow's milk. So she stopped drinking cow's milk and started drinking goat's milk, but then she became sensitive to goat's milk. Now she's back to cow's milk again and she's feeling just fine."

Ironically, some doctors believe that frequent cravings for a specific food might mean that you're sensitive to that food. Though no one knows exactly how common food allergies and food sensitivities are, Dr. Werbach estimates that perhaps 3 percent of us have classic allergic reactions to specific foods, and he suspects that many more of us may be food-sensitive, at least some of the time.

An Elimination Diet Can Pinpoint Culprits

Blood and skin tests for allergies aren't always reliable, says Dr. Werbach. So if you suspect that you're reacting to something you're eating, he suggests that you try an elimination diet instead. Here's how.

Avoid foods that you eat more than twice a week. This usually includes wheat, dairy products, yeast and corn, says Dr. Werbach. That means that you'll have to become a devoted label reader during that time and stay away from bakery items and packaged foods that contain these ingredients.

Give it two weeks. Problems such as headaches will clear up within a few days if the eliminated food is to blame. Some symptoms, such as joint pain, could take much longer to fade. So one to two weeks of elimination is optimal to figure out what's causing most problems, says Dr. Werbach.

If in doubt, avoid. To make sure that you're not getting ingredients that you're trying to avoid, you might have to do more than read ingredient lists closely. Sometimes those lists are vague or incomplete, or they have chemical names that aren't familiar to you. If you don't know exactly what's in a particular food, avoid it, advises Dr. Werbach.

Reintroduce foods cautiously. Once you've started to feel better, add back the eliminated foods one at a time, every three days, to pinpoint the one that troubles you, says Dr. Werbach.

Keep a diet/symptom diary. Write down exactly what you eat and when. Note symptoms, too, and any changes. Rate symptoms on a scale of one to ten and compare them over time. This log should further help you identify (and avoid) foods that cause problems.

Steer clear of prime suspects. Once you've pinned down problem foods, avoid them, says Dr. Werbach.

BONE, JOINT AND MUSCLE PROBLEMS
Help for What Hurts

To an extent, aches and pains are just part of life—little reminders that you're not 18 anymore . . . and haven't been for a long, long time.

But then there's the deep-down lasting hurt of arthritis. Or the recurring agony of tendinitis. Or the often-excruciating aching-muscle pain of fibromyalgia. What can you do when pain takes off its coat and hat and decides to stay for awhile?

You could reach for aspirin, or even prescription medication, but you may wish to consider nondrug pain-relief options. Yoga, exercise, massage and other alternative therapies provide first-line relief for bone, joint or muscle problems.

NATURAL WAYS TO END THE PAIN CYCLE

Medical doctors often prescribe drugs like steroids, but that remedy could prove to be a vicious cycle after awhile, says David Molony, Ph.D., licensed acupuncturist and executive director of the American Association of Acupuncture and Oriental Medicine, who practices in the northern suburbs of Philadelphia.

"Drugs stop any inflammation straight-out, and if nothing else is wrong with the body, it heals itself," says Dr. Molony. "But if there's a functional reason for the pain, which there usually is, the inflammation comes back and the doctor prescribes steroids again. And that can become a problem."

Dr. Molony says that more than 50 percent of the people who come to see him have some kind of muscle, joint or bone problems. By the time that most people turn to alternative treatments, "everyone else in conventional medicine has played with them and they realize they have something that needs more attention," he explains.

Sometimes the body has been "programmed" to do things wrong. Your muscles may be in constant spasm, or you're getting permanent knots in your shoulders simply because you're tensely hunching your shoulders or allowing your back to slump. Over time, you grow used to it, says Dr. Molony.

If habits like these cause a spasm, "it will come back unless you reprogram the muscle and help it heal," Dr. Molony says. "That's achieved with a mixture of acupuncture and Chinese herbs.

"Acupuncture relieves pain by stimulating the release of endorphins, natural pain-relieving substances in the brain that block pain biochemically. It also balances the body and reduces inflammation so that it heals faster." The combination of acupuncture and herbs can reduce inflammation and increase blood flow, Dr. Molony adds.

Acupressure can also help. When someone applies pressure at specific points on the body, it relieves muscle spasms and helps heal what's causing them, reducing pain in the process in most cases, he says.

In addition, here are some other, specific ways to deal with individual bone, muscle or joint problems.

ARTHRITIS: RELIEF FOR JOINT PAIN

If your hips hurt at the mere thought of a hula, or your wrists give up the ship after a few strokes of the canoe paddle, you could have something worse than rebellious joints. You might have arthritis.

This achy-joint condition comes in more than 100 forms, with osteoarthritis and rheumatoid arthritis being the most common. Osteoarthritis, which usually affects people over age 45, is a degenerative joint disease that is caused by the wear and tear of daily life. Rheumatoid arthritis also involves deterioration of joint tissue, but it usually comes earlier in life and is related to an immunity problem rather than a wear and tear on the joints. Two to three times more women than men get the rheumatoid kind, most often between the ages of 30 and 60.

But achy joints don't have to put an end to an active lifestyle. Alternative practitioners offer the following natural ways to help relieve pain and stiffness.

 Get Yourself into Hot Water

Warm water can relieve the pain of stiff joints, says Irene von Estorff, M.D., assistant professor of rehabilitation medicine at New York Hospital–Cornell University Medical Center in New York City. Spending ten minutes in a whirlpool or a warm to hot shower works magic on the joints.

The treatment can also make affected muscles more supple, says Dr. von Estorff.

After the warm soak, you might want to take five minutes or so for limbering stretches, or try some mild exercise. "Heat is very soothing generally—it relaxes the muscles around the joints so that they can move better," she notes.

But this treatment isn't appropriate if you have rheumatoid arthritis. While warm water works well for osteoarthritis, Dr. von Estorff cautions that heat can make an acute attack of rheumatoid arthritis worse by increasing swelling in the joints.

Get Up and Go

Regular aerobic exercise is a great way of improving blood flow and increasing circulation of fluid around the joints, says William Wilkinson, M.D., medical director of the Cooper Institute for Aerobics Research in Dallas. But he has specific advice on how to do it.

Make it low impact. "For women with arthritis, low-impact aerobic and flexibility activities—especially joint-friendly exercise like walking or swimming in a heated pool—help keep the joints mobile," he notes. "It also stimulates the muscles and tendons around it, which improves function and reduces pain." About 20 minutes of walking or swimming three times a week is a good workout. If possible, try to work up to 30-minute sessions five days a week, and avoid exercising when your joints are red, hot or swollen, he advises.

Lift weights—gently. Resistance training can increase range of motion, improve functioning in daily activities and help ease arthritis pain, notes Alan Mikesky, Ph.D., exercise physiologist and director of the Human Performance and Biomechanics Laboratory at Indiana University Purdue University in Indianapolis. Strong muscles help protect the joints from wear and tear. Dr. Mikesky recommends that people with osteoarthritis or rheumatoid arthritis whose pain and inflammation are under control consult their physicians about beginning a low-intensity training program.

The Vegetarian Cure

Vegetarian diets are great natural cures for immune-related conditions such as rheumatoid arthritis, says Andrew Nicholson, M.D., director of preventive medicine for the Physicians' Committee for Responsible Medicine, based in Washington, D.C.

Rheumatoid arthritis is an immunologic process, often in reaction to something foreign entering the body, Dr. Nicholson says. Your immune system can identify the protein in beef, chicken, fish, dairy products and eggs as foreign and attack it. Animal foods, especially dairy products, tend to be among the dietary items that cause the biggest reactions, according to Dr. Nicholson.

By cutting animal food from your diet, you can see improvements in just a few days, says Dr. Nicholson. But other doctors go further than that, he notes. Some precede the change to a vegetarian diet with a medically supervised seven- to ten-day fast using only water or juice, which allows the body to immediately flush out the substances considered troublesome.

How I Healed Myself **Naturally**

Veggies to the Rescue

Lorraine Hoffman, a 37-year-old housewife in Princeton, New Jersey, says a vegetarian diet relieved the severe rheumatoid arthritis that she had since age 19.

"I'd been on every medication that you can think of—gold shots, prednisone, tons of acetaminophen and others—up to eight pills a night," says Hoffman. "I had to have blood tests done every month because one of the medications that I was taking can ruin your liver and kidneys. X-rays of my joints show that, except for my knees, hips and right ankle, much of the cartilage is gone. In fact, most are just bone on bone.

"I got to the point where I could barely walk from my apartment to the car," says Hoffman. "My husband had to do the wash and clean and help with our baby.

"Then, one day I was talking to an acquaintance on the phone and she said, 'Have I got the doctor for you!'" The doctor that Hoffman consulted put her on a diet that was free of meat, wheat and dairy. The diet also excluded vegetables in the nightshade family, such as potatoes and tomatoes.

"Within five days, I felt a difference in my arthritis," Hoffman continues. "After a year on the vegetarian diet, I was a new woman. I lost 60 excess pounds, and I went off all my medications, including acetaminophen.

"I wish I'd found this diet ten years ago," adds Hoffman. "It won't rebuild my ankle, but it helps me stay medication-free."

Visualize Yourself Pain-Free

Using visualization and imagery to picture your joints smooth and healthy can help ease the pain and even the actual swelling of arthritis, according to Judith Green, Ph.D., professor of psychology and biofeedback in the Department of Behavioral Sciences at Aims Community College in Greeley, Colorado, and author of *The Dynamics of Health and Wellness.*

"Try to see the joint as a beautiful ball bearing that's smooth and perfect. Picture that several times a day, whenever you have a free minute to visualize the joint as healthy," she advises.

BACK PAIN: FLEX AWAY THE PAIN

It's almost as common as the common cold but, unfortunately, back pain lingers a lot longer than a case of the sniffles. In fact, back pain results in so many doctor visits—about six million a year—that it's a wonder how all those snowy sidewalks ever get shoveled. About half of working-age adults suffer from lower-back pain each year.

For women, though, more shoveling may be better than less, since too-little activity may contribute to the problem. Experts say that people who sit in front of computers all day often complain of lower-back pain. Before offices went paperless, you had to get up and walk across the room or down the hall every time you needed to retrieve a file or talk to someone. Now all you have to do is click a button or two on a keyboard. The result: no exercise and more stiff backs.

Another troublesome problem for women is pregnancy. The growing fetus puts a heavy burden on backs. Changing hormone levels trigger aches. And after pregnancy comes all the bending and lifting associated with child rearing.

But before you get too sore at back pain, try some alternative therapies. First of all, ice the area immediately, says Dr. von Estorff. Hold an ice pack on the area for 20 minutes with a thin towel between you and the pack to prevent damage to the skin.

Or you can rub an ice cube back and forth over the skin for 2 to 3 minutes. "When you have spasm, you have an awful lot of pain because of severe tightening of the muscles, so the ice slows the pain signals being sent to the brain," notes Dr. von Estorff.

Once you've addressed the immediate pain, you may be ready to try some other approaches.

Flex Your Back with Yoga

Practicing yoga for at least 15 minutes a day helps loosen and strengthen those all-important back muscles, says John Friend, an Iyengar yoga instructor in Spring, Texas. If you're just beginning yoga, practicing yoga in the middle of an acute attack isn't recommended. But stretching the back muscles can head off problems before they become debilitating.

Bend forward, loosen up. To relieve tightness and stiffness in the back, stand in front of a table, with your feet hip-width apart, says Judith Lasater, Ph.D., a physical therapist and yoga instructor in San Francisco and author of *Relax and Renew: Restful Yoga for Stressful Times.*

Bend forward from where your torso meets your thighs and rest your torso on the table. Your torso should be at a 90-degree angle to your thighs. (If the table is too low, stack a few blankets on the table to create a 90-degree angle.) Stretch your arms out in front of you and breathe slowly while you slightly bend your knees. Hold this pose for two minutes, then brace yourself with your arms and stand up straight.

Lift your leg, stretch your back. For a strained back, Friend suggests this yoga move: Lie on the floor on your back. Bend your left leg in toward your chest, while your right leg stays pressed to the floor. Hold this position for 30 to 60 seconds. Then switch legs. Repeat this stretch three times. Try keeping a gentle curve in your lower back, notes Friend.

 Exercise Strengthens a Weak Back

All aspects of exercise are great for back health, notes Nicholas A. DiNubile, M.D., clinical assistant professor of orthopedics at the University of Pennsylvania in Philadelphia and author of *The Exercise Prescription.*

Studies show that people with better aerobic capacities have less incident of back injury. Overall fitness protects the lower back, including its strength and flexibility, notes Dr. DiNubile. That means doing a 30-minute aerobic activity at least three times a week. In addition, strong abdominal muscles are extremely important, he notes. He warns, however, that rowing machines can be a problem for someone prone to back problems.

Do three sets of 15 to 20 stomach crunches a day. To correctly do a stomach crunch, lay on the floor with your legs bent. Be sure to press your lower back toward the floor so that no space exists between your back and the floor. As you contract your abs, your torso will lift slightly off the ground. Use slow, controlled movements and point your chin toward the ceiling.

Lie and lift. To strengthen the back extensor muscles, Dr. DiNubile suggests the following: Lie on your stomach with your arms out in front of you, like Superman flying. Lift your arms, head, shoulders and legs so that only your stomach is still touching the ground. Hold for three to five seconds. Repeat ten times.

Stretch your hips and hamstrings. Flexibility is also important. Dr. DiNubile recommends the pelvic tilt for the lower-back area and the hamstring stretch for the back of the thighs. (For illustrated instructions for these stretches, see pages 106 and 108.)

 ## Get Manipulated

Visiting a chiropractor can do wonders for a hurting back, says Scott Haldeman, D.C., M.D., Ph.D., associate clinical professor in the Department of Neurology at the University of California at Irvine and editor of *Principles and Practice of Chiropractic.* "We use chiropractic manipulation—putting pressure on the spine and moving the bones of the spine as well as pushing on the surrounding tissues and joints. It works very well for back pain."

The average number of visits for back pain is around six or eight, with visits lasting anywhere from 15 minutes to an hour. Some people need more treatments than that, while others may get better after just one treatment, says Dr. Haldeman.

 ## Visit a Hellerworker

Going in for the standard 11 Hellerwork sessions is good for the whole musculoskeletal system, but the back especially reaps benefits, says Sandra Sullivan, a certified Hellerworker and director of practitioner relations at Hellerwork International in Mount Shasta, California. Each Hellerwork session focuses on a different part of the body. Because the back is so important to how the rest of the body feels and moves, every Hellerwork session includes some work on the back. And session six is exclusively for the back.

BURSITIS AND TENDINITIS:
SOOTHE PINCHES AND TWINGES

Your body is actually very chatty. It's shouting, "Hey, take it easy!" when your elbow starts to ache after that fifth set of tennis. And after your third mile of running uphill, it's saying, "Lighten up, buddy!" as your Achilles tendon gets painful and tight.

Tendinitis is caused by inflammation of the tendons, which connect muscle to bone. Bursitis is inflammation in the bursas, or fluid-filled sacs that decrease friction in the body's joints. Both of these problems may be brought on by a sudden increase in activity. And both can be so painful that they sideline you for awhile. Luckily, alternative therapies can help.

 ## Put Your Pain on Ice

When it comes to pain and swelling, ice is the name of the game, notes Dr. von Estorff. "Usually, cold reduces pain more than heat does, so applying ice is best," she says. "Once the pain and swelling have gone away, you can do exercises to help make those muscles strong and less likely to become injured again."

For both bursitis and tendinitis, you want to hold an ice pack on the site of inflammation. Apply the pack for no more than 20 minutes at a time, Dr. von Estorff advises. You can apply the ice pack as often as every hour until the pain or inflammation goes away. Just make sure that you don't resume your normal workout routine until the swelling is gone, she cautions.

 ## Massage: Rub It the Right Way

Tendinitis responds especially well to massage, says Ben E. Benjamin, Ph.D., muscular therapist and president of the Muscular Therapy Institute in Cambridge, Massachusetts. Friction massage is especially effective, according to Dr. Benjamin.

"Rub the tendons very gently, and you'll slowly wear down the scar tissue in the tendon itself," he notes. Such a massage usually takes 10 to 15 minutes. The massage therapist will want to work on you a couple times a week for at least three to four weeks.

For bursitis, however, it's a whole different procedure. A massage therapist won't directly massage the site of your bursitis because that could make the swelling worse, says Dr. Benjamin. "But a massage in the general area can help increase circulation there." (For details on massage therapy, see page 214.)

 ## The Alexander Technique: A Perfect Solution

Because it teaches you how to use your body more efficiently, the Alexander Technique is perfect for bursitis and tendinitis, says Deborah Caplan, physical therapist and teacher of the Alexander Technique in

New York City. "Tendinitis, especially, is caused by repeated strain on the tendon and by using the body when it's out of alignment," she notes. "You need to learn to use your body more efficiently so that there's less pull and strain on the tendons."

Caplan shows women new injury-minimizing ways of carrying out daily activities, from sitting at a computer to playing the violin or painting the ceiling. Because bursitis flares up when the bursa is irritated, you're less likely to have the problem if you learn new ways to move. For bursitis in the shoulder, for example, you may want to work on improving the alignment of your head, neck and spine. This can include learning to sit more upright rather than rounding your shoulders and jutting your head forward.

Feldenkrais Restores Balance

A few sessions with a Feldenkrais practitioner might be just what your sore body is aching for, says Mark Reese, Ph.D., certified Feldenkrais practitioner and trainer in San Diego.

"We work on helping you to balance both sides of your body better," Dr. Reese notes. "A lot of people stand primarily on one leg or put their weight on one sitting bone when they sit. Or one arm doesn't swing as they walk, which can throw the whole body out of alignment."

A lot of the problems in your extremities and joints come from not moving from the center of your body, Dr. Reese says. For example, if your tennis swing isn't coming from your pelvis, you could be putting undue stress on your elbow or shoulder.

"Feldenkrais teaches you to swing so that the force originates from the center of your body and out through your arm, reducing stress to the arm," Dr. Reese explains.

FIBROMYALGIA: NEW HOPE FOR MYSTERY ACHES

Explaining fibromyalgia is even harder than spelling it. A painful condition that involves your muscles and connective tissues but not your joints, fibromyalgia leaves you hurting all over and so exhausted that the simplest tasks are impossible. The condition can be depressing as well as debilitating. Experts link fibromyalgia to not being able to sleep well at night. Lack of all-important sleep that produces deep relaxation, they say, causes muscle fatigue.

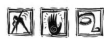 ## A Trio of Remedies: Stretching, Massage and Meditation

If fibromyalgia has you down for the count, experts recommend these natural remedies.

Stretch it out. Just moving those stiff, sore muscles can go a long way toward making you feel better, says Donald Goldenberg, M.D., chief of rheumatology at Newton Wellesley Hospital in Newton, Massachusetts, and professor of medicine at Tufts University School of Medicine in Boston. "Muscles tighten severely in response to the pain of fibromyalgia, so stretching makes sense," he says. "Focus on stretching the whole body, including the neck, shoulders and lower back." (For illustrated instructions on stretching, see page 104.)

Schedule regular massages. Getting a massage is another sure way to help ease muscle pain, says Dr. Benjamin. "In fibromyalgia, your body is very tense and there is pain throughout," he says. "A very gentle overall body massage helps reduce muscle tension and increases your body's circulation in general. Massage could help make it easier for those with fibromyalgia to cope with everyday tasks."

Be mindful. Meditating is a great prescription for unwinding—and for thwarting the tension that makes fibromyalgia worse, notes Dr. Goldenberg.

Dr. Goldenberg studied a group of men and women with fibromyalgia who meditated for 20 minutes a day for ten weeks. "We compared 79 people with fibromyalgia who meditated and 42 people with fibromyalgia who didn't. Overall, the people who meditated improved about 60 percent. The others, who didn't meditate, didn't get any better."

KNEE PAIN: HOBBLE NO MORE

It's the prime spot for all kinds of painful dislocations, sprains, bursitis, fractures, arthritis and just plain pain. The knee is so overworked from kneeling, running and walking that about 50 million Americans hobble to the doctor in pain every year, say experts.

But you may not have to suffer if you take these steps recommended by practitioners.

 ## Muscle Up with Exercise

Build up strength in your quadriceps (the front thigh muscles) and your hamstrings at the backs of the thighs, says Owen Anderson, Ph.D., exercise physiologist and editor of *Running Research News* in Lansing, Michigan. By strengthening those muscles, you'll take the load off overworked knees, he advises.

Start with five squats. When you can do these comfortably, move on to doing another five while holding hand weights down at your sides. The weights can be anywhere from 1½ to 5 pounds each.

Another method that you can try is to work your way up to doing the squats with a barbell balanced on the back of your shoulders, Dr. Anderson says.

Yoga for Stronger Knees

Yoga helps to bring optimal range of motion to the knees by strengthening all of the muscles around the knees and creating flexibility in the muscles, says Friend.

Friend recommends the warrior posture: Stand with your feet parallel about four feet apart (about even with your wrists when your arms are outstretched). Then, turn your left foot slightly in and turn your right leg and foot out about 90 degrees. You'll wind up in a pose similar to a lunging fencer's. Keep your chest facing straight ahead while you turn your head and look out over your right knee. Stretch your arms out to your sides and bend your right knee. Look over your right knee to make sure that it is in line with your right foot and vertical over your ankle. Hold that pose for 20 to 45 seconds. Repeat it three times on each leg.

How I Healed Myself **Naturally**

Herbs for Knee Pain

Jeanne Rose, a practicing herbalist and aromatherapist in San Francisco, relieves knee pain with herbs and exercise.

"Ever since a bad skiing accident 40 years ago, I've had bad knees," says Rose. "I tried taking aspirin and prescription medicines for the pain, but medications didn't help very much. When I got involved in herbalism in 1967, I wondered if herbs could help my knees.

"I started weight training and decided to mix one drop of basil and one drop of sage with eight drops of carrier oil and rub them on my knees as an anesthetic. It works. I don't feel the pain at all. So now I can lift weights to help make my knees stronger, and I have no pain. It's really amazing."

MUSCLE CRAMPS: UNKINK THOSE KNOTS

If your muscles were telephone cords, a cramp would be that annoying knot that develops smack in the middle of it, making it impossible to pick up the receiver without a lot of contortions; except that, with a muscle cramp, your muscle has tightened and shortened, usually as a result of overexertion and dehydration. An imbalance of electrolytes—minerals such as magnesium, calcium, sodium and potassium—is often the culprit.

  ## Stretch It, Ice It

Drinking plenty of fluid before and during exercise can help prevent cramps. To unkink a muscle once a cramp occurs, experts recommend these strategies.

S-t-r-e-t-c-h your calf. For a cramp in your calf, which may strike after exertion or in the middle of the night, Dr. Mikesky recommends that you do this: With your hands against a wall or object for balance, put your non-cramping leg forward with the cramping leg out behind you. Lean forward, keeping your heels on the floor and your toes pointing straight ahead, until you feel a stretch in the cramped calf, and hold that position for 20 to 30 seconds. Then lower yourself, bending the knee of your noncramped leg so that you stretch the cramp out even farther.

Unkink your hamstring. Keeping your cramped leg straight, sit on the floor or your bed and bend your other leg so that the sole of the foot is on the inside knee of the cramped leg, says Dr. Mikesky. Lean forward at the waist until you feel the stretch in the muscle running from the back of your knee to your buttock. That muscle is the hamstring. Hold the stretch for 20 to 30 seconds.

Be nice with the ice. If your muscles are locked into a contraction that just won't relax, try an ice massage. Rub an ice cube back and forth on the affected spot for 2 to 3 minutes, says Dr. von Estorff. Or, you can place an ice pack wrapped in a towel on the area for 20 minutes. Ice slows the pain signals going from the muscles to the brain, so the hurt won't seem as bad, she says.

 ## Homeopathy Helps

Two homeopathic medicines can be very helpful for muscle cramps, says Robert Ullman, doctor of naturopathy and a physician at the Northwest Center for Homeopathic Medicine in Edmonds, Washington.

"*Magnesia phosphorica* is a general remedy for muscle cramps, especially abdominal cramping that gets better with heat or when you bend over," Dr. Ullman says. For hand and foot cramps, he recommends *Cuprum metallicum*, which is homeopathically prepared (diluted) copper.

MUSCLE SORENESS: BYPASS THE PAIN

If you wake up in the morning and your muscles are sore, most likely you did more physical activity than you're used to or worked muscles that you normally don't. When that happens, tiny tears or bruises occur within the muscle tissues, and you feel sore. Here are some paths to relief.

 ### Moist Heat, Soothing Oil

Though sore muscles heal on their own, you'll get faster relief with hydrotherapy, aromatherapy and massage.

Warm yourself up. Holding a warm, moist towel on your aching muscles is a quick way to feel better, says Dr. von Estorff. Or, spend some time in a hot shower or bath. The hot water helps relax the muscles and undo the spasm.

Treat yourself to an aromatic massage. Inhale the scent of essential oils as you also massage them onto your body, suggests Jeanne Rose, a practicing herbalist and aromatherapist in San Francisco. She recommends a blend of herbs, barks and spices, including cypress, sage, juniper, basil and lemon peel. Use two drops of each in a one- to two-ounce bottle of vegetable oil. Apply the oil when you start feeling sore. Repeat the application before bedtime and when you wake up, Rose suggests.

Master the massage. Try a compression massage, which involves squeezing the muscle rather than rubbing it, recommends Dr. Benjamin. "Muscle soreness results from lactic acid, a waste product that accumulates in the muscles. Compression massage pumps the blood and helps you get rid of that lactic acid." Just one or two massages will help, he says.

OSTEOPOROSIS: PREVENTION IS PREFERRED

Osteoporosis, a condition marked by weak, brittle, porous bones, is responsible for 1.5 million fractures suffered every year and poses a major public health threat for 25 million Americans, 80 percent of whom are women. That's because after menopause we produce the female hormone estrogen much more slowly. And when estrogen declines, bones regenerate much more slowly. As a result, bones are weakened and more likely to break on impact.

All too often, women don't know that they have osteoporosis until they get a fracture. At that point, their doctors may prescribe Fosamax, a prescription drug designed to help slow the breakdown of bone. By then, much of the damage is done, although further fractures may be avoided.

Experts offers these strategies for taking matters into your own hands.

Get on Your Feet with Exercise

Probably the best prescription for osteoporosis is doing regular weight-bearing exercise, says Susan Bloomfield, Ph.D., assistant professor in the Department of Health and Kinesiology at Texas A&M University in College Station.

After age 35, women start losing bone mass every year, with a cumulative bone-mass loss of 10 to 20 percent over 20 years, Dr. Bloomfield says. "If you are regularly exercising, you can slow that loss or conserve that bone mass. You may also add bone mass," she says.

Work your bones 30 minutes a day. Weight-bearing exercise such as jogging or weight lifting puts mechanical stress on the bone, which helps maintain it, she says. "If you don't exercise, you lose muscle mass and strength. And with bone, it's the same," observes Dr. Bloomfield. She recommends 30 minutes of exercise a day.

Train with weights. Weight training is the best way to build bone mass, Dr. Bloomfield says. "High-force muscular contractions provide the greatest stimulus to the bone by putting force on it," she says. (For illustrated instructions of weight-training exercises, see page 96.)

Work in aerobics. Walking, running, cycling and rowing are especially good for the arms and back, says Dr. Bloomfield.

A Bone-Sparing Diet

Since calcium is an important component of bone, conventional medical wisdom advocates getting lots of extra calcium, mainly from dairy foods, to stave off bone loss. Yet a growing number of researchers say that the problem isn't too little calcium, but too much protein. The kidneys excrete excess protein into the urine and protein pulls calcium right along with it. The solution, then, is to eat less protein-hearty meat, not more calcium-laden dairy products, says Dr. Nicholson.

Sticking to a vegetarian diet can prevent valuable calcium from being stolen from your bones, says Dr. Nicholson. To reduce calcium loss, he recommends getting excess salt and protein out of your diet.

As for overindulging in protein, meat-eaters usually get 100 grams of protein a day as opposed to vegetarians who often get less than 50 grams a day, Dr. Nicholson notes. Only 10 percent of calories need to come from protein, which is easily available from grains and beans, he adds. So by eliminating things like pork, beef, chicken and dairy from your diet, you reduce protein intake and help eliminate calcium loss.

Make friends with calcium. Women need extra calcium and magnesium in their diets because they're at higher risk than men for developing osteoporosis, notes Alan Gaby, M.D., professor of therapeutic nutrition at Bastyr University of Naturopathic Medicine in Seattle and author of *Every Woman's Essential Guide to Preventing and Reversing Osteoporosis*. Shoot for at least 1,200 milligrams of calcium and 300 to 500 milligrams of magnesium daily, Dr. Gaby says.

If your multi and your diet do not give you those amounts, make up the difference with individual supplements. And eat plenty of calcium- and magnesium-rich foods like leafy greens, seeds and tofu. Though the Daily Value for magnesium is 400 milligrams, research suggests that taking 500 milligrams a day may provide added benefits for your bones, Dr. Gaby says.

REPETITIVE STRAIN INJURY: HEAL THE HURT

There's a certain comfort in routines, but sometimes doing the same old–same old can do a number on your body. Repetitive motions, such as working a cash register or entering data on a computer, can end up hurting your wrist, arm, elbow and hand muscles. Some people are so disabled by a repetitive strain injury (RSI) that they may require surgery.

  Try an Aromatherapy Massage

Of course, the first thing that you want to do, if you can, is lay off the task that caused the problem. But after that, you have some effective options that don't involve taking pain pills, say experts. Here are a few.

Massage your wrist with herbal infused oils. A mix of aromatherapy and massage can shorten carpal tunnel's stay, says Rose. She recommends using herbal oils that contain either of the essential oils Roman chamomile (*Chamaemelum nobile*) or a combination of rosemary and ginger for their anti-inflammatory and painkilling effects. "Put some oil on your hand, work it into the elbow and massage it from there down into the wrist and hand," she says.

 ## Custom Stretches for Wrist Pain

For a repetitive strain injury caused by doing activity improperly, moving your wrist the right way could be the cure, says Sharon Butler, certified Hellerworker in Paoli, Pennsylvania, and author of *Conquering Carpal Tunnel Syndrome and Other Repetitive Strain Injuries*. The following stretches work the inside of the wrist, the base of the thumb and the muscles of the inside of the forearm.

• Place your hands on your hips with your fingers pointing straight forward. Slowly roll your elbows forward to create a deeper bend in your wrists. You'll feel a sensation called the stretch point, the first sign that a stretch is taking place. Sometimes you'll even feel a light aching sensation, usually in the deeper muscles. Pause at each stretch point and wait until you feel the sensation fade. For variation, try pointing your fingers in a slightly downward direction and notice the difference in the sensations that you feel in your muscles.

• To stretch the finger muscles and tendons, press your fingertips against the edge of a desk or table, bending at the base of your fingers and keeping your wrists straight. Press gently until you feel the stretch point and then hold that position until you feel a change in sensation. You can vary this exercise by doing it with your fingers spread apart.

 ## Fight Back with Yoga

"For most people with an RSI, the top of the forearm is really tight and overused and the underside is underused," says Friend. For relief he recommends the yoga position called downward facing dog. "This posture creates the best skeletal alignment between the forearm and arm and between the shoulder and upper arm."

To do this pose, stand in front of a chair and put your palms flat on the front edge of the chair seat, placed about shoulder-width apart. Walk your legs backward until your arms are straightened and your feet are under your hips. Bend your knees and be sure to point your tailbone toward the ceiling, creating a gentle arch in the lower back. Pressing down on your hands, balance your weight evenly between your upper and lower body and pull your forearms and upper arms toward the chair, up away from the floor.

Keeping your hands flat on the seat of the chair, turn your shoulders out and away from your neck slightly. Take a deep breath, feel the stretch. Hold the pose for 15 to 30 seconds. Repeat three to ten times, says Friend.

SCIATICA: STEP UP TO RELIEF

Sciatica pain really gets on your nerves, in more ways than one. Not only does this condition send pain shooting from your back or your buttocks down to your leg, but it makes standing, sitting or even lifting things a giant . . . well, pain in the butt. It's caused by a pinched nerve in the spine, and when that nerve screams "ouch," it sends electrical impulses from your back to your buttocks and down one leg, experts say. Often, sciatica lasts a relatively short time, as little as a month or so. But the pain is so intense, the less you have to endure it, the better. Here are some top alternative ways of bidding pain adieu.

  Stretch That Spine with Bodywork and Yoga

In the Awareness through Movement classes that are part of the Feldenkrais Technique, you learn exercises that could help take the pres-

---

 How I Healed Myself **Naturally**

Hellerwork Relieved Her Wrist Pain

Sharon Butler, 47, from Paoli, Pennsylvania, reports that applying the principles of Hellerwork relieved her repetitive strain injury.

"I was completely incapacitated and couldn't work at all," says Butler, a certified Hellerworker who treats people with this specialized form of therapy and author of *Conquering Carpal Tunnel Syndrome and Other Repetitive Strain Injuries.* "I'd been giving bodywork treatments, which was stressful to my forearms."

Butler stopped using the repetitive movements that were aggravating the problem and instead used Hellerwork on her own wrists, hands and arms. She also practiced stretching. "I found that stretches help every time that a symptom flares up," says Butler.

Now, Sharon recommends Hellerwork to others with repetitive strain injuries. "We see remission in about four sessions," she says.

sure off the sciatic nerve, says Dr. Reese. He says that sciatica often results when the sciatic nerves don't have enough space and mobility and that the best way to increase that space is to make the lower back longer and more flexible. Here's how.

Work the pelvis. Sit on the forward part of a chair with your feet flat on the floor and your back straight. Then follow these steps.

Slowly tilt your pelvis backward a bit so that your lower back is slightly rounded or flexed, and then return to the starting position.

Tilt your pelvis forward very slowly so that your lower back arches or extends a bit, and then return to the starting position.

Alternate between the two movements, tilting your pelvis forward so that your back arches or extends slightly and then slowly tilting your pelvis backward a bit so that your back rounds slightly. Then return to the starting position.

Tilt your pelvis toward your left knee so that your weight shifts to the forward part of your left buttock, and then return to the starting position. Repeat this with your pelvis tilting to your right knee.

Repeat each movement four to eight times before you move on to the next movement, reducing your effort with each repetition, Dr. Reese recommends.

Practice the cobra. Another good exercise for sciatica is called the cobra, says Friend. Lie on your stomach with your hands flat on the floor, next to your armpits. Stretching your legs straight back, turn your thighs inward so that your heels move apart. Your buttocks will broaden, releasing tension in your lower back. Then draw your tailbone deeper into your buttocks, pressing your lower abdomen onto the floor. (Avoid clenching the muscles in your buttocks, which will pinch nerves further.) Holding your lower body in this position, lift your head and chest upward toward the ceiling. Keep your hipbones on the floor—don't push up with your arms. Hold this position for 30 seconds or so to really stretch your spine.

TEMPOROMANDIBULAR DISORDER: MAKE SHOOTING PAIN DISAPPEAR

Temporomandibular disorder (TMD) is a painful disorder affecting the jaw joint and chewing muscles and can be caused by overstraining when you clench or grind your teeth. For some people, the symptoms of TMD are headaches and neck, face and shoulder pain. Others get clicking sounds in the jaw that signal TMD.

Experts recommend the following tips.

Bodywork for Jaw Pain

If you've seen a dentist or doctor and still have trouble with your jaw, these alternatives may help.

Consult a Hellerworker. In session number seven, Hellerwork practitioners focus on the head, neck and jaw, says Sullivan. "We manipulate the connective tissue to bring the muscles of the jaw into balance. It's deep-tissue muscle therapy, but not massage. We work with the whole neck and head in conjunction with the jaw muscles." In a one-hour session, about ten minutes are spent on the jaw, she notes.

Learn to move it. An Alexander Technique instructor will work with you to see what you may be doing to cause chronic jaw pain, says Caplan. "Many people learn a better way of balancing the head and neck. When you're chronically slumping with your head jutting forward, your jaw can't hang in proper alignment in relation to your skull." As a result of re-learning, your head and neck become more aligned with your torso, and your jaw can hang more loosely, which eases tension and pain, she says.

Get rubbed the right way. To ease the pain and tightness of TMD, a massage is just what the doctor should have ordered, says Dr. Benjamin. "Massage therapy is very good for jaw pain because of how it relieves the tension in the area," he explains. "If you grind your teeth at night, it makes your jaw tired, achy and sore. Massage helps to relax the jaw muscles." Dr. Benjamin recommends going to someone who has been trained in working the jaw or face area. The massage needed in these areas for TMD requires a bit more forcefulness than other types of massage, he notes.

BREAST PROBLEMS
Soothing Tactics for Pain, Tenderness and Worry

Few things in life are as unnerving as feeling a lump or pain in your breast. You may be the most unflappable of women, without a hypochondriac's aching bone in your body, yet still find yourself thinking the worst.

"Women wonder, 'What is this I'm feeling? Is it cancer?'" says Linda Dyson, doctor of naturopathy and professor of gynecology and obstetrics at Bastyr University of Naturopathic Medicine in Seattle.

It probably isn't. Most lumps aren't cancerous, says Marilyn Mitchell, M.D., a holistic physician in Palatine and Mount Prospect, Illinois, and associate professor of clinical obstetrics and gynecology at Northwestern University School of Medicine in Chicago. And pain is rarely a sign of breast cancer, she says.

Truth is, normal breast tissue feels lumpy and may feel painful at various points during your menstrual cycle. So before you rush out for a consultation with your doctor, it's wise to look at a few facts about your monthly changes.

ANATOMY OF A LUMP

If you could look inside your breasts, you'd see a network of milk glands, milk ducts and connective tissue surrounded by fat. The size and shape of pumpkin seeds, the milk glands and ducts can swell so that they feel like small, hard lumps.

Breasts are at their lumpiest about a week before your period. "Most women have normal lumps," says Dr. Mitchell.

How do you know that they're normal? The trick is getting to know your breasts through a self-exam so that you're better able to detect unusual changes. Because every woman has lumps during the second half of her cycle, the best time to do a self-exam is right after your period, during the first half of your cycle. That way, you'll get to know what's normal for you during that time of the month.

RELIEF FOR LUMPY, PAINFUL BREASTS

Two conditions—fibrocystic breast disease and what doctors call fibroadenoma—are associated with changes in the breast.

If it's a fibrocystic condition, your breasts will feel both lumpy and painful before your period. The milk glands in your breasts may enlarge and feel like hard lumps, your breasts' connective tissue may thicken and feel ropey or the glands may get blocked and filled with fluid, forming cysts, Dr. Mitchell says. Both the pain and lumpiness usually go away once you

Sagging Breasts: Exercise and Restraint

Legend has it that Marie Antoinette's breasts were so perfectly formed, they served as the inspiration for the classic saucer-shaped champagne glass.

Had the French Revolution not intervened, though, even her imperious bosom would have bowed eventually—to the force of gravity.

Ligaments are the tissues responsible for holding up the breasts. Unfortunately, they aren't very strong and can lose elasticity with pregnancy, nursing and age. Although some of these changes are unavoidable, it helps to get support with a bra—a garment not yet available to the eighteenth-century Antoinette but now readily available. Look for bras that allow minimal bounce and offer good support, says Gina Lombardi, a personal-training coach and owner of the Trainers, in Tarzana, California.

If your breasts are already sagging, exercise won't build them up, since breast tissue is mostly fat. But certain exercises will build the pectoral muscle underneath. And that'll make your breasts look perkier.

Lombardi, chairwoman of the personal trainer committee of the National Strength and Conditioning Association, suggests this breast-lifting push-up.

1. Get down on your hands and knees. Position your hands so that your wrists are directly under your shoulders, your elbows are pointing to the sides and your fingers are pointing slightly inward. Cross your ankles. Make sure that your back is straight, not arched, and your stomach muscles are tight, not sagging.

2. Bending your elbows, slowly lower yourself until your chest is about two inches from the floor. Then straighten your arms slowly and push yourself back up to the starting position. Repeat. Aim for three sets of 12 repetitions each.

get your period. Though a higher than usual estrogen-to-progesterone level during the second half of your cycle makes it worse, no one knows exactly what causes the condition in the first place.

With a fibroadenoma, your milk glands enlarge, forming a nodule that feels like a solid, rubbery lump. No one knows exactly what causes fibroadenomas, either, Dr. Mitchell says. If you have a fibroadenoma, you won't have pain, and the lumpiness won't change over the course of your cycle.

Though most lumps are benign, you should always have a doctor check any new ones that you discover during your monthly exams. If your doctor thinks that the lumps are unusual in any way, she may follow up with a number of different tests. Your physician may do a mammogram (a breast x-ray) or an ultrasound scan (a test that uses sound waves to produce an image of the inside of your body) to make sure a lump isn't cancerous. She may also perform a fine-needle aspiration test, inserting a thin, hollow needle into the lump. If the lump is a cyst, she may do a needle biopsy, which involves withdrawing fluid from it and causing the lump to collapse and disappear. If the lump is solid, she'll remove some cells and examine them under a microscope (also called a biopsy).

Should the examination turn up cells that look suspiciously like cancer, your doctor will recommend removing the lump.

If, on the other hand, your doctor feels that the lump is harmless, you don't necessarily have to have it removed, says Adriane Fugh-Berman, M.D., former head of field investigations for the Office of Alternative Medicine at the National Institutes of Health in Bethesda, Maryland.

NATURALLY SOOTHING ALTERNATIVES

Alternative remedies can help shrink noncancerous lumps and prevent new ones. And various alternatives to prescription and over-the-counter painkillers can help relieve breast tenderness and pain and keep lumps at bay, says Dr. Dyson. "I don't tell women who try these remedies to expect relief in the first menstrual cycle," she says. "It may take several cycles. But definitely by the second cycle they should be seeing some improvement."

 What Naturopathic Medicine Has to Offer

One of the first things that you should do if you have breast pain or lumps is scrutinize your diet, says Dr. Dyson. What you eat or drink may be the culprit.

Call a moratorium on methylxanthines. Cola, chocolate, tea and coffee all contain methylxanthines—naturally occurring substances that

(continued on page 364)

A Diet to Prevent Breast Cancer

In Asian countries, breast cancer rates are lower than those in the United States. Research suggests that the Asian diet, which includes less fat and meat and more soy food than ours, offers significant protection.

Diet has a considerable effect on breast cancer risk, according to Steve Austin, naturopathic physician in Portland, Oregon, and co-author of Breast Cancer: What You Should Know (but May Not Be Told) about Prevention, Diagnosis and Treatment. So, one of the simplest ways to cut your risk is to change your diet, he says. Here is his list of the breast cancer–fighting dietary changes that you can make today.

Avoid alcohol. The more you drink, Dr. Austin says, the higher your risk of breast cancer. Why? Alcohol seems to interfere with your liver's ability to clear excess estrogen from your body. That's bad. The higher your exposure to estrogen, research finds, the higher your breast cancer risk.

Shun fat. "Population studies show that every country where the diet is low in fat has a low risk of breast cancer, and every country where the diet is high in fat has a high risk," Dr. Austin says. Research suggests that a diet high in saturated animal fats (bacon, butter, cheese and so forth) in particular may prompt your body to produce more estrogen. Unfortunately, moderate reductions in fat intake don't seem to help much. Think "major cuts," he suggests. If you want more suggestions, see the low-fat menus beginning on page 129. There, you'll see that it is possible to slash fat.

Switch to olive oil. Mostly monounsaturated fat, olive oil doesn't affect your body the way that saturated fat does, Dr. Austin says. A study of more than 2,000 women in Greece suggests that those who used olive oil more than once a day had a 25 percent lower risk of breast cancer than women who used olive oil less often.

Befriend fatty fish. Substances known as omega-3 fatty acids are found in fish like tuna and salmon. In the laboratory, mice injected with human breast cancer cells developed smaller, less invasive tumors when fed these fatty acids.

Serve soy. Soy foods such as soybeans, soy nuts and soy milk are rich in phytoestrogens, plant chemicals that seem to protect against breast cancer. As these chemicals latch on to your body's estrogen receptor cells, they crowd out your body's own estrogen, a suspected "fuel" for breast cancer. Women who live in countries where people eat lots of soy have lower rates of breast cancer. Shoot for one to two ounces of soy nuts, a four-ounce serving of tofu or a couple cups of soy milk daily, Dr. Austin says.

Sprinkle on flaxseed. These tiny edible seeds contain substances called lignans that seem to help fight off breast cancer. Studies at the University of Toronto suggest that flaxseed both inhibits and slows the progression of breast cancer. Grind the seed in a coffee grinder or food processor for a few seconds so that it's easier to digest. Then sprinkle the seed on your cereal or salad, Dr. Austin suggests. Flaxseed oil won't do, though—it doesn't contain enough lignan, he says.

Pick brightly colored organic produce. Fruits and vegetables are good sources of cancer-fighting vitamin C and beta-carotene. This is particularly true of the bright orange, yellow, red and green fruits and vegetables, such as butternut squash, oranges, peaches, red peppers and spinach.

Cabbage, broccoli, brussels sprouts, kale and collard greens are also high in phytochemicals (chemicals naturally found in plants), which may inhibit estrogen synthesis and guard you from estrogen overload. In one study, women who ate the most fruits and vegetables were least likely to get breast cancer. Shoot for at least five servings a day, Dr. Austin says. And look for organic produce, since certain chemicals sprayed on crops can have adverse estrogen-like effects on your body.

Refuse refined foods. "A high-fiber diet may help the body cleanse itself of excess estrogen," Dr. Austin says. It'll also help you control your weight because bulky, high-fiber food fills you up before you can pack in lots of calories. Weight control is key since body fat actually manufactures a type of estrogen. So choose brown rice over white rice and whole-wheat pasta over refined. And remember those fruits and vegetables.

Season with garlic. This savory, aromatic herb seems to stimulate the immune system functions. Garlic appears to protect against a wide variety of cancers, including breast cancer, according to Dr. Austin.

Sip green tea. "Asian societies in which women consume a lot of green tea tend to have less breast cancer—and less cancer in general," Dr. Austin says. Plant chemicals called polyphenols seem to be responsible. You can also get polyphenols (although in small amounts) in black tea.

may contribute to lumpiness and pain, says Dr. Dyson. "Sometimes just cutting out foods and beverages that contain methylxanthines can get the pain to go away."

Scope out fat. High estrogen levels seem to aggravate breast pain and lumpiness. That's why you're likely to have these problems in the middle of your cycle, when your endocrine system boosts estrogen production, says Christiane Northrup, M.D., in her book *Women's Bodies, Women's Wisdom*. Dr. Northrup is also a practitioner of obstetrics and gynecology in Yarmouth, Maine, and assistant clinical professor of obstetrics and gynecology at the University of Vermont College of Medicine in Burlington.

Since a high-fat diet seems to boost estrogen levels even further, cutting back on fat should help alleviate and prevent pain and lumpiness. "Try to get less than 20 percent of your daily calories from fat," says Dr. Dyson. "Getting 5 to 10 percent of calories from fat would be ideal."

How I Healed Myself **Naturally**

Evening Primrose Oil for Fibrocystic Breasts

Elizabeth Bauer, a 28-year-old photographer from Smethport, Pennsylvania, started to experience breast discomfort in her early twenties.

"Two weeks before my period, my breasts would get lumpy and swollen and painful," says Bauer. "They'd be so tender that it would hurt when I walked downstairs or ran. After my period, the symptoms would go away for two weeks, then come back.

"I talked to gynecologists—they said I had fibrocystic breasts," says Bauer. "They mentioned that caffeine and chocolate could make fibrocystic breasts worse and suggested that I cut back. I tried, but I still had the symptoms every month."

Bauer decided to look into some herbal remedies. "I tried evening primrose oil, which comes in liquid form in a little bottle with a dropper cap and is available at most health food stores. It's simple: I add three drops to a beverage and drink it."

Evidence suggests that evening primrose oil works by acting as an anti-inflammatory, reducing pain and swelling in sensitive breast tissues.

"When I use evening primrose oil regularly, I can really feel a difference," says Bauer. "I can go through the whole month with no breast discomfort."

To do this, you'll have to stop adding fat when you cook and when you sit down to eat. (For tips on cutting fat, see page 136.) Research suggests that similar cuts in fat can reduce your risk of breast cancer as well.

Fill up on fiber. Eat a high-fiber diet and your body's estrogen levels will fall, notes Dr. Northrup.

What's considered high fiber? Shoot for two servings of fruits, four servings of vegetables and three to four servings of whole grains daily, suggests Leslie Axelrod, a naturopathic physician in Phoenix and a supervising physician at the Southwest Naturopathic Medical Center clinic in Scottsdale, Arizona.

Go vegetarian. "Researchers have found that women who eat vegetarian diets excrete more estrogen, which is probably because vegetarian diets tend to be higher in fiber," says Dr. Axelrod. (For more information on vegetarian diets, see page 286.)

Buy organic. Many farmers feed their animals and spray their crops with chemicals that act like estrogen in the human body, says Steve Austin, naturopathic physician in Portland, Oregon, and co-author of *Breast Cancer: What You Should Know (but May Not Be Told) about Prevention, Diagnosis and Treatment.* If you choose to eat meat and dairy, buy beef and poultry that has been fed organic grain (look for it on the packaging), and milk from organically fed herds, he suggests. Also, look for organically grown produce.

Soothe with evening primrose. An effective anti-inflammatory, evening primrose oil can soothe pain and help shrink lumps, says Dr. Dyson.

Look for evening primrose oil in health food stores, and add a tablespoon to your morning oatmeal or sprinkle it over your salad. Or take one or two capsules two or three times a day, says Dr. Fugh-Berman.

Caution: If you're pregnant, wait until after your baby is born, since the oil can cause miscarriage and premature birth.

 ## Help from Vitamins and Minerals

Certain nutritional supplements can help your body eliminate excess estrogen. They soothe symptoms because excess estrogen contributes to breast pain and lumpiness.

Other supplements reduce inflammation and breast pain in other ways, says Dr. Dyson. But whatever your breast problem, here are some things that can help.

Add extra E. Some practitioners believe that vitamin E encourages your body to excrete excess estrogen. "At least one-third to one-half of fibroadenomas show some improvement with vitamin E," says Dr. Dyson. She recommends starting with 600 international units (IU) a day (20 times the Daily Value) and working up to 800 IU if necessary. But be sure to consult your doctor if you are considering taking doses above 600 IU.

Take C. When pain and lumpiness are at their worst, try 500 milligrams of vitamin C every couple of hours, for a total daily intake of 3,000 to 5,000 milligrams, says Dr. Dyson. She states that doses this high will ease and prevent inflammation. But doses higher than 1,200 milligrams may also cause diarrhea, so be aware of that, and cut back on the dosage if you begin to have a diarrhea problem.

BREAST PAIN AND TENDERNESS: BANISH DISCOMFORT

Sometimes you can have breast pain without the lumps. The culprit may be mastitis, a bacterial infection that's most common in nursing mothers. Or, it may be swelling due to water retention. You'll know you have mastitis if the pain is accompanied by fever, redness and warmth in your breast, says Dr. Mitchell. Here's what to do.

 Naturopathic Solutions

Hot compresses, held to your breast, do a good job soothing most types of pain, Dr. Axelrod says.

Compress with castor oil. Hot compresses soaked in castor oil are particularly helpful, Dr. Axelrod says. To make a castor-oil pack, soak a piece of wool flannel with castor oil. Wrap one side in plastic wrap, then in a towel, and hold the pack against your breast, so that the oil-soaked flannel touches your skin. Finally, cover the pack with a heating pad or hot-water bottle. Dr. Northrup suggests that you repeat this entire procedure for an hour at a time, three times a week over the course of two or three months.

Warning: Castor oil is toxic if ingested and could harm a nursing infant, Dr. Axelrod says. So don't rely on this remedy if you develop mastitis during the time that you're nursing.

Soak in ginger tea. Compresses soaked in ginger tea can also help relieve the pain of mastitis, Dr. Axelrod says. To brew the tea, add four tablespoons of chopped fresh ginger to one quart of water, boil for a half-hour and allow to cool.

While the tea is warm, dip a towel into it. Hold the towel to your breast for 20 to 60 minutes, every few hours. If the pain doesn't diminish within 24 hours, see your doctor for treatment.

DIABETES
New Choices for Balancing Blood Sugar

Diagnosed with diabetes at age 30, Sandra Panchak had more or less resigned herself to a lifetime of daily insulin injections when she heard about an alternative.

Like other women with diabetes, Panchak has trouble using glucose, the simple sugar that is the body's primary energy source.

Normally, your digestive system breaks carbohydrates such as pasta, fruit, cookies and vegetables into glucose and channels the sugar into the bloodstream. This prompts your pancreas, a gland behind your stomach, to secrete insulin. A hormone, insulin ferries the sugar into cells throughout your body, where it's used for fuel.

If you have diabetes, however, glucose can't get into your cells. Either your pancreas doesn't produce enough insulin or your cells resist insulin's attempts to usher in the sugar, or both. Uncontrolled, this cellular glucose embargo can lead to serious, and sometimes fatal, complications. Sugar can build up in your bloodstream, damaging your blood vessels, nerves, eyes and kidneys. Blood vessel damage that accompanies diabetes can impair circulation, delaying wound healing and increasing risk of infection. Diabetes also raises your risk of heart disease and stroke.

NEW HOPE FOR A STUBBORN PROBLEM

Some women with diabetes can get by with oral medication that stimulates insulin secretion. But others, like Panchak, need daily injections of synthetic insulin to keep blood sugar levels within the normal range. "Normal" is 80 to 115 milligrams of glucose per deciliter of blood.

Initially, Panchak's doctor told her that she might be able to manage her diabetes with oral medication—if she lost weight. Overweight is a key contributor to diabetes. Despite her best efforts, though, Panchak never lost enough weight to make a difference.

"I tried dieting, but it didn't work, so I went straight to using insulin," says Panchak, 53, who lives in Washington, D.C. "I'd almost given up hope of getting off insulin, when I had an opportunity to try an alternative approach."

Panchak learned that researchers at nearby Georgetown University were looking for volunteers to test the effectiveness of a vegetarian diet in the treatment of diabetes. With her doctor's blessing, Sandra signed up for the study. Just three months after she started the diet, Panchak's blood sugar levels were well under control and her doctor lowered her insulin dose.

"By the end of the study, I'd lost 17 pounds, and since then I've lost another five," says Panchak, who continues to eat low-fat vegetarian fare. "My doctor says that if I continue to lose extra weight, I may be able to stop using insulin and rely on oral medication alone. Before, that was out of the question."

A vegetarian diet is just one alternative that can help women manage diabetes, says Jill Sanders, a naturopathic physician practicing in Portland, Oregon. "There are a lot of things you can do that can help."

But first, you need to know where you stand.

HAVE YOU HAD YOUR BLOOD SUGAR CHECKED?

Diabetes is extremely common. One in 20 Americans, many of them women, have the disorder. Unfortunately, roughly half don't know that they do, says Philip Cryer, M.D., endocrinologist, researcher and professor at Washington University School of Medicine in St. Louis and president of the American Diabetes Association. "The problem is, complications can arise even before a women is diagnosed," he adds.

Warning signs include frequent urination and excessive thirst, unexplained weight loss and repeated vaginal infections. Don't ignore these symptoms. Ask your doctor to test your blood sugar levels, says Dr. Cryer. A fasting blood glucose test can usually tell you whether or not you have diabetes. (You'll be asked to go without food overnight and then have your blood tested in the morning before you eat or drink anything.) If this test is normal but symptoms persist, measuring blood glucose levels after swallowing glucose can identify impaired glucose tolerance, a condition that can lead to diabetes.

There are two basic types of diabetes, known as Type I and Type II. With Type I (insulin-dependent) diabetes, which usually develops during childhood, your body can't use glucose because the pancreas makes little or no insulin. If you have Type I diabetes, you'll need daily insulin injections to keep your blood sugar levels in a safe range.

With Type II (non-insulin-dependent) diabetes, which develops in adulthood, your body makes some insulin, but your cells resist it, interfering with insulin's ability to lower blood sugar. If, like Panchak, you have Type II, or what used to be called adult-onset diabetes, you may need to inject insulin or take oral medication.

No one knows exactly what causes diabetes, says Dr. Cryer. Type I seems to be result of a glitch in which immune cells destroy the cells that manufacture insulin. Some research indicates that this wanton destruction may sometimes be triggered by a virus. Type I also seems to run in families.

Besides being overweight, a family history of diabetes also increases your risk that you will develop Type II diabetes. During pregnancy, some women develop gestational diabetes, a temporary but dangerous form of Type II diabetes. If that happens, you're more likely to develop Type II later in life. And for reasons that aren't entirely clear, African-American, Hispanic and some Native American women also run higher risks of Type II diabetes, Dr. Cryer says.

YOU'RE IN CONTROL

Studies suggest that the best way to prevent diabetes may be to drop excess weight, improve your diet and exercise regularly. That's also the best way to control your blood sugar levels and limit complications associated with diabetes if you already have Type I or II. If you have Type I and take steps to control it, you may be able to get by using less insulin. If you have Type II, you may be able to get by with less medication, or none, says Dr. Cryer.

Professional health organizations such as the American Diabetes Association offer advice on how to change your diet and work exercise into your life. But some alternative practitioners offer additional ways to manage and prevent diabetes, like switching to a vegetarian diet, taking vitamin or mineral supplements or trying certain herbs. Research suggests that vegetarianism and other alternatives get good results.

Before you modify your diet or activity level or start taking supplements or herbs, however, be sure to check with your doctor, says Dr. Sanders. And if you have gestational diabetes, your obstetrician should monitor your progress throughout your pregnancy. If lifestyle changes aren't enough to bring your blood sugar levels under control, she may prescribe insulin injections until the danger passes.

No matter what type of diabetes you have, trying alternative treatments may change your need for insulin and medication. But never stop taking insulin or medication or adjust the dosages without your doctors consent, says Dr. Cryer.

FOOD THERAPY: INSULIN-FRIENDLY EATING PLANS

As a rule, a high-fiber, low-fat diet that helps you lose weight will improve blood glucose levels and help control Type II diabetes, explains Christine Beebe, R.D., president-elect of health care and education for the American Diabetes Association and director of the Health and Wellness Center at St. James Hospital in Chicago Heights, Illinois. High-fiber, low-fat diets fill you up before you overeat. So you eat less and lose weight, which keeps blood glucose levels comfortably normal.

Another key to blood glucose control is spacing out the carbohydrate-rich foods that you eat during the day since carbohydrates raise blood glucose levels more than fat or protein, says Beebe. If you take insulin, it may mean adjusting your dose to keep your blood glucose on an even keel. So a high-fiber, low-fat diet that assists in weight loss is a good choice whether you're trying to prevent or control diabetes. But specific high-fiber, low-fat diets may be particularly beneficial. Here are your best bets.

Try the vegetarian route. In the Georgetown study, men and women with Type II diabetes saw their blood sugar control improve and their weight drop significantly after they switched to a totally vegetarian diet, free of meat and dairy food. Like most vegetarian diets, the Georgetown diet was high in fiber and low in fat and included adequate, but not excessive, protein.

Because vegetarian diets usually don't contain as much protein as diets that include meat or dairy foods, they may have an edge over other high-fiber, low-fat diets, says Andrew Nicholson, M.D., the researcher who headed the Georgetown study and the director of preventive medicine for the Physicians' Committee for Responsible Medicine, in Washington, D.C.

Extra protein can overburden your kidneys, the organs responsible for ridding your body of excess protein. If you have diabetes, your kidneys are already vulnerable. (Doctors aren't sure why, but diabetes damages the kidneys.) In the Georgetown study, volunteers excreted less protein in their urine after switching to a vegetarian diet, which suggests that the diet helped protect their kidneys from damage, says Dr. Nicholson. (For information on following a vegetarian diet, see page 286.)

Try the Ornish approach. The Ornish diet—a low-fat vegetarian diet designed by Dean Ornish, M.D., cardiologist, assistant clinical professor of medicine at the University of California in San Francisco and director of the Preventive Medicine Research Institute in Sausalito, California—offers another dietary alternative. (To follow the Ornish diet, see page 132.)

Consider the Pritikin diet. If you're not ready to do without meat, you might consider the Pritikin diet. Developed in the 1970s by an engineer named Nathan Pritikin, this diet allows a modest 3½ ounces of animal protein per day and only 10 percent of calories from fat, with generous portions of high-fiber grains, vegetables and fruits.

Like the Ornish diet, the Pritikin diet seems to help control diabetes. In a University of California, Los Angeles, study of more than 600 women and men with diabetes, 71 percent of those taking oral hypoglycemic drugs and 39 percent of those using insulin were able to stop taking medications after switching to the Pritikin diet and starting an exercise program. (For more information on the Pritikin Diet, see page 137.)

Cruise the Mediterranean. Some men and women with diabetes do well on a diet that's slightly higher in fat, provided that the fat is consumed in the form of monounsaturated fat, like olive oil. Unlike animal fats, which are largely saturated, olive oil is composed primarily of monounsaturated fat.

In a study at the University of Texas Southwestern Medical Center at Dallas, ten men with diabetes needed 13 percent less insulin after they started following a Mediterranean-style diet typical of Italy, Greece and Spain. The diet included lots of whole grains, vegetables, fruits, legumes like white beans—and olive oil. The diet got 50 percent of calories from fat.

That's far more fat than the 10 percent supplied by the Ornish or Pritikin diets, says Abhimanyu Garg, M.D., associate professor of internal medicine at the center and the study's chief researcher. He speculates that the individuals in this study needed less insulin because they ate fewer carbohydrates while on the diet. In other words, the calories that came from olive oil took the place of calories that would have otherwise come from carbohydrates. The results imply that men and women alike can benefit from a Mediterranean diet.

"People with diabetes are less able to metabolize carbohydrates than those who don't have diabetes," explains Dr. Garg. "So, if you reduce carbohydrate intake by replacing carbohydrates with monounsaturated fat, that improves diabetes control."

Not only were the individuals in the study better able to control their blood sugar levels, but their low-density lipoprotein (LDL) cholesterol levels dropped, too. Saturated fat such as butter and lard will raise levels of LDL cholesterol, contributing to heart disease.

In contrast, monounsaturated fat such as olive oil lowers blood levels of LDL cholesterol—a significant benefit to people with diabetes, who are at higher risk for heart disease. (For information on following the Mediterranean diet, see page 159.)

How I Healed Myself **Naturally**

On a Vegetarian Diet, She Needs Less Insulin

At age 43, Pamela Crutchfield, a nurse in Potomac, Maryland, learned that she had Type II, or adult-onset, diabetes. Following a medically supervised vegetarian diet, Crutchfield was able to cut her insulin needs in half.

"I have a family history of diabetes," says Crutchfield. "My mother had Type II diabetes, my brother has it and I was also overweight. That was a big part of the problem.

"My doctor told me to lose weight, and he hooked me up with a nutritionist who gave me tips on dieting and exercise," recalls Crutchfield. "I tried and I tried to exercise, but I didn't lose weight.

"My doctor prescribed oral medication to control my blood sugar levels, then he increased the dosage," she says. "But even with medication, my blood sugar levels kept escalating."

Crutchfield says that she ended up needing insulin injections, just like her mother and brother—something she'd hoped to avoid.

"When I started using insulin, I'd get episodes of hypoglycemia, low blood sugar caused by overly high doses of insulin," she says. "I wanted to get off insulin.

"One day I was reading the newspaper, and I saw an ad inviting people with Type II diabetes to participate in a study at Georgetown University in Washington, D.C. I called immediately," says Crutchfield.

Along with other volunteers, Crutchfield was prescribed a vegan diet—a total vegetarian diet that includes no meat, fish, eggs or milk. For comparison, other women in the study followed a diet commonly recommended by the American Diabetes Association.

"It was my first experience with a vegan diet," recalls Crutchfield. "A nutritionist at the university worked with me to come up with a plan that fit my lifestyle. I was able to cut out meat and dairy foods and cut back on fat and sugar.

"Cutting out dairy was hard," she confesses. "I was a big ice-cream lover. But it paid off: After three months, I was able to get my blood sugar into a healthy range and cut the amount of insulin that I needed in half. Plus, I lost 20 pounds without feeling hungry."

Other women on the diet fared equally well. And at age 47, Crutchfield continues to follow the vegan diet. Her doctor says that if she sticks with it, she should be able to get off insulin entirely.

Cook with onions and garlic. Some research suggests that onions and garlic—members of the lily family—may lower insulin resistance and help control blood sugar. When researchers at the University of Kerala, India, treated diabetic rats with an active compound isolated from garlic, their blood sugar levels stayed under control. These researchers believe that onions may have a similar benefit.

To enjoy these benefits, add garlic to sauces, soups and stews, says Dr. Sanders. Sprinkle sliced onions on salads and use them in sandwiches, soups, stews and casseroles.

HERBAL HELPERS

A number of herbs can help prevent and control diabetes, Dr. Sanders says. Try incorporating some of them into your diet.

Benefit from ginseng. In a Finnish study, people with non-insulin-dependent (Type II) diabetes had more stable blood sugar levels when they took on a daily basis 200 milligrams of ginseng, a fleshy root widely used for its medicinal properties. Look for ginseng (*Panax ginseng* or *Panax quinquefolius*) in health food stores.

Get gymnema. The leaves of this woody plant, which grows in the tropical forests of central and southern India, seem to help control blood glucose levels, says Dr. Sanders. She recommends 400 milligrams of gymnema (*Gymnema sylvestre*) a day. This herb is available as an extract made from the leaves. You may have to shop around to find it or special order it through health food stores.

Add bilberry and ginkgo. A relative of blueberry, bilberry (*Vaccinium myrtillus*) may help improve your circulation and, if you have diabetes, lower your risk of eye damage, says Dr. Sanders. The same goes for ginkgo (*Ginkgo biloba*), a tree native to China. You can find both bilberry and ginkgo in freeze-dried or tincture form at health food stores. Follow the manufacturer's directions.

VITAMINS AND MINERALS OFFER PROTECTION

Research suggests that women with diabetes may be falling short in certain vitamins and minerals that can help ward off some of the complications associated with the disorder. To avoid deficiency, include these in your diet.

Add some C. "Vitamin C can help prevent the damage to blood vessels that accompanies diabetes," says Dr. Sanders. She recommends at least

1,000 milligrams of vitamin C a day. Take 500 milligrams in the morning and another 500 milligrams at night.

Get extra E. In an Italian study, daily doses of vitamin E helped people with Type II diabetes make better use of insulin. Dr. Sanders recommends 400 international units of vitamin E every day.

Check out chromium. In a U.S. Department of Agriculture (USDA) study, people with Type II diabetes had more stable blood sugar levels when they took supplemental chromium. Some USDA research suggests that the mineral may help prevent diabetes. Dr. Sanders recommends 200 micrograms. (People with diabetes who take chromium should be under medical supervision since their insulin dosage may need to be reduced as blood sugar drops.)

 EXERCISE: TRAINING THE PANCREAS TO BEHAVE

Whether you have Type I, Type II or gestational diabetes, regular exercise can help keep your blood sugar levels in the normal range.

Exercise seems to make all your cells more sensitive to insulin and allow more glucose to enter. Regular exercise also helps control your weight, which reduces insulin resistance, says Dr. Cryer. Consequently, exercise can help control diabetes and possibly prevent Type II diabetes in the first place.

Aim for a half-hour workout. Shoot for at least 20 minutes of moderately intense physical activity, such as jogging, brisk walking or swimming, three or four times a week, says Dr. Cryer.

"Start slow if you've been inactive," says Dr. Sanders. "Do as little as five minutes of exercise a day for the first couple of weeks. Then add ten minutes a week. Walking, swimming and low-impact aerobics are good choices for beginners," she says.

Have fun. Pick an activity you like, adds Dr. Sanders. If you enjoy your exercise routine, you're more likely to stick with it.

Adjust accordingly. If you have diabetes, remember to use your home blood glucose meter to test your blood sugar before and after exercising, Dr. Sanders says. This way you will be able to anticipate a drop in blood sugar and adjust your medication or food intake.

Blood sugar levels that are too low can cause symptoms of hypoglycemia, or low blood sugar, says Dr. Cryer. These symptoms include confusion, shakiness and, in extreme cases, unconsciousness and coma.

Map out a plan with your doctor. Like insulin and medication, exercise will make your blood sugar levels drop. To keep sugar levels within the safe range, then, you need to strike a balance among eating, exercising and taking either insulin or oral medication. If you step up your exercise regimen, you may need to cut back on insulin or your medication. You may also need to eat occasional snacks before, during or after exercise to keep your blood sugar in a safe range, says Dr. Cryer.

Be kind to your hard-working feet. If you have diabetes, you may not feel pain in your feet, due to nerve damage. Untended sores and cuts can get badly infected, and unchecked infections can destroy skin and blood vessels, says Dr. Cryer. So check your feet for sores every day, especially on days you don't exercise. If you find a sore, see your doctor. If the sore is infected, she may prescribe an antibiotic.

BETTER BLOOD SUGAR WITH BIOFEEDBACK

Stress triggers the release of adrenaline and other hormones that interfere with your body's blood sugar control mechanisms, raising or lowering blood sugar levels. But stress-fighting techniques like biofeedback, which teaches you to control your body's response to stressful events, can even your blood sugar levels out again, when used with your medication, says Angele Mc-Grady, Ph.D., professor of psychiatry and physiology at the Medical College of Ohio in Toledo and past president of the Association for Applied Psychophysiology and Biofeedback, based in Wheatridge, Colorado.

In a study headed by Dr. McGrady, men and women with Type I diabetes who used biofeedback to relax were able to lower their blood glucose levels. In another study, biofeedback also enabled people with diabetes to increase circulation to their feet. (For information on where to find a health professional trained in biofeedback, see page 65.)

DIGESTIVE AILMENTS
Cures for Irregularity, Upset Stomachs and Other Ills

Nausea. Vomiting. Diarrhea. Constipation. Indigestion. Heartburn. Abdominal pain. Hemorrhoids.

No matter how healthy you are, chances are you've endured a gut-wrenching bout with digestive trouble sometime or another. Doctors say that the most disruptive is irritable bowel syndrome, or IBS, a constellation of abdominal upsets that affects 20 million men and women. But whether or not you have IBS, you're likely to have some close encounters with intestinal distress that will send you hunting for a cure.

Doctors don't know why, but far more women than men are beset with digestive problems. If the problem is stress-related—as it often is—it can be gently eased with natural medicine, says Michael Gershon, Ph.D., professor of anatomy and cell biology at the Columbia-Presbyterian Medical Center at Columbia University in New York City.

"People totally underestimate the impact of stress on the digestive system," states Kathleen Maier, a physician's assistant, herbalist and director of Dreamtime Center for Herbal Studies in Flint Hill, Virginia, and former adviser on botanical medicine to the National Institutes of Health in Bethesda, Maryland. Alternative healers like Dr. Gershon and Maier, among others, say that stress-reducing natural therapies such as yoga and meditation have proved helpful to many women.

A BAROMETER OF OVERALL HEALTH

Knowing how your digestive system is supposed to work is the first step in helping yourself prevent problems or heal them when things go wrong, says Maier. For instance, digestive problems can start when we don't take time out for simple rituals such as chewing our food properly and savoring what we eat, she explains. "So if your grandmother nagged you about chewing each bite of your food 100 times, she had good reasons," says Maier. Saliva contains specific enzymes that help break down complex carbohydrates. Without this enzymatic breakdown, food hasn't begun the proper digestive process.

But, of course, assiduous chewing isn't the only answer. Digestive problems have a wide range of possible causes. Many kinds of medications, including antibiotics and prescription steroids, can disturb intestinal peace; so can recreational drugs and alcohol. Any of these substances can wipe out beneficial bacteria, causing vague, unpleasant symptoms.

Natural approaches to digestive ills generally tackle problems from more than one angle, involving food therapy, vitamin and mineral therapy, herbal medicine and some form of mind-body therapy, like yoga or meditation.

CONSTIPATION: EASING ELIMINATION NATURALLY

You probably know the feeling only too well. You're bloated and you haven't, um, evacuated, for a couple of days. And now, you're getting pretty darn edgy. Constipation will do that to you.

Estimates suggest that at least once in a while, 50 million Americans get that internal going-nowhere-fast feeling, while 18 million are often troubled by it. And in another nod to the gene fairy's lack of fair play, twice as many women as men report being frequently constipated.

Happily, nature has ways to ease things along. Here are some of the best natural remedies for irregularity.

Give it time. The simplest thing that you can do to ease constipation is to give your body enough time to do its job, says Maier. "There's a psychological component to constipation for many women who subconsciously fear letting go of things," she explains. "Rampant in our culture, too, is the hurry-it-up factor. I say, relax! Give yourself sufficient time while you're sitting in the bathroom. For some women, time alone may be all that's needed."

To move your bowels, move your body. Exercise is an ideal way to jog your system into action. "The good muscle tone that results from a regular exercise program is important for optimal bowel function," says Maier. She recommends a brisk walk of a mile or two each day.

Forage for fiber. "Most women, even those who eat wholesome diets, can benefit from a daily fiber supplement," says James Scala, Ph.D., nutritionist and author of *Eating Right for a Bad Gut*. On average, women get about 12 grams of fiber each day, says Dr. Scala. They should be getting 30 grams a day.

Dr. Scala advises the women that he treats for constipation and other intestinal ills to take up to two tablespoons of fiber supplements three times each day. He suggests a generic natural-fiber laxative made from psyllium seed, stirred into water and swallowed about a half-hour before meals.

It's best to work fiber supplements into your diet gradually. Suddenly increasing your fiber intake can cause gas, cramps and diarrhea, says Adriane Fugh-Berman, M.D., former head of field investigations for the Office of Alternative Medicine at the National Institutes of Health in Bethesda, Maryland.

Drink early and often. Constipation is often a sign that you're not drinking enough water. So along with regular exercise and more fiber, drinking eight or more eight-ounce glasses of water a day can help provide relief, according to Maier.

Add in some apple juice. Apple juice works wonders because it contains sorbitol, a natural sugar with laxative properties. So a glass a day may be just what you need to get things moving again, according to Dr. Scala.

DIARRHEA: TOO MUCH GET UP AND GO

There's nothing subtle about the symptoms of diarrhea. The cramps are sharp, and the urge to go is frequent. But if diagnosing diarrhea is easy, tracking down its cause may not be.

An episode of diarrhea is often caused simply by eating foods to which you're sensitive. Some people have lactose intolerance or gluten sensitivity, so they will have problems eating wheat or dairy foods. A sudden increase in fiber intake or high-sugar foods can also cause problems, as can gas-producing vegetables such as brussels sprouts and cabbage. Viral or bacterial infections can also irritate the intestine, causing the runs.

You've ruled out those suspects? Sudden stress, even subtle distress, can loosen your bowels; so can antacids, caffeine, antibiotics and beverages sweetened with sorbitol, a calorie-free sugar substitute.

You might even get diarrhea from your children—and not just because they delight in pushing your stress buttons. Mothers of tots in day care are 10 to 25 percent more likely to acquire the runs than are moms of stay-at-home children, according to one study. That's because it's easy for diarrhea-causing bacteria or viruses to spread among groups of yet-to-be-toilet-trained toddlers. Your kids pick up the germs and pass them to their caregivers—and to you.

With any luck, though, your particular blast of diarrhea won't last more than three days, especially if you try these natural remedies.

Roll some slippery elm. "Slippery elm is my favorite diarrhea remedy," says Susun S. Weed, an herbalist and teacher from Woodstock, New York, and author of the *Wise Woman* herbal series. She also speaks widely on the medicinal use of herbs at medical gatherings.

"Take a few spoonfuls of slippery elm bark (*Ulmus fulva*) powder, found at health food stores, and blend it with honey till you can roll the mixture into small balls. Dust the balls with additional slippery elm powder, store in a closed container and use as needed.

"I like to store them in little cough-drop tins," says Weed. "At the first sign of diarrhea, let a ball dissolve slowly in your mouth, and repeat as necessary." Slippery elm works because it contains a nutritive mucilage, which soothes intestinal irritation, she says.

Dry up some blueberries. In Europe, dried blueberries are highly recommended as an effective cure for simple diarrhea, notes Varro E. Tyler, Ph.D., professor emeritus of pharmacognosy at Purdue University in West Lafayette, Indiana, and author of *Herbs of Choice: The Therapeutic Use of Phytomedicinals*. They contain pectin, a binding agent that helps dry up the problems. The antidiarrheal work is done largely by astringent tannins formed during the drying process, he adds.

In his book, Dr. Tyler suggests chewing and swallowing three tablespoons of dried blueberries. Or, boil the crushed dried berries in water for about ten minutes and drink the strained tea.

If you can't find dried blueberries in a gourmet or health food store, you can dry fresh berries in the sun or on a tray in a low-heat (150°F) oven overnight. Depending on the intensity of the sun and the temperature, drying time varies. Dry until no moisture oozes out when you squeeze a berry. But don't eat fresh blueberries for diarrhea, cautions Dr. Tyler. They may actually have a laxative effect.

GALLBLADDER PROBLEMS: NO STONES, NO PAIN

You may not even know where your gallbladder is, exactly. But if you have gallstones, you'll get a fast anatomy lesson—the hard way.

Linked by ducts to the liver and the duodenum, which is just below the stomach, the gallbladder stores bile, a fluid that helps your body digest fat.

Gallstones form when the bile becomes concentrated and crystallizes. The stones may lodge themselves in several different nearby ducts, causing severe pain and other problems. Gallstones are three times more common in women than in men.

Once a gallstone has gotten stuck somewhere, surgery is often recommended. But some changes in your diet can help prevent their formation, say healers.

Food Therapy: The Easiest Cure

A diet high in animal fat and low in fiber could be a prescription for getting gallstones, says Melvyn Werbach, M.D., assistant clinical professor of psychiatry at the University of California, Los Angeles and author of *Healing with Food* and *Nutritional Influences on Illness*.

Conversely, a nutritional plan that lowers your fat intake and increases your fiber intake could make you stone-free for life. Here are Dr. Werbach's recommendations.

Consider vegetarianism. Gallstones are linked to eating animal foods such as meat and dairy. And you're less likely to get gallstones if you eat plenty of fiber. For these reasons, he advocates a vegetarian diet for women who've had gallbladder problems.

Say no to fats and sweets—and yes to fiber. If giving up meat and dairy foods is too restrictive for you, consider switching to a low-fat, low-sugar, high-fiber diet. What would a high-fiber diet look like? You might start out with a whole-grain cereal like bran flakes for breakfast, have beans for lunch (bean salad or chili) and high-fiber vegetables like corn on the cob and a baked potato with dinner.

Don't skip breakfast. To prevent stones, eat breakfast every day, says Dr. Werbach. Other than whole-grain cereal, you can try whole-grain toast, whole-grain pancakes or cooked oatmeal topped with bran and raisins.

Lose a few pounds. As soon as you weigh 25 pounds more than you should, you're increasing your risk for developing gallstones. Losing excess pounds seems to help reverse the process, says Dr. Werbach.

HEMORRHOIDS: SHRINK THE NASTIES

If you've had hemorrhoids, you know only too well why hemorrhoids are so very hated. Not only do hemorrhoids cause pain that's often severe but also they bleed sometimes. And when you see bright red blood in your stool, you may think that you're in serious trouble.

Even when they are painful, you don't need to be alarmed. "Hemorrhoids are swollen veins found in the anal canal below the rectum," says Max M. Ali, M.D., in his book *Hemorrhoids: No Laughing Matter*. Describing them as "little balloons filled with blood," Dr. Ali says that hemorrhoids are caused by constipation, bad bowel habits or pregnancy. In fact, hemorrhoids are almost an inevitable condition of pregnancy because the fetus exerts extraordinary pressure on the rectum.

If you have hemorrhoids, here's how to ease them naturally.

Bulk up. Eat plenty of vegetables and grains or use psyllium-based fiber supplements, say doctors. Fiber adds bulk, which contributes to larger, softer stools, and soft, bulky stools are easier on your hemorrhoids than hard, dry ones.

Dab on some witch hazel. Distilled witch hazel (*Hamamelis virginiana*) extract is a natural astringent, and astringents help shrink swelling. "Put witch hazel on a plain cotton pad, or use a cotton pad like Tucks that are presoaked in witch hazel. Apply to your hemorrhoids as often as needed to ease discomfort," suggests Maier.

Make an herbal sitz bath. Make two strong herbal infusions from dried comfrey leaves (*Symphytum officinale*) and dried calendula flowers (*Calendula officinalis*). Both herbs are known for their healing, anti-inflammatory and soothing properties, says Maier. Mix 1 tablespoon per cup of boiling water using ½ tablespoon calendula and ½ tablespoon comfrey, she recommends.

To make an infusion, pour hot water over the herbs and let them steep. In a one-quart canning jar, add 4 tablespoons of the blend to 4 cups boiling water; cover and steep for a half-hour. Strain the herbs, then add the infusion to a bathtub half-full of warm water. Sit in the bath for at least 20 minutes, recommends Maier. Do this once a day, or twice a day if hemorrhoids are very painful.

Smooth on an herbal salve. Like witch hazel, horse chestnut (*Aesculus hippocastanum*) salve has astringent properties that soothe and shrink swollen hemorrhoidal tissues, says Maier. It's available at health food stores.

INDIGESTION AND HEARTBURN: PUT OUT THE FIRE

That burning sensation. That way-too-full, I-can't-believe-I-ate-the-whole-thing sensation. That gassy, bloated feeling. Welcome to indigestion, an all-too-familiar discomfort that most women, especially most pregnant women, have felt on at least a few occasions.

Indigestion is a catchall word for problems with digestive functions. Symptoms can include heartburn (a burning feeling felt near your breastbone), nausea, cramps, belching and flatulence. Stress is probably a catalyst for indigestion, though scientists aren't exactly sure why. Eating too much or too fast is also commonly to blame.

One fast way to take the edge off indigestion is to use herbs, say natural healers. Here's what they recommend.

Sip herbal teas. "Chamomile and peppermint teas are wonderful for soothing tension-induced digestive troubles," says Andrew Weil, M.D., professor of herbalism and director of the Program of Integrative Medicine at the University of Arizona College of Medicine, near Tucson, and author of *Spontaneous Healing* and *Health and Healing*.

"When you make the tea, be sure to keep the teapot and your cup covered so that the vapor can't evaporate. A travel mug with a lid works well. The volatile oils in the vapor make the teas work," explains Dr. Weil. To be certain that you are getting pure chamomile, he advises buying the herb from an established health food store or other reputable source.

How I Healed Myself **Naturally**

Yoga, Herbs and Fiber Cured Her Digestive Woes

Carrie Havranek, a 23-year-old college graduate from Medford, New Jersey, turned to natural remedies for her digestive problems—with outstanding results.

"I've had a sensitive stomach for as long as I can remember," says Havranek. "Foods like garlic, tomato sauce, cucumbers and coffee disagreed with me.

"I was getting these sharp, shooting abdominal pains on a regular basis," she continues. "I'd wake up in the morning hungry, but I couldn't even finish my breakfast because of the pain. A couple hours later, I'd be starving again."

Havranek's problems worsened during the fall of her senior year in college when she had to decide between getting a job or going to graduate school. The pressure was intense.

"It got to the point where everything I ate bothered my stomach," she explains. "Pretty soon, I was only eating bland things like turkey sandwiches and bagels."

Havranek suspected her stomach trouble was hereditary—she says that her mother also has a very sensitive stomach.

"My mother is in her forties, and she has always had digestive problems. Her doctor told her to change her diet. She's now on a high-protein, low-carbohydrate diet and eats fewer fattening foods. It has really helped. She's doing much better."

Try marshmallow tea. Teas made from the soothing herb marshmallow (*Althaea officinalis*) are excellent aids for your digestive system, says Maier. To make marshmallow tea, use a tablespoon of dried herb to a cup of boiling water steeped for a minimum of 40 minutes. Drink a cup of this once a day.

Slip slippery elm into your food. Powdered slippery elm (*Ulmus fulva*) soothes irritated mucous membranes and eases many digestive complaints, says Maier. Whenever you're troubled by indigestion, sprinkle a spoonful or two into your morning oatmeal or add it to stir-fry. Slippery elm also makes an easy addition to fruit smoothies—bananas or other fruit blended with milk or yogurt.

So Havranek wondered if she, too, could benefit from a dietary change. She was diagnosed with irritable bowel syndrome (IBS), which is typically characterized by abdominal pain and irregular bowel movements.

"The practitioner prescribed an antispasmotic, a type of medicine that is typically used for IBS, but also said that stress plays a big role in digestive problems, and she said that yoga could help reduce my stress levels," adds Havranek. "So I signed up for a yoga course at school."

The practitioner also recommended herbal teas—including chamomile, mint and ginger, known to soothe stomach distress—and more fiber, to relieve abdominal pain and irregularity associated with IBS.

"I became a fiber junkie," she admits. "I try to eat foods like fresh spinach at least once a day, and I drink Metamucil, a commercial fiber supplement, mixed with water.

"If stress seems to be getting the best of me and I can't get down on the floor to do a yoga position, I just take a nice, long walk or go to the gym."

Havranek says that she feels a whole lot better. Her irritable bowel syndrome is under control.

IRRITABLE BOWEL SYNDROME:
ALL QUIET BELOW THE BELT

"Irritable bowel syndrome is a catchall word for all sorts of digestive problems," says Dr. Scala. Often it's alternating constipation and diarrhea. "For women who have irritable bowel syndrome, certain foods and stressful conditions can cause incredible abdominal pain, diarrhea and even rectal bleeding." And the problem tends to be frequent or constant.

Because it has so many forms, IBS is known by a multitude of other names, such as spastic colitis, mucous colitis, spastic colon or functional bowel disease. If you have true colitis, the lining of the bowel is inflamed, infected or even ulcerated. There's none of these specific problems with IBS, even though the symptoms may resemble those of colitis.

Symptoms of IBS vary from woman to woman and will usually begin during the teen years or young adulthood.

 ## Eating Right When Your Gut's Gone Wrong

The best ways to heal an irritable bowel are to modify your diet and your lifestyle.

"Women who follow special diets, manage stress and take nutritional supplements stand a good chance of easing their IBS symptoms for up to two years," says Dr. Scala. "You have to make a commitment to making some major lifestyle changes, but I promise you that you'll be richly rewarded when your symptoms start easing off."

Here's what Dr. Scala recommends.

Help yourself to flaxseed oil. Scientists have discovered that oils like flaxseed oil and fish oils are rich in the omega-3 fatty acid called EPA (eicosapentaenoic acid), which is valued for its anti-inflammatory effects.

"Studies show, quite convincingly, that one of the best things that women with IBS can do for themselves is to add oils containing omega-3 fatty acids to their diets on a regular basis," says Dr. Scala. He recommends taking two tablespoons of flaxseed oil every day. It's all right to slurp it right from the spoon, but the oil is pretty tasteless. Instead, just add the two tablespoons of oil to your morning cereal. Or, take two or three fish oil capsules once a day before a meal, he adds.

You can even make salad dressing out of flaxseed oil, says Dr. Fugh-Berman.

Shun red meat. Women with IBS should follow a vegetarian diet or at least avoid red meat, says Dr. Scala. Fish is fine. Or, have some skinless turkey or chicken breast. You can also have the meat from game animals such as rabbit and deer that were raised on grasses instead of corn, he adds.

Make those veggies well-done. Your cookbook may tell you to steam green, yellow and orange vegetables till they're crisp-tender or al dente. But if you have IBS, Dr. Scala says, "Cook your vegetables till they're soft. You want to eliminate any sharp edges that can cause irritation." And, of course, completely raw vegetables are not advisable.

Go soft on hard foods. Be wary of chunky, sharp-edged foods, such as nuts. "Hard foods like nuts and seeds are more irritating than softer foods," says Dr. Scala.

If your love of hard foods makes eliminating them from your diet too difficult, then make sure that you chew them well, says Dr. Fugh-Berman.

 Watch your Bs. Medications prescribed for IBS can increase a woman's need for B vitamins. "A good multivitamin/mineral supplement, one that includes all the B vitamins, is helpful to any woman who has IBS," says Dr. Scala.

Choose soluble fiber supplements over bran. Bran or a high-fiber diet is routinely recommended for people with IBS. But according to a study conducted by researchers in the Department of Medicine at the University Hospital of South Manchester in England, bran and other soluble fiber-rich foods may make IBS symptoms worse.

In the study, 100 men and women with IBS were questioned about their response to various forms of fiber. Fifty-five percent reported that their symptoms worsened after eating bran. After taking soluble fiber supplements such as psyllium, however, 39 percent reported an improvement in their IBS symptoms. Only 10 percent of those who took bran reported an improvement. Based on this evidence, the researchers say that soluble fiber supplements may be a better option than bran.

Mind-Body Therapy for Digestive Bliss

What happens in your head can have an impact on what's happening in your belly and below, say experts. "Your brain sends signals to your digestive system and influences activity there," says Dr. Gershon. And the reverse is true, too. Any distress that you feel in your bowel can also cause mental distress.

For women with IBS, learning to retrain the brain—and soothe the belly—is a key part of finding relief. Likewise, soothing the belly can bring profound relief to the mind.

Consider cognitive therapy. "When you have unpredictable, disruptive pain, as do many women who suffer from IBS, you can be overwhelmed by a profound sense of vulnerability," says Douglas A. Drossman, M.D., gastroenterologist, psychiatrist and associate professor of medicine and psychiatry in the Division of Digestive Diseases at the University of North Carolina School of Medicine in Chapel Hill. "Cognitive therapy allows women to focus on their IBS symptoms and to gain control over them."

In cognitive therapy, you'll probably be asked to keep a diary noting your symptoms and how they make you feel. During sessions, the therapist will examine your thoughts and feelings to help you reframe your ineffective responses. According to Dr. Drossman, women who successfully complete a 12-week treatment program using cognitive therapy can feel even better a year later. In other words, both the women and the doctors who tested them agreed that these were long-term, positive results.

Get a handle on stress. "Women who internalize stress, who 'implode' rather than 'explode,' have a harder time with digestive diseases because stress is definitely a precipitating factor," says Dr. Scala. He suggests that women with symptoms of IBS try yoga, massage, meditation, exercise or other stress-busting strategies.

Hypnosis may also be very helpful since it has been shown to help irritable bowel syndrome, adds Dr. Fugh-Berman.

NAUSEA AND VOMITING: FIGHT THE URGE TO PURGE

There's nothing quite like vomiting to make us realize how little control we have over the physical shell we inhabit. No matter what its cause—illness or tainted food, motion sickness or drinking too much—once the wave of nausea overtakes you, vomiting is almost sure to follow.

But sometimes vomiting doesn't follow, and you're stuck with the nausea, that queasy, not-quite-but-almost-dizzy feeling that starts in your stomach. When nausea lingers, you'll know exactly why cartoon characters who feel nauseated are colored green.

For very welcome relief from nausea, turn to the world of natural remedies. **Try a wristband for relief.** Acupressure, the ancient Chinese healing art, is the basis for a modern remedy that scientists say can control nausea and vomiting.

A simple wristband, called Sea-Band, presses a bead into the P6 meridian point called nei-guan on the underside of your wrist, a spot associated with relief of nausea by those who practice the oriental arts of acupressure and acupuncture. The effectiveness of the wristband was supported by a German research team that found that women who wore the bands for 24 hours after minor gynecological surgery were able to reduce postsurgical nausea and vomiting by 50 percent. You can find Sea-

Bands in health food stores and in some drugstores.

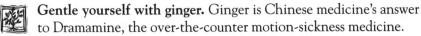 **Gentle yourself with ginger.** Ginger is Chinese medicine's answer to Dramamine, the over-the-counter motion-sickness medicine.

"It's a wonderful antinausea remedy," says Maier. "Whenever you feel queasy, grate a teaspoonful of fresh gingerroot into a hot cup of tea or eat some crystallized gingerroot candy." You can find this candy in gourmet or health food stores.

Consider homeopathic help. "If you can match your symptoms to the correct remedy, using homeopathy at home can stem sudden, severe vomiting and nausea," says Michael Carlston, M.D., assistant clinical professor at the University of California, San Francisco, School of Medicine.

"In my experience, some over-the-counter homeopathic medicines can relieve nausea and vomiting, especially if they contain the proper remedy for your specific symptoms," says Dr. Carlston. He recommends reading labels carefully to find out whether the OTC remedy fits the symptoms that you're having.

For motion sickness that's more dizziness than nausea, Dr. Carlston suggests trying Cocculus, a homeopathic remedy derived from *Anamirta cocculus*, known as the Indian cockle. If the nausea outweighs the dizziness, use Tabacum, a remedy made from the tobacco plant. With both remedies, follow the label directions and look for potencies of 6c or 12c, suggests Dr. Carlston. The "c" indicates a homeopathic remedy's level of concentration.

EMOTIONAL PROBLEMS

Coping with Stress and Negative Emotions

It's noon in New York City and the yoga class at Crunch Fitness, a trendy Manhattan health spa, is packed. While traffic groans by on 13th Street, two dozen women and men, oblivious to the lunch-hour bustle, quietly follow along as Dana Flynn, the instructor, demonstrates a handstand.

Usually, Flynn says, people sign up for her class because they've heard that yoga can make them more flexible or stronger. But they keep coming back for a different reason, she says.

"People who take the class—and about three-quarters of them are women—notice that they feel less stressed, less anxious and less depressed," says Flynn. "They feel better because yoga cultivates self-acceptance, and a lot of women feel stress, anxiety and depression because they don't accept themselves."

Women, studies show, report considerably more emotional problems than men do—more anxiety, more panic attacks, more phobias, more mood swings and more depression, including seasonal affective disorder, a type of depression common in fall and winter. Some researchers speculate that this is because the hormonal changes that we experience premenstrually, during pregnancy and at menopause widen the arc of our emotional swings.

Other experts say societal factors predispose us to emotional wear and tear. We're still doing most of the work at home and just as much of the work at the office, though for less pay than our male colleagues, they note. Still other researchers say it's possible that men have just as many emotional troubles but are less vocal and less likely to seek help than we are.

DON'T LET NEGATIVE EMOTIONS ERODE YOUR HEALTH

Whatever the cause of women's angst, emotional problems can exact a heavy toll on our physical health. Research suggests that sustained anxiety and stress, for instance, can trigger physiological changes that raise your blood pressure and heart rate. Too much stress or anxiety over too long a period, it seems, can make you more susceptible to serious conditions like heart disease.

You don't have to let negative emotions get the best of you, however. If you have milder symptoms, an apothecary of nondrug therapies—from yoga, aromatherapy and exercise to meditation, imagery or simple cognitive therapy—can help. If the anxiety or depression or stress that you're feeling is so overwhelming that you no longer enjoy yourself or can't do the things that you need to do, self-help methods may not solve the problem, says Annabelle Nelson, Ph.D., psychologist in Prescott, Arizona, professor at the Fielding Institute in Santa Barbara, California, and author of *Living the Wheel: Working with Emotions, Terror and Bliss through Imagery*. That's especially true if there's a physical reason for the way you feel.

So if you feel overwhelmed or severely distressed, it's a good idea to consult a medical doctor or professional psychotherapist. She may recommend biofeedback, professional cognitive therapy, breath therapy or light therapy or long-term psychotherapy, alone or in combination with medical treatments.

Whatever route you take, the idea isn't to use these techniques to chase away your bad feelings and forget about them, says Judith S. Beck, Ph.D., director of the Beck Institute for Cognitive Therapy and Research, clinical assistant professor of psychology in psychiatry at the University of Pennsylvania in Philadelphia and author of a textbook on cognitive therapy. Feelings—good and bad alike—can tell you something, says Dr. Beck. "Negative moods may be telling you that there's a problem you need to solve," she explains. If you're depressed, you may need to make some changes in your life. Therapy, whether it's drug therapy or professional psychotherapy, can help you feel better so that you can take a clear-eyed look at your life, decide if and how you might change things and then move on.

ANXIETY, PANIC AND PHOBIAS: UNFRAZZLE YOUR NERVES

At the Monmouth Medical Center in Long Branch, New Jersey, staff members regularly prescribe personal, portable headset stereos for women awaiting gynecological surgery. The wait before surgery normally makes most women very anxious. But women who listen to music before surgery report less apprehension and worry and have lower heart rates and blood pressures (also a sign of lower presurgical jitters).

Apprehension, worry and rapid heart and breathing rates are all classic symptoms of anxiety. A state of arousal triggered by the threat of danger, anxiety can also bring on stomachaches, restlessness, dizziness and difficulty concentrating.

Sometimes you know exactly why you're anxious—because you have an upcoming job review, for instance. At other times, you may feel anxious, but the danger may not be immediately apparent, says Dr. Beck. You may feel worried and not know why. If you ponder a bit, though, you can usually discover what's triggered your anxiety, she says. You might get anxious awaiting surgery, for instance, because you're afraid there will be complications, or because you're worried that you'll have a great deal of pain and a long recovery after.

Anxiety isn't necessarily bad. Rather, it's a warning that you need to take action, to prepare for, say, an upcoming presentation. When anxiety is ongoing or so intense that it interferes with your ability to concentrate, to sleep or to enjoy yourself, you need relief. Here's what works—and why.

How I Healed Myself **Naturally**

Biofeedback and Deep Breathing Help Her Relax

Anna Bennett, a 62-year-old librarian from Toledo, Ohio, says biofeedback enabled her to control her blood pressure and overcome stressful feelings of anxiety and panic.

"I had always been anxious as a child," says Bennett (who asked us not to use her real name). "As an adult I started taking Xanax, an anti-anxiety drug, which I took only in extremely stressful situations, such as a plane flight. Then, three years ago, things got worse. During a routine medical checkup, my internist discovered that my blood pressure was extremely high. I didn't think much about it because my blood pressure always went up when I went to the doctor, even though I was taking blood pressure medication. Nevertheless, the doctor decided to put me on a second blood pressure medication.

"Well, he tried four different medications, and with each I had side effects, including extreme nervousness and panic," recalls Bennett. "I developed full-blown panic attacks. They were scary—each time, I thought that I was having a heart attack. So, in addition to Xanax, my doctor prescribed the antidepressant drug Zoloft.

"After two days on this drug combination, I began to hallucinate," says Bennett. "So I stopped taking Zoloft, and my doctor said that I should try Prozac, another antidepressant drug. But I refused. Instead, I went to a cardiologist, who determined that I didn't need all those

Stop and think. Cognitive therapists like Dr. Beck teach the men and women whom they counsel to identify troubling thoughts and evaluate them. A basic premise of cognitive therapy is that erroneous beliefs contribute to emotional problems and counterproductive behavior. You can try some basic cognitive techniques on your own, Dr. Beck says.

Next time you're feeling anxious, ask yourself, "What thought just went through my head?" Perhaps you thought, "I'll blow the budget presentation, and my boss will fire me!" Ask yourself, "How likely is it that this will happen?" If you've been working diligently on the budget presentation, you probably won't blow it. And if your boss has been happy with your work, it's unlikely that she'd give you the boot even if the presentation didn't go perfectly. Thinking things through this way can help alleviate anxiety and other emotional problems, says Dr. Beck.

---

blood pressure medications. He took me off all medications except the Xanax, which I was taking in large doses at the time. Eventually, I was able to cut back on it."

Meanwhile, Bennett looked for and found another internist. Her new doctor suggested that she consider biofeedback as a way to control her blood pressure and anxiety without drugs and relieve the panic attacks. He referred her to a psychologist who used biofeedback, combined with breathing exercises and relaxation tapes, and cognitive therapy to talk about the causes of her stressful emotions.

"I've been going to biofeedback sessions for a year," notes Bennett, who says that the treatments have helped. "I still have occasional panic attacks, but they're not nearly as frightening. My blood pressure is still on the high side when I'm in a doctor's office, but it's normal when I measure it at home.

"The breathing exercises and relaxation tapes that I use with biofeedback have been a great help. And my discussions with the counselor have helped me to put things in perspective and understand why I have these reactions. She taught me not to take life so seriously, to laugh more and to be more relaxed and less anxious," says Bennett.

"I'm still taking very low doses of Xanax. My goal is to get off it completely and, instead, use relaxation exercises when I feel anxious."

See and conquer. Imagining yourself pulling through a difficult situation with ease can help take the edge off your anxiety, says Dr. Nelson. "Imagery talks to the part of your brain called the limbic system, which is the threshold between your mind and body," she explains. "Relaxing imagery affects the limbic system in such a way that your heart rate slows and your blood pressure drops."

Still worried about that budget presentation? Close your eyes and image yourself giving a calm, cool, dazzling presentation. Make it vivid. See the managers' smiling faces, feel the conference room carpet under your feet, smell the coffee in the pot in the middle of the table.

Maybe budget presentations aren't your problem. But mentally rehearsing a positive outcome can help defuse anxiety about other high-pressure situations.

Try yoga. If you're struggling with anxiety, practicing a series of four calming yoga postures can help, says Richard C. Miller, Ph.D., a yoga instructor and psychologist in San Rafael, California, co-founder of the International Association of Yoga Therapists and founder of the Marin School of Yoga.

Start with a forward bend from a standing position posture. Inhaling, raise your arms overhead. As you exhale to a count of eight, bend down at your waist. Then, straighten up slowly, to a count of four or six, as you inhale. Repeat eight times.

Follow with the two-legged table posture. Lie on your back, feet on the floor, knees bent and arms by your side. Inhale to a count of six as you slowly lift your pelvis. Hold the position for a count of one. Then, exhaling, lower your pelvis to the floor to a count of eight. Repeat eight times.

Now try the child posture. Kneel on the floor with your arms overhead and feet straight out behind you. Exhale as you slowly count to six while bending at the waist. Bring your arms down behind you as you lower your buttocks to your heels and bring your forehead to the floor. Relax, then inhale as you straighten up to a count of eight. Repeat eight times.

Finish with yoga Nidra, or quiet contemplation. Shut off the lights, lie on the floor and close your eyes. Spend three to five minutes simply observing how you feel, paying particular attention to your breathing. When you're ready to stop, tell yourself that you're going to resume your day. Then take a deep breath, stretch, open your eyes and get up.

Panic Attacks: Stop Out-of-Control Anxiety

Sometimes, anxiety escalates into a panic attack, a sudden episode of intense anxiety. Symptoms may include heart palpitations and disorientation, along with shortness of breath, dizziness, chest pain, nausea, smothering sensations and bouts of sweating. The experience can be terrifying.

"In the middle of a panic attack, you think that you're facing some kind of catastrophe," says Dr. Beck. "If you're having chest pain, you may think that you're going to have a heart attack. If you feel disoriented, you may think that you're going to go crazy."

Panic attacks can trigger a vicious cycle. Convinced that they're experiencing warning signs of heart attacks or bouts with madness, women who experience panic attacks try desperately to control the symptoms.

"They stop whatever they're doing," says Dr. Beck. "If they're at the mall, they go home. If they're out walking, they sit down. When the symptoms go away—and they usually do—they're convinced that leaving the mall or sitting down was what averted catastrophe. So they stop going to the mall or they avoid going out to walk, to try to avoid repeat episodes."

Some women who experience panic attacks put so many limits on what they can do that they become agoraphobic—irrationally afraid of leaving home and going out in public.

Panic attacks can be treated with intensive therapy—and sometimes medication—with the guidance of a health care practitioner. If you have panic attacks and your doctor has told you that you do not have some other medical problem, remind yourself that they're not warning signs of a catastrophe, says Dr. Beck. The symptoms will go away on their own, usually after less than 20 minutes. You don't have to stop what you're doing or give up the things that you need and like to do, she says.

"If you have panic attacks, you need to stop trying to control the symptoms and prove to yourself that, no matter how bad the symptoms, the catastrophe won't happen," she says. Here's what practitioners suggest.

Calm yourself with self-talk. Cognitive therapy can help you revise the erroneous thinking that contributes to panic attacks, says Dr. Beck. While you're feeling calm, ask yourself, "What catastrophe am I afraid will happen? Why has it never happened?" Then ask yourself, "What can I do to prove to myself that the catastrophe won't happen?"

Say your panic attacks trigger a fear that you're having a heart attack at the mall. Chances are, you've never had a heart attack at the mall and you're not likely to. Rather, you've had panic attacks at the mall. You can prove this to yourself by going to the mall, experiencing the symptoms and coming out of the experience perfectly fine.

Try soothing angelica oil. For panic attacks, Jane Buckle, R.N., a certified aromatherapist and aromatherapy teacher in England and author of *Clinical Aromatherapy in Nursing*, often recommends the essential oil extracted from the herb *Angelica archangelica*, available at health food stores. Keep a small bottle handy, add a drop to a hanky and sniff the aroma whenever you feel a panic attack coming on.

Phobias: Rational Solutions for Irrational Fears

So you know what claustrophobia is. But what about agoraphobia? Or acrophobia?

These phobias—irrational fears of enclosed spaces, leaving home, and heights, respectively—are fairly common. But you can have a phobia of virtually any object, activity or situation that frightens you so much that you'll go out of your way to avoid it. Faced with whatever you fear, your heart races, you sweat, blush and want to flee.

Think of a phobia as an intense fear that interferes with daily life. A normal fear—say, a fear of wandering alone into a sinister neighborhood after nightfall—is often well-founded and useful. By contrast, a phobia can keep you from doing perfectly safe things that you want or need to do.

"A phobia is an irrational fear that exerts control over your daily living," explains Eileen F. Oster, registered occupational therapist and meditation instructor from Bayside, New York, and author of *The Healing Mind: Your Guide to the Power of Meditation, Prayer and Reflection*. "You try to avoid feeling overwhelming anxiety or panic, so you avoid the thing that makes you afraid."

Some phobias stem from past trauma. You might be able to trace your fear of animals, for instance, to the day your neighbor's dog gave you a nasty bite. The origin of other phobias may be more difficult to trace.

Deeply entrenched phobias that interfere with your life require professional help, says Angele McGrady, Ph.D., professor of psychiatry and physiology at the Medical College of Ohio in Toledo and past president of the Association for Applied Psychophysiology and Biofeedback based in Wheatridge, Colorado. For milder phobias, you can try the simple anxiety-relieving techniques described earlier. Here's what else to try.

Imagine yourself victorious. The classic remedy for phobias is a process called systematic desensitization. Basically, you confront the thing that you're phobic of very gradually. To make this easier, imagine yourself confronting the person or thing that you fear before the actual confrontation, says Judith Green, Ph.D., professor of psychology and biofeedback in the Department of Behavioral Sciences at Aims Community College in Greeley, Colorado, and author of *The Dynamics of Health and Wellness*.

Say you're afraid to ride in elevators. Before you actually set foot in an elevator, imagine yourself approaching the elevator and feeling fine. When you can imagine yourself doing this and actually feel fine, imagine yourself getting into the elevator. And once this mental image no longer makes you uneasy, imagine yourself riding up one floor, without a hitch. Again, when you're able to imagine this without sweating it, imagine yourself riding far-ther, without incident. Repeat, slowly adding floors, until you can see yourself riding to the top of a tall building without panicking.

Next, approach an elevator while staying calm and relaxed and using positive imagery. First, ride it up one floor, repeating the trip until you're comfortable. Then ride to a second floor and repeat, and so forth. Finally, ride to the top floor. You may want to take a companion with you.

You can use desensitization to gradually overcome other common phobias, such as tunnels, crowded spaces or other close environments.

Think things through. It's often helpful to systematically expose yourself to feared situations, says Dr. Beck. Before you get on the elevator, ask yourself, "What am I so afraid of?" Maybe the answer is, "I'm afraid the elevator will crash." Now ask yourself, "How likely is it that the elevator will crash? How many times has this elevator gone up and down without crashing?" Realistically assessing the risk in this way should help calm your fear, says Dr. Beck.

DEPRESSION: YEAR-ROUND HELP FOR THE BLUES

Everyone gets the blues from time to time, when ambitions fail, for example, or when relationships end. While the blues are relatively short-lived, though, in true depression, individuals suffer moderate to severe symptoms for at least two weeks. If not treated, feelings of sorrow and hopelessness may last weeks, months and sometimes years.

Often, depression is accompanied by other changes: You can't sleep, or you do nothing but sleep. You can't eat, or you overeat. Or you lose interest in sex and other activities that once brought pleasure, have difficulty concentrating, feel restless or tired or develop headaches or back pain. When depression is severe, it can lead to suicidal fantasies, even suicide.

Prolonged depression that won't let up calls for professional help, says Dr. Beck. Your doctor may recommend antidepressants, psychotherapy or a combination of treatments. If you're mildly depressed, and you're not having any thoughts of harming yourself, the following alternatives may help you feel good enough to figure out what's troubling you and how to deal with it.

Talk your way out. When you're depressed, you may tend to have distorted, negative thoughts, like "Nobody cares about me anymore," says Dr. Beck. Ask yourself, "Is there any evidence that this is true?" Odds are, there's little evidence that no one cares. Perhaps you feel this way because family members aren't offering you the help that you need to get everything done. If that's the case, you have to find a solution. "You'll need to ask for help or do less," says Dr. Beck.

"Do less" doesn't mean do less for yourself, however. "When women get depressed, they tend to isolate themselves from others, say no to plans or drop things that they've done that gave them a sense of accomplishment or pleasure. They don't play tennis anymore or ask people to lunch," says Dr. Beck. "Instead of telling yourself, 'Once I feel better, I'll do these things,' tell yourself, 'In order to feel better, I need to start doing these things now.' "

Turn into a cobra. In a German study, women who practiced yoga regularly reported better emotional health—less anxiety and less depression—than nonpractitioners.

When combined with the forward bend from a standing position and the child posture, used to relieve anxiety, the cobra position can stimulate you and lift depression, says Dr. Miller.

First, do the forward bend from a standing position and the child posture, described on page 392. Then do the cobra: Lie on your stomach with your elbows by your sides and your palms flat on the floor by your shoulders. As you inhale, lift your chest to a count of six, keeping your hands on the floor. Now lower yourself back down to the floor as you exhale to a count of eight. Repeat eight times. Then follow with the yoga Nidra, also described on page 392.

Meditate with sound. To boost your energy level and your spirits, Oster suggests "sounding meditation."

Choose any short word that has syllables and consonants in it, like ohm, and repeat it, focusing on nothing but the word. Let the sound of the word

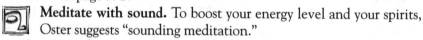

How I Healed Myself **Naturally**

Meditation Keeps Depression at Bay

Ellen Kauffman, 33, a certified personal trainer and yoga instructor from California, used meditation and visualization to overcome deep depression prompted by a divorce.

"It was very bad," recalls Kauffman (who asked us not to use her real name). "I had all the symptoms of depression, including loss of interest in all of the things that normally interested me. I stopped exercising. I didn't read a magazine for a year."

A two-day hospital stay and a brief course of antidepressants helped pull Kauffman out of the depression. But meditation and visualization, she says, help keep her out. "That's what keeps me mentally well."

vibrate throughout your body, imparting energy, Oster explains. "The act of sounding is putting forth energy. When you're depressed, you have trouble harnessing energy. A sounding meditation helps you gather some energy."

Imagine relief. Visualization is often used to relive physical pain, but it can also be used to heal emotional pain. If you're feeling depressed, Dr. Nelson suggests that you visualize the feeling. "Ask yourself 'Where do I feel pain?' and 'What does it look like?'" she says. "Maybe the image that comes to mind is of a dark blanket that's smothering your heart." Now imagine some relief. "See yourself removing the blanket and freeing your heart," she says.

Try St.-John's-wort. Working with researchers in Germany, a research team at Audie L. Murphy Memorial Veterans Hospital in San Antonio reports that St.-John's-wort (*Hypericum perforatum*) is effective as a standard antidepressant drug for treating mild to moderate depression—and causes fewer side effects. The researchers based their conclusion on an analysis of 23 trials involving 1,757 men and women. Most of the trials took place in Germany, where herbal medicines are prescribed extensively by psychiatrists, internists, obstetricians and gynecologists for treatment of anxiety, depression and sleep problems.

St.-John's-wort doesn't work overnight. The herb needs two to four weeks to take effect. Follow package directions.

Postpartum Depression: Take It Seriously

It arrives soon after the baby does, but it's no joyous delivery: Postpartum depression leaves many new moms feeling very low.

Roughly three-quarters of new mothers get the postpartum blues. They may feel teary, anxious, tense, moody or angry—or all of the above. Some feel guilty about feeling low when they think that they should be ecstatic. Others worry that they're ill-equipped to care for their infants. In rare but severe cases, new moms begin to toy with the idea of harming themselves or their babies.

A number of things appear to contribute to the postpartum blues, says Dr. Beck. Hormonal changes seem to play a role, as does the stress of adjusting to life with a completely dependent, very demanding new person.

Postpartum depression usually lifts after a week or two, though some women suffer for months if they don't get help. You should see your doctor if you're thinking about harming yourself or your child or if the depression gets worse instead of better, says Dr. Beck. Your doctor may recommend a short course of antidepressants or psychotherapy, or both. For milder postpartum blues, other tactics against depression may help. Practitioners also offer these suggestions.

Foresee good times with your baby. Imagine yourself happy and coping well with your baby, suggests Dr. Green. That way you program yourself for a positive experience.

Help yourself to aromatherapy. If you find yourself feeling blue after delivery, try inhaling the essential oil extracted from *Pelargonium graveolens*—a species of geranium, suggests Buckle. The aroma affects your adrenal cortex, the part of your brain that is responsible for establishing hormonal balance, she explains. So it can be particularly helpful if you're suffering from postpartum blues, she says.

Seasonal Affective Disorder: Climb with the Light

Stockholm, Sweden, gets less than 12 hours of sunlight a day in early October, a mere 6 hours a day in December and ekes out 8 hours of sunlight a day by the time February rolls around.

That makes Stockholm an ideal place to study seasonal affective disorder (SAD), a type of depression that settles in when days grow short in autumn and doesn't lift until the sunlight hours lengthen in spring. Research finds that SAD is more common in darker, northern climes. It's more widespread in Stockholm than Boston, for instance, but more common in Boston than Miami.

The severity and symptoms of SAD can vary from person to person. But most of those who are affected experience some combination of sadness, crying spells, fatigue, irritability, headaches, difficulty thinking and carbohydrate cravings. Women and men with severe SAD may become suicidal.

Fortunately, a growing body of scientific evidence points to a simple and effective cure. In a study at the Institute of Clinical Neuroscience at St. Göran's Hospital in sun-spare Stockholm, for instance, more than half of a group of 68 male and female volunteers with SAD improved markedly after a short session of light therapy. After just ten sessions of treatment, which involved spending two hours a day in a very brightly lit room, most felt considerably better.

Why does bright light help? Researchers aren't sure. Nor is it clear why some people get SAD in the first place. The hormone melatonin, which regulates many seasonal responses in animals, may play a role, says Brenda Byrne, Ph.D., director of the Seasonal Affective Disorder Clinic at Jefferson Medical College of Thomas Jefferson University in Philadelphia. Bright light suppresses the body's production of melatonin, she explains.

In the Stockholm study, participants spent two hours in bright light. But you may get the same benefit by spending half an hour in front of a light box, says Dr. Byrne. Light boxes are specially designed lamplike devices that emit a wide spectrum of intense light, mimicking sunlight.

"In my experience, about two-thirds of people with definite seasonal affective disorder feel better with light treatment," says Dr. Byrne. (For details on how to use light therapy, see page 210.)

MOOD SWINGS: EVEN OUT THE HIGHS AND LOWS

"A woman is always a fickle, unstable thing," griped the Roman poet Virgil, one in a long line of men to accuse women of changing their minds and moods too often.

Women do report more mood swings—more dips into depression and more free falls into anxiety—than men. While guys may be just as moody and simply more tight-lipped than we are, the hormonal changes that we undergo after childbirth and before menstruation can affect our moods, says Dr. Beck.

"The trigger may be hormonal," she says. "Or it could be situational—that is, prompted by what is going on in your life."

If you're bothered by mood swings, you may benefit from many of the techniques that help depression and anxiety. Cognitive therapy may also help. When you find yourself slipping into anxiety or depression, ask yourself, "What just went through my mind?" suggests Dr. Beck.

Maybe your mood swing occurred after a friend stood you up for lunch, for example. Perhaps that made you think, 'She doesn't like me anymore. No one does.' Test that hypothesis, says Dr. Beck. Ask yourself if there's any evidence behind that belief. Have all your friends suddenly abandoned you? Probably not. Now ask yourself whether there might be some other explanation for her failure to appear. Maybe she got caught in traffic or her car broke down.

Finally, ask yourself what you might do if the worst scenario were true and your friend didn't like you any longer, she continues. For starters, you could talk to her about the rift. Testing the validity of your thoughts with basic questions like these should help temper your mood swings. (For information on mood swings associated with menopause, see page 437.)

STRESS: ANTIDOTES FOR WHAT LIFE DISHES OUT

Jane Buckle crosses time zones the way most of us cross city limits, jetting between Europe and the United States, teaching and lecturing on aromatherapy. No matter what her destination, Buckle heads for an aromatic bath when she lands.

"Whenever I finish a flight that crosses a time zone, I check into my hotel and have a bath with one drop of geranium oil and one drop of

How I Healed Myself **Naturally**

Light Therapy Cured Her Depression

Irene Dalton, a mother of two grown daughters in Pottstown, Pennsylvania, had suffered from depression since her twenties. She says that light therapy changed her life.

"Before, I'd literally take to my bed from November till springtime," says Dalton. "I couldn't hold a steady job or even take care of my family."

Dalton's depression was so severe that doctors had prescribed powerful medications such as Prozac and Zoloft. "The drugs had terrible side effects," says Dalton.

In addition, during her most depressed times, she craved carbohydrates and gained weight, which added to her depression. "I didn't know how I was going to live out my life," she says.

One day, Dalton saw a TV news report about a condition called seasonal affective disorder (SAD). The broadcast mentioned the work being done by Brenda Byrne, Ph.D., director of the Seasonal Affective Disorder Clinic at Jefferson Medical College of Thomas Jefferson University in Philadelphia.

"I had never heard of SAD before, but its symptoms fit me to a T," says Dalton. "As soon as I realized that there was a name and a treatment for what I had, I sped off to Philadelphia for an appointment with Dr. Byrne. She saved my life."

Now, instead of wanting to crawl back under the covers each winter morning, Dalton turns on a special light box, puts on her headphones and hops on her exercise bike for half an hour.

"I use my light-box time to my advantage," says Dalton. "I can return work calls or listen to tapes from my church and get the exercise that my doctor says is important when you have SAD."

Today, Dalton is happily holding down her first permanent job. And she effortlessly lost 25 pounds during her first few months of treatment. "I could have gone my entire life living a normal life only six months out of the year. I thank God now that I don't have to—and so does my entire family."

lavender oil," says Buckle. "When I do that, I don't get too stressed."

Stress is what we feel when we have more to do than we can comfortably manage, explains Dr. Miller. A little stress can be a good thing, since it makes us feel challenged and energized. Too much stress for too long a period of time is another matter, though.

Different people respond differently to stress overload, says Dr. Beck. Some get anxious. Others grow depressed. High levels of stress can also cause physical symptoms, such as rapid heartbeat, increased blood pressure, difficulty concentrating, overeating, irritability, headaches, backaches and neck aches. And unrelenting high stress can raise your risk for heart disease and weaken your immune system.

Since stress is most overwhelming and damaging when it's unrelenting, stress relievers like aromatherapy, meditation and imagery can help. Sometimes, though, you need to make changes in the way that you schedule your time—and in your expectations—to protect yourself from chronic stress overload, says Dr. Beck. Here's a list of short- and long-term stress-fighting alternatives.

Imagine calm. If you're really stressed, pause for a moment and put your palms over your eyes. "Then imagine yourself in a place that you really enjoy," like a beachfront cottage or mountain cabin where you once vacationed, says Dr. Nelson.

Build relaxation breaks into your schedule. Imagery breaks and other antistress techniques can help revive you so that you don't feel so overwhelmed. Regular relaxation can also build your tolerance to stress, says Dr. McGrady. "The negative effects of stress accumulate over time. But the positive effects of relaxation also accumulate. If you practice techniques like deep breathing, imagery and yoga over time, you'll find that you become a little more resilient to stress."

Use your time wisely. If you have so much to do that you always feel stressed out, ask yourself, "What's necessary and what's not?" says Dr. Beck. Then, eliminate some of the unnecessary demands. It helps to ask yourself, "What do I need to do in order to do a reasonable job, as opposed to a perfect job?"

"If you're always aiming for perfection—always trying to do an A-plus job—your expectations are too high, and you're going to be under too much stress," explains Dr. Beck. If you're reluctant to lower your expectations, she suggests that you ask yourself, "What are the advantages and disadvantages of always trying to do an A-plus job?"

"You need to make it clear to yourself that you're paying a price for perfectionism," Dr. Beck explains. "You may look extremely competent, but you may not be enjoying your life. You may have no time to swim or walk, you may always be eating on the run or you may be too tired to have sex."

Finally, ask yourself, "What does it mean to me to do grade-B work sometimes?"

"Frequently, women will say, 'If I do grade-B work, it means that I'm not living up to my potential,'" says Dr. Beck. "They ascribe all kinds of pejorative meanings to anything less than grade-A work." If you do the same, ask yourself a final question, "If my best friend did grade-B work, would I think badly of her?" The answer is probably no. So give yourself the same break that you'd give a friend.

WHOLE-BODY TECHNIQUES FOR EMOTIONAL CALM

Some techniques are useful for day-to-day emotional health or more than one negative or stressful emotion. Practiced regularly, these tips can help keep you feeling emotionally well-tuned.

Take deep, slow breaths. Studies find that rapid, shallow breathing can contribute to anxiety, panic attacks, phobias, stress and even depression, says Robert Fried, Ph.D., professor of psychology at Hunter College, City University of New York, director of the Stress and Biofeedback Clinic at the Institute for Rational Emotive Therapy in Manhattan and author of *The Breath Connection*. That's because shallow breathing leaves your body starved for oxygen and triggers physiological changes that affect mood, says Dr. Fried.

Certain exercises help you to breathe more slowly and deeply, from down in your abdomen, counteracting negative emotions and stress, says Dr. Fried. One simple way to correct your breathing is to lie down, put a book on your stomach and watch it carefully. If you're breathing deep down from your abdomen, the way that you should, the book should rise when you inhale and fall when you exhale.

Sweat it out. Women who exercise seem to enjoy better mental health than those who don't. In a study at Baylor College of Medicine in Houston, women who exercised reported less depression than those who didn't exercise. In another study, conducted by researchers at Hofstra University in Hempstead, New York, exercisers reported less anxiety than nonexercisers.

Further study reveals that sustained exercise—more than 20 minutes of walking, running, swimming, cycling and the like—triggers the release of mood-enhancing brain chemicals. But even a walk around the block can help, says Jody Wilkinson, M.D., exercise physiologist and medical director for the clinical research division at the Cooper Institute for Aerobics Research in Dallas.

Still your mind, improve your mood. Meditation—quiet, relaxed contemplation—can help you manage anxiety, depression, stress and other emotional problems, says Oster. Research bears that out. In a study at the University of Massachusetts Medical Center in Worcester, men and women complaining of anxiety and panic attacks had significantly fewer attacks after taking an eight-week meditation course.

"Meditation helps ease you into a state of relaxed wakefulness," explains Oster. "It provides you with the space and time to tend to your emotional needs and nurture yourself." Oster suggests that you reserve five to ten minutes for meditation once or twice a day.

Before you start meditating, take a few moments to take stock of your feelings. "Acknowledge them," Oster says. "You might say to yourself, 'I'm feeling sad, but that's not inappropriate. I'm a healthy person for being aware that I have these feelings and not denying them. This is temporary. Right now, I'm going to meditate and get some rest and nurturing. Then I'll come back to my feelings and think about what to do.' Then take a few deep relaxing breaths and begin your meditation."

Stop to smell the lavender. Many women find that the scent of a particular species of lavender, *Lavandula*, enhances their moods, says Buckle. Make sure that you're using *Lavandula angustifolia* because other species of lavender can produce a completely different effect. And make sure that you have pure essential oil of lavender, not chemically treated oil, which can cause subtle changes in scent and effect.

Even with pure essential oil of *Lavandula angustifolia*, not everyone responds to the same scent in the same way, says Buckle. She suggests that you give lavender a test sniff before buying, to see if it leaves you feeling more relaxed.

Once you've found the right stuff, you can use it in a number of ways, Buckle says. Add one to five drops of the oil to a few tablespoons of cold-pressed vegetable oil and massage yourself with it. Or add one to five drops to a half-cup of milk (essential oils aren't soluble in bath water but will dissolve in milk). Then add the mixture to your bath and relax.

Doodle, sketch or paint what you feel. Sometimes it's hard to know what you're feeling, let alone how to respond. You're upset, but in what way? Are you angry? Scared? Art therapy can help you sort things out, says Doris Arrington, Ed.D., an art therapist, licensed psychologist and professor and director of the Art Therapy and Marital and Family Therapy Program at the College of Notre Dame in Belmont, California.

Dr. Arrington suggests that you keep what she calls a doodle diary, a small spiral-bound notebook with blank pages, in your purse, along with some colored pencils. Every day, use the pencils to render your feelings in the diary. Draw whatever represents your feelings—abstraction is fine.

For the analytical part of this process, Arrington recommends a technique developed by Lewis Savary, Ph.D., from Washington, D.C., and author of several books on spirituality. First, give your work a title. It looks like a black tornado? Call it Storm.

Now describe the theme. Maybe the theme is "I'm upset today." So consider your feelings: What does the work say about how you feel? Maybe that black tornado that you just drew is a sign that you're angry. What overall effect (emotion) does the art represent?

Finally, ask yourself, "What question does this piece of artwork pose?" In this case, the obvious question is: "Why am I angry today?" If you think about it, you may realize that you're angry with your husband for forgetting your birthday. The thing to do in this case would be to talk to your inner self first to clarify your feelings, and then talk to him, explains Dr. Arrington.

Tune in to your favorites. Music can affect your mood by triggering a variety of physiological changes, like altering levels of stress hormones in your blood or changing your breathing and heart rates. The right music can soothe you if you're anxious or lift your spirits if you're low, observes Suzanne Hanser, Ed.D., chairperson of the music therapy department at Berklee College of Music in Boston.

What's right for you, though, isn't necessarily what's right for another woman. You have to experiment to find out what kind of music mellows you out and what kind revs you up, says Barbara J. Crowe, a registered music therapist and director and professor of music therapy at Arizona State University in Tempe. If you find that Sinatra's love songs are cathartic when you're blue, give them a listen the next time that you're down.

Build confidence with biofeedback. Biofeedback training incorporates emotionally and physically soothing techniques like deep breathing and visualization. Learning these skills can help you monitor how well you manage anxiety or stress.

If you consult a professional trained in biofeedback therapy, she will hook you up to equipment that monitors your heart rate, muscle tension or other indicators of your stress and anxiety levels. Then she'll have you practice deep breathing and other stress- and anxiety-reducing techniques while you get feedback from the monitors to help you learn. If you're using relaxation techniques effectively, the machines will show your breathing and muscle tension heading from "red alert" to the normal range.

Biofeedback is a valuable tool for practicing mood-enhancing relaxation techniques, and the training gives you a sense of control. "And that is going to help with any emotional problem," says Dr. Green. "With a sense of control comes a greater confidence in your ability to manage life and emotions. This works against depression, anxiety and other negative feelings."

HEADACHES
Stop the Pain That Drains Your Brain

They pound, throb, ache or bug you just enough that your day is ruined. They can make your head feel like it's filled with 100 pounds of wet concrete or make it painfully buzz as if a sadistic bumblebee were doing figure eights on your frontal lobe.

The two most common types of headaches are tension (or muscle contraction) headaches and migraines. With tension headaches, you usually feel a steady, uncomfortable pressure, but not enough to completely disable you from your daily routine. A migraine, by comparison, is an intense, throbbing pain that can last for a few hours or even days, sometimes accompanied by vomiting, nausea and sensitivity to light and noise.

Not only do many women get stuck dealing with menstrual pain and bloating every month, but they also get stuck with a lot worse headache pain than most men. That's probably due to the changes in estrogen levels that rule their monthly cycles: Women prone to headaches are more likely to get them during their periods and at midcycle, during ovulation.

Other triggers common to both sexes are nervous tension or stress, sinus congestion, certain foods (like aged cheese), caffeine withdrawal, environmental factors like pollen or pollution, muscle tension, light, loud noise and being overly tired or hungry. And headaches tend to run in families, so if your mother or grandmother got these head-splitters, then you're more likely to get them, too.

DRUG-FREE RELIEF

Whether caused by tension, stress, noise, light, eating the wrong foods or hereditary factors, headaches have one thing in common—they hurt.

Painkillers like acetaminophen, aspirin or ibuprofen often bring relief. But you don't have to automatically down aspirin or other pain medication that can leave you feeling out of sorts. An amazing number of non-drug approaches can bring relief. Here are practitioners' top picks.

Smell your way well. The smell of fresh peppermint is a headache-easer, says Paul Petit, D.C., certified chiropractic sports physician, aromatherapist and naturopath in Poway, California. If you have a tension headache or migraine, you can inhale the peppermint from the bottle for quick relief, he says.

Rub on essential oil of oregano. When massaged on the skin, scents of oregano and lavender (*Lavandula officinalis*) also work well for sinus headaches because they have anti-infectious properties, Dr. Petit notes. "The bacteria offer no resistance to some essential oils. These oils have been on Earth since the beginning of time. Antibiotics have just been here for the last 50 to 60 years." When using oil externally, especially with massages, always dilute them in vegetable oil, such as almond oil, at a concentration of 20 percent to 65 percent, advises Dr. Petit.

Rinse your nose out. Irrigating your sinuses is another good solution for sinus headaches, says Thomas M. Kidder, M.D., associate professor of otolaryngology and human communications at the Medical College of Wisconsin in Milwaukee.

To unclog nasal passages, make a saline solution from one level teaspoon of table salt and 13 ounces of warm water, and then sniff it into your nose through cupped hands. Or take a bulb syringe and squirt into your nose, or use a water pick with a bulb-tip adapter that fits into the nostril. "If you squirt it into the congested nostril and lean forward, the saline will drain out the other nostril. It cleans out the nose and the thick secretions that you get there," says Dr. Kidder.

Give pain the rub. Getting a head massage can be a soothing experience, notes Dr. Petit. It's not always easy to drop everything and head for a massage therapist every time you have a headache. But you can deeply massage the back of your head where the cranium starts and the vertebrae stop, and the temples on either side of your eye, which are definite pressure points during headaches. "I'd say that you need a deep massage of the area for 10 to 20 minutes," says Dr. Petit. "Those points act as an accessory pump to the brain, so this helps get your blood pumping, relaxing constricted blood vessels."

Hit the right spot. Applying reflexology techniques on your toes could lead to headache relief, says Dwight Byers, president of the International Institute of Reflexology in St. Petersburg, Florida, and author of *Better Health with Foot Reflexology*.

For tension headaches, which are often caused by tightness in the neck, back and shoulders, working the reflex areas of the foot that correspond with those body parts is the answer. That's your toes—and all their sides. "You don't want to rub the reflex areas, but use the end and corner of your thumb to apply pressure and work those reflexes. These are really small pressure points the size of a grain of sand, so you have to walk your thumb like a caterpillar that's inching its way along all the toes," he says. "Go up, down and all around, as you see fit."

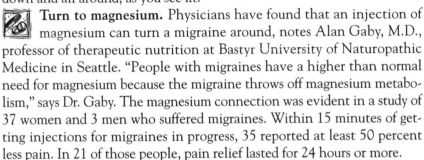 **Turn to magnesium.** Physicians have found that an injection of magnesium can turn a migraine around, notes Alan Gaby, M.D., professor of therapeutic nutrition at Bastyr University of Naturopathic Medicine in Seattle. "People with migraines have a higher than normal need for magnesium because the migraine throws off magnesium metabolism," says Dr. Gaby. The magnesium connection was evident in a study of 37 women and 3 men who suffered migraines. Within 15 minutes of getting injections for migraines in progress, 35 reported at least 50 percent less pain. In 21 of those people, pain relief lasted for 24 hours or more.

How I Healed Myself **Naturally**

Acupressure Relieved Her Migraines—Finally

Anne Savage, a 49-year-old owner of an interactive distribution business in Egremont, Massachussets, credits acupressure with relief of her migraines.

"I've had headaches for most of my life, but I'd been getting migraines more and more frequently," says Savage. "They sometimes came every three weeks or so. Some episodes were worse than others, sometimes disabling me for 12 hours at a time. I had to leave everything, lie down and drop out of life. It's like being possessed—something takes over and there's nothing that you can do about it."

Savage worked with a homeopathic physician for a while but, she says, "it didn't do anything for me. I turned to acupressure when I met a couple who do Jin Shin Do acupressure, a form of acupressure that also works with the emotional cause of headaches.

"It helped me get to the root of my headaches and release the emotions that were being held in," says Savage. "I see a practitioner, and while she's holding points on my body, things about my life come up as we talk. Very deep relaxation occurs as she holds the points. It really does work. You're totally refreshed by it. It's amazing stuff that has changed my whole life.

"Now I only get headaches about three times a year, and they're not nearly as violent," says Savage. "I press certain points on my hand and around my eyes. It makes the energy flow through the places where it's blocked, and you can feel that happening."

A smart preventive step is to add magnesium—about 200 to 500 milligrams a day—to your diet, Dr. Gaby says. (If you have kidney or heart problems, it's a good idea to check with your doctor before taking supplemental magnesium.)

Cool it with calcium. Some women with migraines have found help when calcium was added to a magnesium injection, says Dr. Gaby. "Some patients who don't respond to magnesium respond to the other vitamins. I'm not sure anyone knows how that works, but it definitely works faster and better than chemical drugs."

In one report, two women with a history of menstrual migraines experienced a major reduction in headaches after two months of treatment with a combination of 1,200 milligrams of calcium and 1,200 to 1,600 international units (IU) of cholecalciferol, a prescription-only form of vitamin D.

Caution: Vitamin D can be toxic above 600 IU. Use it only with a doctor's supervision. (For details on locating a physician experienced in treating health problems with higher-than-over-the-counter dosages of vitamins or minerals, see page 306.)

Leaf your pain behind. Eating a single leaf of the herb feverfew every day may help keep migraines and chronic headaches at bay, says Ethan Russo, M.D., a neurologist at the Western Montana Clinic in Missoula, academic adjunct professor in the Department of Pharmacy at the University of Montana in Missoula and clinical assistant professor in the Department of Medicine at the University of Washington School of Medicine in Seattle. "It's unknown how it works but it's an anti-inflammatory and painkiller."

Although you can buy feverfew capsules in health food stores, Dr. Russo says that you can't be sure of their quality. "I usually recommend growing a plant of your own," he notes. "You can get seeds anywhere that you can get herbs. Your best bet is to try to find a local supplier of fresh herbs, or look through seed catalogs. It's not a hard plant to grow."

Try nature's cure. In their book *The Complete Guide to Homeopathy*, Andrew Lockie, M.D., and Nicola Geddes, M.D., suggest the following homeopathic remedies for migraines, depending on your symptoms.

If the migraine is worse on the left side, with severe nausea and vomiting and pain that extends to the face, mouth or teeth, the remedy is taking 6c of ipecac every 15 minutes for up to ten doses. (Homeopathic remedies are available in different potencies, or concentrations, expressed by a number and commonly followed by the letter "c".)

If it's a blinding, throbbing migraine that begins with numbness and tingling in the lips and tongue and the pain is severe and pulsating, the remedy is taking 6c of nux vomica every hour for up to six doses.

If it's a migraine that settles over the right eye, usually starting in the morning at the back of the head and spreading up to the forehead, the remedy is sanguinaria, which should be taken at the fist sign of an attack, in a dosage of 6c every 15 minutes for up to ten doses.

Note: If you don't improve within the time period noted on the remedy package or you experience chronic migraines, see a physician. If a headache follows a head injury or it's severe and associated with a fever or lasts more than a few days, seek immediate medical assistance.

HEAD GAMES FOR HEAD PAIN

Sometimes, the pain in your head can be cured by the same thing—your head, says Joseph P. Primavera III, Ph.D., psychologist and co-director of the Comprehensive Headache Center at Germantown Hospital and Medical Center in Philadelphia.

Relaxation techniques such as self-hypnosis, biofeedback, imagery and meditation all help to calm the autonomic nervous system, the network that connects your brain, spinal cord, nerves, blood vessels and organs. So

How I Healed Myself **Naturally**

Traditional Chinese Medicine for Facial Pain

Peg Horan, a 40-year-old social work student, found relief for trigeminal neuralgia, or facial pain, through Traditional Chinese Medicine.

"It began as a little numbness and a tingle in my face," recalls Horan. "Flashes of pain would jet around my cheekbones, fly to my ears and stab me in the eyes and forehead. My doctor could find no cause for the pain, so he sent me to an ear, nose and throat specialist, who sent me to a dentist, who sent me to a neurologist, who sent me to another neurologist. No one could get rid of the pain, although they were able to finally name it: trigeminal neuralgia."

Horan says that the pain threatened to ruin her life, but she was determined not to let that happen. "Someone steered me to a medical doctor who practices acupuncture. She performed a classic Traditional Chinese Medicine exam, treated me with acupuncture and gave me special herbal preparations in capsule form. The pain and numbness lessened. The best news is that I was able to stop taking prescription medication for the pain."

each of these can cut down on headaches, notes Dr. Primavera.

"Anything that can relax you is a different way of getting to the same place—being pain-free," he says. "So if someone enjoys prayerful meditation, I don't tell them to do something else. The most important thing is that you choose a method that works for you."

Take a breather. Sometimes, stopping everything that you're doing and simply breathing deeply can work wonders for tension headaches, says Dr. Primavera. "Stop doing whatever you were doing that was stressful. Take slow, deep, rhythmic breaths. Breathing this way alters your carbon dioxide level and sends a message to your brain to slow your heartbeat and promote the relaxation response."

A quick way to take a breather is by slowly taking a deep inhalation through your mouth, filling up your lungs and then taking a full respiration through your nose and breathing out nice and slow, Dr. Primavera says. "It makes you pay attention and breathe slow and rhythmically."

Learn to relax. If you have tension headaches, biofeedback (a technique that measures your muscle tension and body temperature) is a good way to learn to read your body, says Angele McGrady, Ph.D., professor of psychiatry and physiology at the Medical College of Ohio in Toledo and past president of the Association for Applied Psychophysiology and Biofeedback based in Wheatridge, Colorado.

In about eight to ten visits to a biofeedback specialist, you can learn to detect clues that your body gives off, before succumbing to tension, says Dr. McGrady. Use deep breathing exercises or imagery recommended by the specialist. For instance, you might imagine yourself walking along the beach and listening to sounds of the ocean to relax yourself whenever you feel tension setting in. "So once you become aware of when a headache is coming on, you'll be able to do something about it," she says.

HEART DISEASE
Control Tactics for Angina, Blood Pressure and Cholesterol

A mere generation ago, most doctors told women with advanced heart disease to go home and rest, take their medicines and expect to undergo coronary bypass surgery at some point or another.

And that was it. No advice on what to eat or foods to avoid, whether or not to exercise or how to deal with stress or other risk factors. Preventing heart disease was a pretty revolutionary concept.

A maverick named Nathan Pritikin saw matters differently. In his groundbreaking book, *The Pritikin Program for Diet and Exercise*, Pritikin argued that sitting around resting and eating high-fat, circa-1960 American cuisine clogged the arteries leading to our hearts, causing heart disease.

Pritikin was more or less written off as an extremist, until research proved him right. These days, many mainstream medical organizations such as the American Heart Association (AHA) recommend a low-fat diet, exercise and stress management to both treat and prevent heart disease. What was once alternative has become conventional.

ROOM FOR IMPROVEMENT

Despite a sea change in medical thought and practice, heart disease is still the number one cause of death among American women. Women tend to get heart disease later in life than men do. Research suggests that the female sex hormone estrogen helps protect our hearts until menopause, when production of this hormone declines and our risk for heart disease climbs. Despite the odds, women tend to underestimate their risks and pay less attention to heart health than they should.

"While the average woman has a 1 in 11 chance of contracting breast cancer, her chances of contracting heart disease are 1 in 2," says Bruno Cortis, M.D., a cardiologist in River Forest, Illinois, and author of *Heart and Soul: A Psychological and Spiritual Guide to Preventing and Healing Heart Disease.*

Controllable risk factors for heart disease include smoking, high blood pressure and high blood cholesterol. You also have a greater risk of getting heart disease if you don't exercise or if you have a sedentary job, which contributes to one of the leading factors—being overweight. Women with diabetes and those with stress may also be in the higher-risk category.

Risk factors that you can't change include a family history of heart disease and race. African-American women are twice as likely as white women to develop heart disease, for example.

ANATOMY OF HEART DISEASE

Heart disease is the end result of a series of events that take place in your arteries. Frequent or ongoing exposure to norepinephrine and other stress hormones, coupled with high blood pressure, damage the inner lining of the arteries leading to your heart. Once your blood vessels are damaged, they begin to accumulate deposits of low-density lipoprotein (LDL) cholesterol, a sticky blood fat manufactured by the body. As this arterial plaque forms, it obstructs blood vessels and limits the blood flow to your heart.

A diet high in dietary cholesterol, found in animal foods like meat and butter, accelerates heart disease, as does a diet high in saturated fats, found in animal fats and some vegetable fats. Saturated fat prompts your body to produce exceptionally high levels of LDL cholesterol. Saturated fat also lowers blood levels of high-density lipoprotein (HDL) cholesterol. This adds insult to injury, since HDL cholesterol can actually help clean cholesterol from your arteries. Refined sugars and starches can also lead to high cholesterol, according to Glenn S. Rothfeld, M.D., clinical instructor in the Department of Community Health at Tufts University School of Medicine in Boston, a practitioner in Arlington, Massachusetts, and co-author of *Natural Medicine for Heart Disease.*

A reduction in blood flow to your heart, caused by plaque buildup in your arteries, can trigger chest pain, or angina. It can also lead to arrhythmia, or erratic heartbeat. Both symptoms are warning signs of heart disease. Unfortunately, some women have no warning signs at all. The first tip off that they have heart disease can be a heart attack, says Dr. Rothfeld.

If you have a heart attack, a combination of two things could be going on. Artery plaque can continue to build up until it completely seals off your arteries, shutting off the flow of blood. Or plaque can rupture and prompt blood to clot, which can completely block blood flow in narrow arteries. (If the clot travels to blood vessels leading to your brain, you can experience a stroke.)

Any interruption in blood flow deprives your heart of oxygen and can seriously damage your heart muscle. That's why heart attacks can be deadly.

Standard treatment for heart disease focuses on risk factors that you can change. If you have heart disease, your doctor has probably told you to keep a lid on stress and to eat less saturated fat and cholesterol. She has probably also mentioned that exercise can help control your blood pressure and LDL cholesterol levels and help prevent or slow the buildup of plaque in your arteries. And if you smoke, she has most likely told you to quit, especially if you take birth control pills. Like high blood pressure, smoking damages your arteries, triggering plaque buildup, says Dr. Rothfeld. It also makes your blood stickier and more likely to clot, as does taking the Pill, although the Pill by itself isn't a big risk factor. Smoking and taking oral contraceptives, however, puts you in double jeopardy for heart disease, he says.

But how little fat should you eat? Are there any vitamins or minerals that can help? How often should you exercise? What kind of exercise should you do? Exactly how can you relieve stress? Alternative practitioners have some very specific advice on all counts.

A MENU OF HEART-HEALTHY DIETS

To protect against heart disease in the first place or reverse existing disease, alternative practitioners offer the dietary options described below. R. James Barnard, Ph.D., professor of physiological science and medicine at the University of California in Los Angeles, suggests that you choose a very low fat diet plan that best suits your tastes.

Order what Dr. Ornish eats. For people at risk for heart disease, the American Heart Association recommends a diet deriving less than 30 percent of calories from fat. But Dean Ornish M.D., cardiologist, assistant clinical professor of medicine at the University of California in San Francisco, director of the Preventive Medicine Research Institute in Sausalito, California, and author of *Dr. Dean Ornish's Program for Reversing Heart Disease,* says that to truly protect against heart disease, you need to limit fat intake to 10 percent of calories from fat, with minimal amounts of saturated fat.

The Ornish program consists of a very low fat, low-cholesterol vegetarian diet combined with daily exercise and stress reduction programs.

The diet consists mostly of vegetables, grains, fruits and beans. Dr. Ornish published studies proving his program could reverse the progression of heart disease.

The AHA considers the Ornish diet to be too austere, calling it impractical for most people. Yet women who try the diet are proof that it can and does work. In a study conducted at the University of California in San Francisco, both men and women with heart disease did significantly better on the Ornish plan than they did following a more liberal diet consisting of about 30 percent of calories from fat. Their LDL cholesterol and blood pressure levels dropped, and plaque deposits were reduced. In comparison, men and women following the conventional diet got worse. (For information on how to follow the Ornish program, see page 132.)

Follow the Pritikin diet. Low in fat, sparing with meat and generous with grains, vegetables and fruit, the Pritikin diet is similar to the Ornish diet—with one exception. You can eat roughly three ounces of very lean meat a day. In a study conducted at the University of California in Los Angeles, men and women with heart disease saw their cholesterol levels drop when they followed the Pritikin diet and exercised regularly. (For information on how to follow the Pritikin diet, see page 137.)

Try a traditional Asian diet. Based on traditional Asian diets, the Asian Diet Pyramid is also similar to the Pritikin plan in that it's mostly vegetarian. Population studies show that most Asian countries have lower heart disease rates than the United States, supporting the use of the Asian Food Pyramid diet in protection against heart disease. (For information on how to follow a traditional Asian diet, see page 154.)

Dine as the Mediterraneans do. Modeled after the cuisines of Italy, Spain and Greece, the traditional Mediterranean diet is also sparing with meat and generous with grains, fruits and vegetables. But compared to the Ornish and Pritikin diets, the Mediterranean diet derives a somewhat generous 25 to 35 percent of calories from fat. Nonetheless, studies show that men and women who eat the Mediterranean way have relatively low rates of heart disease.

Researchers suspect that the benefit comes from olive oil, the primary source of fat in Mediterranean diets. Olive oil is low in saturated fat, so it's less likely to raise blood levels of artery-clogging LDL cholesterol. But olive oil is also rich in monounsaturated fat, which lowers blood levels of harmful LDL cholesterol while it raises blood levels of helpful HDL cholesterol. (For information on how to follow a Mediterranean diet, see page 159.)

Invite garlic to dinner. Savory and kind to your heart, garlic helps lower blood pressure and cholesterol and makes your blood less likely to form unwanted clots, says Varro E. Tyler, Ph.D., professor emeritus of pharmacognosy at Purdue University in West Lafayette, Indiana, and author of *Herbs of Choice: The Therapeutic Use of Phytomedicinals*.

"The best way to consume garlic and maintain your close friends is to eat enteric-coated capsules containing dried garlic powder," says Dr. Tyler.

How I Healed Myself **Naturally**

A Vegetarian Diet for Out-of-Control Blood Pressure and Cholesterol

Madge Wilson lives in Newark, New Jersey, and works for a nonprofit community organization. Wilson credits a vegetarian diet and fasting for reining in her high blood pressure and lowering her cholesterol, thus lowering her risk for heart attack and stroke.

"I developed high blood pressure and high cholesterol when I was 39," says Wilson. Her blood pressure was 160/98. Doctors consider blood pressure readings higher than 140/90 to be too high. And her cholesterol was 290 mg/dl (milligrams per deciliter). Cholesterol levels over 240 are considered high.

Wilson knew that her family history of heart and artery disease put her health at risk. "My mother and dad both died of strokes," she says. "My mother was 50 when she died. My father was 43. I felt like I was sitting on a time bomb.

"I'd been going from one doctor to another, and every one put me on some kind of medication." None of the drugs worked well, so Madge consulted Joel Fuhrman, M.D., a physician in nearby Belle Mead, New Jersey, and author of *Fasting—And Eating—For Health*.

"Dr. Fuhrman put me on a fast, which he supervised, for 12 days," says Wilson. He told her that fasting is a useful treatment for decreasing blood pressure without the use of drugs. "After the fast, Dr. Fuhrman told me exactly what to eat: vegetables, fruits, legumes, grains, nuts—and nothing else. It's a vegetarian diet. Dr. Furhman told me to cut out all meat and dairy. And he told me not to eat sugar, salt or anything containing sodium.

"My new way of eating is really working," says Wilson, who at age 64 has already outlived her mother by 14 years. "I check my blood pressure every day, and it's great—120/80. I haven't needed to take medication for high blood pressure since the fast. Plus, my cholesterol is fantastic—195. And I lost ten pounds.

"I exercise every day," she adds. "Every morning at 6:30, I spend half an hour to 45 minutes in the gym. I feel like a new person."

The coating on these handy capsules keeps them from dissolving until they reach your small intestine. During digestion, your body converts the key ingredient in garlic, a sulfur compound called alliin, into an active form, allicin and related compounds, that comes to your heart's aid. The capsules are more or less odor-free, Dr. Tyler says. They are available in health food stores.

How much garlic should you take? Robert I-San Lin, Ph.D., executive vice-president of Nutrition International in Irvine, California, and chairman of the First World Congress on the Health Significance of Garlic and Garlic Constituents, has reviewed many garlic supplements on the market and says that most will provide significant health benefits if sufficient amounts are taken—usually two to four times the dosage recommended on the label. Look for garlic supplements in health food stores, supermarkets and drugstores.

CARDIO-FRIENDLY VITAMINS AND MINERALS

Evidence suggests that vitamin and mineral supplements can lower heart disease risk in various ways. The American Heart Association doesn't endorse vitamin and mineral therapy. But some alternative practitioners do.

Certain supplements can help treat and prevent heart disease, says Bobbi Lutack, a naturopathic and homeopathic physician and professor of cardiology at Bastyr University of Naturopathic Medicine in Seattle. She suggests that women begin by taking the Recommended Dietary Allowance of most essential vitamins and minerals (excluding iron, unless you're anemic). In addition, she offers the following advice.

Bolster your intake of antioxidants. Evidence suggests that vitamins C and E and the trace mineral selenium protect your heart in three ways. Collectively known as antioxidants, studies suggest that these nutrients come to your heart's defense by neutralizing highly destructive molecules called free radicals. In that way, antioxidants protect your artery walls from the damage that triggers plaque accumulation. They also help inhibit chemical changes that make LDL cholesterol stickier and more likely to clog arteries. And they inhibit blood clots.

Researchers at Boston University have found that 2,000-milligram doses of vitamin C improved blood flow to the heart. And in a British study, men and women with angina were less likely to have heart attacks if they took 400 to 800 international units of vitamin E daily.

Based on this evidence, Dr. Lutack advocates taking at least 1,000 milligrams of vitamin C, 400 international units of vitamin E and 200 micrograms of selenium. (Because we get about 100 micrograms of selenium in our diets, taking more than 100 micrograms in supplement form should be done under medical supervision.)

Don't forget your Bs. Research shows that vitamins B_6, B_{12} and the B vitamin folate help prevent chemical changes that lead to hardening of the arteries. In a Canadian study that followed about 5,000 men and women for 15 years, for example, those with high blood levels of folate were less likely to die of heart attacks than those with low levels. So, make sure that your daily supplements include these B vitamins.

Supplement with magnesium and calcium. These two minerals relax your arteries, lower blood pressure and help regulate heartbeat, Dr. Lutack says. In a portion of the Nurses Health Study, an ongoing study of about 87,000 women, those with the highest magnesium intakes were least likely to have high blood pressures. Dr. Lutack suggests that women take 250 to 500 milligrams each of magnesium and calcium. If you have heart or kidney problems, check with your doctor before taking supplements of these minerals.

Consider coenzyme Q_{10} and L-carnitine. Studies show that coenzyme Q_{10}, a lipidlike substance found in practically all cells, may help to lower blood pressure, increase the strength of heart muscle contractions and benefit those suffering from mitral valve prolapse (the most common valve disorder in women), especially when combined with L-carnitine, an amino acid, according to Dr. Lutack. So she recommends a daily dose of 30 to 60 milligrams each of coenzyme Q_{10} and L-carnitine. Look for these supplements in health food stores.

Savor some omega-3 fatty acids. Found in fish oils, walnuts and flaxseeds, omega-3 fatty acids lower LDL cholesterol levels and help prevent blood clots, says Michael Janson, M.D., director of the Center for Preventive Medicine in Barnstable, Massachusetts, in his book *The Vitamin Revolution in Health Care*.

To increase omega-3 fatty acids in your diet, add ground flaxseed in muffins. Researchers at Incarnate Word College in San Antonio, suggest substituting ground flaxseed for up to half the flour in your favorite muffin recipes. Look for ground flaxseed in health foods stores.

 EXERCISE: MORE THAN A STROLL IN THE PARK

The American Heart Association recommends 30 minutes of aerobic exercise, such as swimming, running, brisk walking or cycling, three or four days a week.

Aerobic exercise helps your heart in a number of ways. For one thing, aerobic exercise burns an average of 300 to 400 calories per hour and helps you lose weight. That's important because excess weight puts an excess burden on your heart.

Aerobics also strengthens your heart muscle. When you exercise hard enough to raise your pulse and breathing rate, you also increase the amount of oxygen your blood can carry to your heart. And aerobics lowers both your blood pressure and your LDL cholesterol levels while boosting your HDL cholesterol levels.

Research suggests that to truly protect your heart, you need more than 30 minutes of exercise a day, at least three days a week.

A study at the University of Washington in Seattle finds that exercise may even help dissolve blood clots in coronary arteries before they can cause heart attacks, but you'll have to do more than 20 minutes of aerobics to see similar results. In the study, men and women who walked, jogged or biked three times a week had increased levels of clot-dissolving chemicals in their blood.

To reap this benefit, though, they exercised long and hard. Each session lasted a total of 90 minutes, including a 20-minute warm-up and 20-minute cooldown. "And we had them exercise strenuously enough so that they were at 60 to 80 percent of their maximum heart rates," says Wayne Chandler, M.D., who headed the study and is an associate professor of laboratory medicine at the university. Heart rate is a standard method of gauging exertion.

A growing body of evidence suggests that exercise may be one of the most important steps that a woman can take toward long-term heart health. A strenuous workout, it seems, is a prerequisite for an increase in levels of clot-dissolving chemicals, says Dr. Chandler.

Chest Pains? See a Doctor

If you have unexplained chest pain or irregular heartbeat, call your doctor immediately. If you have chest pain, pressure or heaviness accompanied by sweating, shortness of breath, nausea or heart palpitations, go to a hospital emergency room. It might not be a heart attack, but you're better off in the emergency room until you know for sure, says Glenn S. Rothfeld, M.D., clinical instructor in the Department of Community Health at Tufts University School of Medicine in Boston, a practitioner in Arlington, Massachusetts, and co-author of *Natural Medicine for Heart Disease*.

Even if you've had a heart attack, exercise is beneficial. S
that women who have had heart attacks live longer if they st

And in addition to aerobic exercise, you need to inclu
training and some form of flexibility exercise in your routine, say
Rothfeld. Resistance training—strengthening exercises using dumbells and
barbells or weight-training machines—is important because it builds
muscle. Since muscle burns more calories per hour than fat does, weight
training helps you keep your weight in line more than aerobics alone. And
stretching will keep you flexible so that you're less likely to strain your
muscles and joints when you work out. (For information on starting a program of aerobic exercise, resistance training and stretching, see page 85.)

YOGA OFFERS MULTIPLE BENEFITS

Yoga offers all the benefits of stretching and then some. Like stretching,
practicing yoga postures daily or several times a week keeps you flexible so
that you're less likely to strain your muscles and joints in the midst of your
heart-healthy aerobic workouts, says Dr. Lutack.

Yoga also helps you to relax, counteracting the effects of stress hormones
that raise your blood pressure and trigger spasms in your coronary arteries.
And yoga improves circulation, says Dr. Rothfeld.

For heart-healthy benefits, Dr. Rothfeld recommends a yoga posture
called the expansion pose. While standing, hold your arms out at your
sides and slowly move them backward until you can interlace your fingers.
(You'll have to bend your elbows to do this.) Hold your trunk straight and
without straining, slowly raise your arms. Gently arch your back as you
begin to lift your locked hands toward the ceiling. Hold for five seconds.
Then slowly bend your body farther forward, lowering your head and
raising your arms to shoulder level for ten seconds. Then return to an upright position, drop your arms to your sides and relax.

MIND-BODY THERAPY FOR YOUR HEART

Dr. Ornish's program for reversing heart disease goes beyond diet and
exercise to include yoga, meditation and other stress-reduction techniques.
For total heart protection, more and more doctors are recommending some
form of mind-body therapy to the men and women that they counsel.

"To protect your heart, it's not enough just to watch your diet and exercise," says Dr. Cortis. You also have to tend to your mind and spirit, he
adds, since your emotional and physical well-being are interdependent.

"Imagine that health is like a stool with three legs," he says. "One leg is your physical body. The second is your mind—the way that you think. And the third is your spirit. You have to care for each."

Diet and exercise take care of your physical requirements. Here's how to care for your mental and spiritual needs.

Jettison stressful thought patterns. Cognitive therapy is a technique that effectively combats stress created by distorted perceptions or negative thinking. A counselor trained in cognitive therapy can help you change the way that you react to stresses that are beyond your control, such as difficult people, demanding jobs or worries about the future. (For more information on cognitive therapy, see page 79.)

Take a meditation break. Meditation reduces levels of stress hormones, decreases blood pressure and reduces the likelihood that your coronary arteries will go into spasm. In an Iowa study, African-American women and men who learned meditation lowered their blood pressure significantly. Since the release of stress hormones can also contribute to angina, meditation may help alleviate chest pain as well.

Imagine a healthy heart. If you have heart disease, you can aid treatment by visualizing your heart as healthy, Dr. Cortis says. Sit quietly, close your eyes and relax. Form a mental image of your heart, surrounded by clear, open arteries and beating regularly and powerfully. Picture the artery walls as smooth and wide, flowing abundantly with oxygenated blood. For best results, repeat daily.

Breathe away tension. Slow, rhythmic breathing can also help you relax when you're stressed out, says Jeff Migdow, M.D., holistic medical doctor and director of yoga teacher–training at the Kripalu Center for Yoga and Health in Lenox, Massachusetts, and co-author of *Take a Deep Breath*. He recommends the following exercise.

To begin, take five to ten deep breaths, making sure that your stomach expands with each inhalation and falls with each exhalation. Continue this deep abdominal breathing. With each inhalation, imagine that you're breathing into a tense or painful part of your body. Then, with each exhalation, imagine that tension streaming out of your nostrils. Continue for a few minutes or longer.

Give your heart a lift with aromatherapy. Certain scents can reduce heart-hurting stress. Others appear to stimulate circulation, calm heart palpitations and lower blood pressure, says Dr. Rothfeld. Though scents have different effects on different people, he says, most people find chamomile and marjoram oils to be beneficial. Rub the essential oils on your wrist or a hanky and periodically take a whiff.

INFECTIONS
Ward Off Pesky Invasions

Becky Hieter, a 37-year-old mother of two from Ames, Iowa, is no stranger to earaches, sore throats, pinkeye and other infections that frequently plague kids and their parents.

When infection strikes, however, Hieter doesn't turn to over-the-counter medicines like antihistamines. And her kids rarely need to take antibiotics for ear infections. Instead, she relies primarily on herbs, vitamins and other natural remedies known for their infection-fighting powers. "I swear by mullein oil, echinacea and vitamin C," says Hieter.

Over-the-counter drugs like antihistamines and prescription drugs like antibiotics can help treat and ease ear and other infections. But they can also cause unpleasant side effects. Antibiotics, for instance, can cause rashes and diarrhea. Yet alternative treatments such as vitamin and mineral therapy, herbal medicine and homeopathy can get equally good results without the side effects, says Keith DeOrio, M.D., a homeopathic physician in private practice in Santa Monica, California.

Here's the rundown on what works and why.

EAR INFECTIONS: GET RID OF THE ACHE

If you have kids, odds are that you've dealt with your share of ear infections. Or, you've had one yourself.

The most common types are middle ear infections, the kind that torment kids, and outer ear infections, also known as swimmer's ear. Both can be quite painful.

Middle ear infections are usually caused by a proliferation of bacteria in a narrow tube—the eustachian tube—that runs from the ear to the throat and nose.

"Middle ear infections are more common in children. Their eustachian tubes are not fully developed, so saliva and bacteria in their mouths back up through their tubes," says Dr. DeOrio. Ear infections often come on the heels of colds because colds cause inflammation that blocks the eustachian tube, trapping saliva-borne bacteria inside.

With swimmer's ear, the culprit may be bacteria found in inadequately chlorinated water in public pools, hence the name. Excessive amounts of this bacteria-laden water in the ear can then trigger pain and inflammation.

A severe ear infection of either type can lead to hearing loss, so you should see a doctor if an earache is excruciating or your ear hurts for no apparent reason, says Dr. DeOrio. Doctors usually prescribe antibiotics for both middle ear infections and swimmer's ear, especially if the infection is severe.

If you're not in a lot of pain and you don't have a high fever, Dr. DeOrio suggests that you try alternative remedies for a day or so and turn to antibiotics only if you see no improvement or if your condition worsens. Experts offer these alternatives.

Try a drop or two of mullein oil. Mullein flowers have antibacterial properties, making them useful for treating both middle and outer ear infections, explains Dr. DeOrio. Mullein also offers potent pain relief, says Susun S. Weed, an herbalist, teacher from Woodstock, New York, and author of the *Wise Woman* herbal series.

You can buy mullein oil drops at most health food stores, says Dr. DeOrio. Place the bottle in a small pan of water and heat until the oil is warm but not hot. Test the temperature of the oil as you would a baby's bottle: Shake the bottle gently and then put a drop or two of the oil on your wrist. Then add a drop to each infected ear and cover the opening of the ear with a wad of cotton. Repeat the drops two or three times daily, until the infection clears.

Add garlic oil. If you don't have mullein oil on hand, you can use garlic oil instead. Like mullein flowers, garlic fights bacteria, says Weed. To make the oil, chop several cloves of garlic and put them in a small jar. Cover with olive oil and leave overnight. After straining the garlic, says Weed, add a few drops of the oil to each ear a couple of times each day, until the infection clears.

Sip some elder flower tea. Elder flowers help reduce inflammation and open clogged eustachian tubes, says Deb Soule, an herbalist in Rockport, Maine, and author of *The Roots of Healing: A Woman's Book of Herbs*. To brew elder flower tea, add two to three teaspoons of dried elder flowers to a cup and fill with boiling water. Steep for half an hour, then strain before drinking it. You can find dried elder flowers at your local herbary and some health food stores. Elder flowers have a shelf life of only one year, so make sure that you're buying products that haven't expired.

Eliminate food triggers. Middle ear infections can also be a symptom of food allergies, says Chris Meletis, doctor of naturopathy and clinic director, chief medical officer and medicinary director at the National College of Naturopathic Medicine in Portland, Oregon. Allergies to bananas, citrus, cow's milk, wheat, egg whites, corn and peanuts are often to blame. In one study, children who tested positive for these food allergies had far fewer ear infections once they stopped eating the offending foods.

To determine if one or more of those common culprits is a problem, eliminate bananas, citrus, cow's milk, wheat, egg whites, corn and peanuts for two to three weeks, Dr. Meletis says. Then add each food back one at a time, allowing at least one week between reintroductions, and see if infections recur. For example, if nothing happens when you start eating bananas again, but you start getting infections as soon as you reintroduce wheat, then wheat may be the culprit.

If you think that your child is allergic to milk, be sure to talk to a doctor or nutritionist about substitutes that will supply bone-building calcium. For most children, milk is the main source of this essential nutrient, so they'll need a fill-in if they're no longer having dairy products.

Rinse with vinegar, alcohol and peroxide. If swimmer's ear is your primary problem, try this: Mix an ounce each of vinegar, alcohol and peroxide in a bottle with a dropper top. After swimming, give the bottle a shake and add a few drops of the mixture to each ear. The alcohol will help evaporate any water left behind in your ears, and the peroxide and vinegar will kill lingering bacteria, says Dr. DeOrio.

PINKEYE: RELIEF FOR A COLD IN YOUR EYES

An inflammation of the conjunctiva, the film covering parts of your eye and inner eyelid, acute contagious conjunctivitis leaves your eyes pink, swollen and smarting. More commonly called pinkeye, this type of conjunctivitis is often accompanied by a sticky discharge. If you have conjunctivitis, you may find that your eyelids are "glued" together with this discharge when you wake up in the morning.

Pinkeye can be the result of either an allergy or an infection, says Dr. DeOrio. Viruses, including those that cause colds, can cause pinkeye—so can bacteria.

Both bacterial and viral conjunctivitis are extremely contagious and spread by hand-to-eye contact. Though pinkeye is most common in children, adults get it, too, says Dr. Meletis.

If you have symptoms of pinkeye, you should see a doctor, says Dr. DeOrio. If a bacterial infection is to blame, she'll probably prescribe antibiotic eyedrops. If a viral infection or allergy is the problem, she'll likely prescribe an antihistamine or steroid eyedrops to reduce the inflammation and itching.

At that point, Dr. DeOrio suggests that you try alternative remedies and take the prescription medicine only if necessary. Here are two remedies recommended by experts.

Swab with chickweed. Chickweed helps fight infection, yet it's mild enough to use on your eyes, says Weed. She suggests that you brew a pot of chickweed tea and let it cool until it is comfortable to the touch. Then dip a clean cloth into the tea and hold the cloth to the closed affected eye for as long as possible, up to an hour, rewetting the cloth periodically.

You can buy chickweed at your local herbary and some health food stores. Or better yet, pick fresh chickweed from your garden or lawn, boil briefly and when it reaches a safe temperature, apply to the outside of the eye as instructed, Weed advises.

Apply hot and cold compresses. If you don't have any chickweed handy, soak a clean washcloth in very warm water, wring it out and hold the damp cloth to your eye for a minute, says Dr. Meletis. Then soak the cloth in cold water, wring it out and again hold it to your eye for a minute. Repeat the process two or three times, being careful not to contaminate your unaffected eye with the washcloth.

By alternating hot and cold compresses, you stimulate circulation, bringing more blood and more infection-fighting white blood cells to your eye, explains Dr. Meletis.

Give it two days. "If you try natural remedies and see no improvement after 48 hours or feel that your condition is getting worse, take any medicine that your doctor has prescribed for your pinkeye," says Dr. DeOrio. You can continue using natural remedies as well, he says.

SORE THROAT: REACH FOR HERBAL SOOTHERS

A sore, inflamed throat can be a symptom of an allergy, a viral infection like a cold or a bacterial infection such as streptococcus (strep throat).

For some people, strep infection can lead to rheumatic fever, a more serious condition that can damage your heart or kidneys. So if you have a sore throat that's not clearly the result of an allergy or cold, you should see a doctor, says Dr. DeOrio. Strep throat calls for different treatment than sore throats due to a cold or allergies. Should your doctor determine that you have strep throat and need antibiotics or other medication, you can still use alternative remedies, in addition to your medication, says Dr. DeOrio.

Here's what nature has to offer.

Suck on zinc lozenges. "Regardless of why your throat is sore, zinc lozenges can help reduce inflammation and soothe the pain," says Dr. DeOrio. "They can also help stimulate the immune system so you can better fight an infection."

In a study at the Cleveland Clinic in Ohio, men and women who sucked an average of five zinc lozenges a day during a cold got rid of their colds, including related sore throats, an average of three days earlier than people not using the lozenges. (You can find zinc lozenges at most health food stores. Look for zinc gluconate on the list of ingredients.)

Dr. DeOrio recommends sucking on two or three lozenges a day whenever your throat hurts.

Take the lozenges with food, Dr. Meletis says, since zinc on an empty stomach can cause nausea. Take note of how many milligrams of zinc are delivered in each lozenge and then make sure that you don't take more than 50 milligrams of zinc lozenges a day for longer than a month.

Higher doses can deplete your body of copper, a mineral that works in balance with zinc, says Shari Lieberman, Ph.D., clinical nutritionist and certified nutrition specialist in New York City and co-author of *The Real Vitamin and Mineral Book.*

 ## How I Healed Myself **Naturally**

Zinc Lozenges Cured Her Sore Throat

Maureen Elmaleh, 34, an advertising executive in New York City, relies on zinc lozenges to head off sore throats at the first sign of trouble.

"I used to get sore throats that would lead into colds," says Elmaleh. "The sore throat would be the first sign.

"I heard about zinc from a pharmacist," she says. "He told me about a study that found zinc lozenges helped with cold symptoms like sore throat. I tried the lozenges and they worked."

Elmaleh starts sucking on zinc lozenges whenever she feels a sore throat coming on. "I probably take one lozenge four times a day. I take them after meals, since taking them on an empty stomach makes me queasy. The lozenges don't taste that great—they're kind of chalky—but they really soothe my throat. And sometimes, if I take lozenges at the onset of a sore throat, I won't even get a cold. And if I do get a cold, it's much shorter than my colds used to be."

Pick the right homeopathic remedy. For sore throats, Dr. DeOrio often recommends three homeopathic remedies: belladonna, mercurius sol (merc. sol) or lachesis. "These remedies can work no matter what's causing the sore throat. But be sure to match the symptoms to the remedy."

- If pain and redness are worse on the right side of your throat or you have difficulty swallowing and your tonsils appear enlarged, a 30c potency dose of belladonna three or four times daily is the homeopathic remedy for you, he says. (Concentrations, or strengths, of homeopathic remedies are expressed by a number followed by the letter c.)
- If you have raw, burning pain extending from the middle of your throat to your ears, bad breath and both swelling and white or yellow discharge appearing in the back of your throat, the ticket may be merc. sol at 30c potency three or four times a day.
- If your throat feels constricted, looks red and burns and the pain is stronger on the left side and extends to your ear, take a dose of lachesis at 30c potency three or four times daily.

Continue the remedy until the symptoms subside, typically two to four days, but no longer, says Dr. DeOrio. If you continue to take homeopathic treatments, the symptoms can return.

ALL-PURPOSE INFECTION FIGHTERS

In addition to specific remedies for specific infections, other natural remedies can help you fend off and recover from infections in general, including the common cold, earaches, pinkeye and sore throats.

Enlist echinacea, the herbal helper. Also known as purple cone-flower, echinacea reportedly perks up your immune system, helping it fight both bacterial and viral infections. So echinacea may help you, whether you're up against an ear infection, sore throat or pinkeye, says Weed.

You can find echinacea capsules and tinctures at most health food stores and drugstores. (When given a choice, Weed strongly recommends opting for a tincture as they appear to be much more effective than capsules.) Try 30 to 60 drops of the tincture or take a 500-milligram capsule three times a day as soon as you start feeling a cold or flu coming on, says Dr. Meletis. If you're already in the throes of a cold, he recommends taking 30 to 60 drops four times a day. (To determine the number of drops you should take, multiply your weight by 60 and then divide that amount by 150, says Dr. Meletis. For example, if you weigh 150 pounds, you would take 60 drops.)

Some believe that echinacea loses its effectiveness if you use it on a daily basis. So, unless otherwise instructed, try not to use it for more than two straight weeks at a time, and then give yourself an additional two weeks before you start taking it again, says Dr. DeOrio. And don't use the herb at all if you have an autoimmune disease such as lupus, since echinacea may further stimulate your overactive immune system.

For strep throat, Weed recommends taking as much as a teaspoonful of echinacea tincture every two hours, day and night, for two or three days until symptoms abate. Then continue with a half-teaspoonful of tincture three or four times a day, for at least seven more days. Continue for up to three weeks if needed.

Boost your intake of C. Vitamin C can also give your immune system a lift, says Dr. DeOrio. In a study at the University of Wisconsin in Madison, researchers asked one group of volunteers to take 2,000 milligrams of vitamin C daily. The other group was given a pill that looked like vitamin C but contained no active ingredients. The researchers then exposed both groups to a virus that causes colds. Those who took the extra vitamin C, it turned out, had much milder symptoms and recovered faster than the other group.

Dr. Meletis recommends 500 to 1,000 milligrams of vitamin C two to three times daily for adults. (Excess vitamin C may cause diarrhea in some people. If this happens to you, cut back the dosage.)

MENOPAUSE
Natural Solutions for Hot Flashes — And More

For many women in their forties and early fifties, the approach of menopause presents one of the biggest health decisions that they'll make at midlife: to take hormone replacement therapy or not to take hormone replacement therapy.

Since puberty, your body has been generously producing estrogen (the female hormone associated with functioning ovaries) and progesterone (the hormone secreted after ovulation, triggering menstruation and enabling the uterus to nourish a fertilized egg). At around age 50, your body begins to secrete fewer and fewer of these hormones, so you no longer menstruate.

Officially, menopause is that moment in time when you haven't had a period for 12 months. Tampons become a thing of the past—but so does your natural protection against heart disease and weakening bones. And beginning several years before your last period, your ovaries produce ever-smaller amounts of estrogen and progesterone. As hormone production wanes and you approach what our mothers called the change, you may experience hot flashes, insomnia, irregular bleeding, mood swings, vaginal dryness and other changes.

NOT A PROBLEM FOR EVERYONE

Menopause doesn't bother everyone. Only about 15 percent of us will experience severe menopausal symptoms, says Margery Gass, M.D., director of the University Hospital Menopause and Osteoporosis Center at the University of Cincinnati. "We estimate that 25 percent of women will sail through menopause with no trouble whatsoever, while some 60 percent will experience hot flashes, mood swings, vaginal dryness and other discomforts associated with menopause." The remainder experience occasional but not significant discomfort.

For women with severe or bothersome concerns associated with menopause, medical science offers hormone replacement therapy (HRT). Both synthetic hormones and "natural" estrogen (collected either from the urine of pregnant mares or from plants) will compensate for the decline in estrogen production at midlife. They're also prescribed after surgical removal of both ovaries. But hormone replacement therapy is not the perfect solution for every woman. Many doctors consider HRT inadvisable for women who've had breast cancer or who are at an increased risk of breast cancer due to their family histories, for example.

Other women resist hormone replacement therapy because they object to taking what they consider "medication" for a condition that is not a disease but a natural transition.

Among women who decide to go on HRT, 38 percent (roughly one out of three) stop using it by the end of the first year, due to side effects. Half of all women who go on HRT experience one or more problems, including menstrual bleeding, bloating, premenstrual irritability, cramps and breast tenderness. Some women also report headaches and weight gain, depression, abnormal uterine bleeding and hair and skin changes. And estrogen use can double your chances of developing gallbladder disease.

WHAT NATURE HAS TO OFFER

Figuring that since menopause is a natural transition, nature just may offer some natural solutions to discomforts associated with the change, many women bothered by menopausal changes started experimenting with the use of herbs, vitamins and other alternative approaches to menopause—with promising results. And a growing number of women's health care practitioners followed suit.

In fact, many natural options are so effective that mainstream women's doctors have begun to incorporate them as part of their treatment programs for menopausal patients. Here's what practitioners say are the best alternative options for treating menopausal problems.

Food Therapy: Soy Makes Sense

Diets abundant in soy products contain a group of natural chemical compounds called phytoestrogens because they possess estrogen-like activity, says Wulf Utian, M.D., Ph.D., director of the Department of Reproductive Biology at Case Western Reserve University in Cleveland and executive director of the North American Menopause Society.

Phytoestrogens come in two general forms: isoflavones and lignans. Isoflavones are found in soy foods like tofu and soy milk; lignans are found in whole grains, flaxseed and, to a lesser extent, fruits and vegetables.

What's their benefit to menopausal women? "If a woman wants to relieve her menopausal symptoms and doesn't want to go on hormone replacement therapy, certainly one or two daily servings of soy products is a reasonable approach," says Mark Messina, Ph.D., nutritionist in Port Townsend, Washington, participant in the Asian food conference and author of *The Simple Soybean and Your Health*. (One small study of six-month duration showed that soy did increase bone strength, adds Dr. Messina. But until phytoestrogens are studied further, he says that women at risk for osteoporosis shouldn't assume that phytoestrogens have the same bone-protecting benefits as hormone replacement therapy.)

"Soy foods, the richest food source of phytoestrogens, may be the reason why Asian women have fewer menopausal symptoms than American women do. I recommend adding two servings of soy foods four or five days a week," says Jane Guiltinan, doctor of naturopathy, clinical professor and medical director of the teaching clinic at Bastyr University of Naturopathic Medicine in Seattle. Dr. Guiltinan also suggests that you add flaxseed, walnuts and oats to your diet for rich sources of plant estrogen.

"There are lots of benefits that we already know about to eating less animal protein," says Gregory L. Burke, M.D., vice-chairman and professor in the Department of Public Health Sciences at the Bowman Gray School of Medicine of Wake Forest University in Winston-Salem, North Carolina. "I say 'go ahead' to women who ask if they should replace animal protein with soy protein as they near menopause."

Experts offer these easy, tasty ways to add soy to your diet.

Add soy milk to your cereal. Admittedly, soy milk doesn't taste like cow's milk. But when chilled, it's perfect for pouring over your cereal. Look for calcium-added nonfat or low-fat soy milk in health food stores.

When cooking, substitute soy milk for cow's milk. Replace cow's milk with equal amounts of soy milk in practically any recipe, including cream sauces, shakes, baked goods and puddings, suggests Dr. Messina.

Whip up a breakfast smoothie. For a delicious, satisfying breakfast treat, combine ½ cup unsweetened orange or apple juice, 1 medium banana and 3 ounces tofu in a blender and blend until smooth. If you like, add frozen strawberries or substitute them for the banana.

Use soy cheese. An excellent substitute for cow's milk cheese, soy cheese is lower in fat and salt and is available in some grocery stores and health food stores in an ever-growing variety of flavors, including mozzarella (try in lasagna or on pizza), Cheddar, American and Monterey Jack.

Try soy protein. Textured vegetable protein is made from defatted soy flour and found in health food stores and some grocery stores. Its meaty texture makes it a ringer for ground beef when used in spicy taco, chili or sloppy-joe recipes. You can substitute some, even all, of the meat in a recipe and your family is unlikely to be the wiser.

Yoga: Assume the Lotus Position

"For many women, menopause is a time of dramatic changes: children leaving home, worries about your sexual attractiveness and changing relationships with your parents and/or spouse—any one of which can be highly stressful," says Judith Lasater, Ph.D., a physical therapist and yoga instructor in San Francisco and author of *Relax and Renew: Restful Yoga for Stressful Times.*

"One of the lovely things about yoga for women in transition is the way that it makes you listen to your body more," says Dr. Lasater. "Our bodies are very wise and when we listen to them carefully, they'll often tell us what to do."

In addition, says Dr. Lasater, with the practice of yoga comes the "awareness of the moment" that allows us to heal ourselves. "You learn to anticipate what tenses your shoulders and how to untense them. You learn to rest when you're exhausted, how to improve your posture when you slouch and how to release anger when it builds up."

TAMING THE WILD HOT FLASH

Of all the changes heralding menopause, most women agree that the hot flash is the most notorious. Most research or experimentation with natural remedies for menopause has focused on this symptom.

Hot flashes arise when estrogen levels fall, says Nancy Lee Teaff, M.D., in her book *Perimenopause—Preparing for the Change.* Estrogen affects the hypothalamus, your brain's "thermostat." When estrogen levels begin to ebb, your body's ability to regulate your temperature goes haywire. As a result, blood vessels may dilate inappropriately.

Starting as a sudden warmth in your face, head or chest, a hot flash can spread like wildfire in just seconds, and as your body tries cooling itself off, you start sweating. The kicker to a reddening, drenching, hot flash can be a bout of shivering chills, as your body reacts to your wide-open pores and dampened skin.

If you're among the estimated 75 to 85 percent of women who experience hot flashes, alternative practitioners offer these time-tested natural strategies for relief.

Vitamin Therapy to Cool the Surge

Vitamin E improves the stability of your blood vessels and wards off the erratic dilation of the superficial blood vessel walls that cause hot flashes when estrogen levels fall, according to Dr. Guiltinan. By taking 400 to 1,200 international units (IU) of vitamin E daily, you may be able to prevent these power surges. (If you are considering taking amounts above 600 IU, talk to your doctor first since high doses can cause side effects in some people.)

Evidence that vitamin E may be useful for menopausal women emerged in the 1940s when women who couldn't take estrogen for their debilitating hot flashes and mood swings were given vitamin E. After treatment, their symptoms were markedly improved.

Start with lower doses and increase gradually. Vitamin E may take a few weeks to a few months to become effective. Also, if you have high blood pressure, diabetes or a rheumatic heart condition, don't take more than 200 IU of vitamin E without checking with your physician, according to Dr. Guiltinan. Vitamin E is absorbed only in the presence of fat, so it should be taken with foods that contain fat.

 ## Herbs Can Cool Hot Flashes and Night Sweats

Certain herbs have a cooling effect on your body and can put a chill on hot flashes and night sweats, says Susun S. Weed of Woodstock, New York, in her book *Menopausal Years: The Wise Woman Way*. Weed, who writes, teaches and lectures extensively about herbs, says that you should work regularly with one herb at a time for three or more months. Some herbs work very quickly, while other herbs work slowly and have a cumulative effect over time.

With that said, here's what herbal medicine has to offer for menopausal discomfort.

Black cohosh. Black cohosh (*Cimicifuga racemosa*) has been proven to be as effective as estrogen for the relief of hot flashes, according to Varro E. Tyler, Ph.D., professor emeritus of pharmacognosy at Purdue University in West Lafayette, Indiana, and author of *Herbs of Choice: The Therapeutic Use of Phytomedicinals*. (You may need to use it for up to four weeks before you feel better, however.)

To find the best dosage, Weed suggests starting with ten drops twice a day and increasing the dose by five drops every other day until you are satisfied with the results. Some women take black cohosh daily, others take it simply when needed and some take it for any two consecutive weeks each month.

Motherwort. Weed calls motherwort (*Leonurus cardiaca*) a magnificent herbal ally for moderating menopausal symptoms such as hot flashes and night sweats. She dilutes 5 to 15 drops of the tincture of motherwort, made from fresh, flowering tops, in a little water or tea. Take it as needed to cool hot flashes—or several times a day to prevent them.

Common chickweed. Weed says chickweed (*Stellaria media*) has provided hot-flash relief for many women. She uses 25 to 40 drops of fresh plant tincture once or twice a day to reduce the severity and frequency of hot flashes. Most women get results within a week or two of regular use.

Elder flower. This herb (*Sambucus canadensis*) specifically resets the body's thermostat, says Weed. For women who have frequent hot flashes or night sweats, 25 to 50 drops of fresh elder blossom tincture several times a day should bring rapid results, she adds.

Violet. Violets (*Viola odorata*) can also cool hot flashes, says Weed. Eat the fresh leaves in your salad (violets grow in many lawns), or brew a strong tea by steeping one ounce (by weight) of dried violet leaves in a quart of boiling water overnight. Strain, refrigerate and drink within 48 hours. She suggests drinking at least a cup a day. (You can find these dried leaves at many herb stores.)

Help Yourself to Exercise

In a study of 79 women, moderate and even severe menopausal symptoms, such as hot flashes and sweating, were reduced when the women exercised for three to four hours a week. But it's wise to start before you're menopausal: Later, unaccustomed exertion may trigger hot flashes.

Breathe Deeply

Researchers speculate that women who don't take hormone replacement therapy may benefit from doing deep breathing exercises. In a small study done among women who had at least five hot flashes a day, participants who practiced slow, deep breathing had half as many hot flashes.

If you want to try this technique, aim for 10 to 20 minutes of deep breathing, says Linda Ojeda, Ph.D., author of *Menopause without Medicine*. Here's how.

- Sit comfortably.
- Close your eyes and relax your muscles.

- Slowly breathe in and out through your nose.
- Become aware of each breath.
- Disregard distractions.

 ## Chill Out with Biofeedback

Thermal biofeedback can help you learn to gain control when you're caught in the midst of a hot flash, says Barry L. Gruber, Ph.D., a psychologist with Health Professionals in Chevy Chase, Maryland. "Women who have hot flashes are taught how to warm their hands via biofeedback, which seems, through some strange mechanism, to actually help them remain cool."

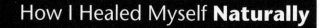

How I Healed Myself **Naturally**

Traditional Chinese Medicine Eased Menopause

Carol Young, a 53-year-old housewife from Chicago, remembers when menopause hit. She was 46, and she went into total "menopause meltdown."

"I hit menopause just as my son hit puberty. For both of us, boarding the hormone roller coaster was the wildest ride in the world," says Young.

It started with physical symptoms. "I started bleeding so heavily during my periods that I had to use three supersize sanitary pads and sometimes even a towel between my legs," remembers Young. "But I didn't realize that it was menopause because I'd always had menstrual problems, as had my mother and sister."

But soon Young was troubled by insomnia, exhaustion, mood swings, bowel problems and weight gain. Worried and wondering what was wrong, she made an appointment to see her doctor.

"My gynecologist told me that I was probably beginning menopause," she says. "He said that hormone replacement therapy (HRT) was the way to go. His wife and his sister were taking HRT, and they were doing just fine, he said. I asked him what would happen if I didn't take hormones, and he went through a whole litany of what could go wrong."

According to Dr. Gruber, learning how to control hot flashes with biofeedback involves weekly sessions for eight to ten weeks, following which biweekly, monthly and finally annual refresher visits are necessary. (For more information on biofeedback, see page 61.)

Traditional Chinese Medicine: Wisdom from the East

Practitioners of Traditional Chinese Medicine (TCM) say that the intricate healing system from the East provides excellent relief for hot flashes and other menopausal problems.

"For many women, a combination of acupuncture and Chinese herbs can ease hot flashes as effectively as estrogen can, yet without the side

---

Nevertheless, Young decided against the hormones. Her mother and sister had sailed through menopause without taking drugs, and that was what she wanted to do, too. She consulted Martha Howard, M.D., co-director of Wellness Associates, a Chicago-based family medical practice, who integrates Traditional Chinese Medicine and other alternative therapies into her practice.

"I had to fill out a ten-page medical questionnaire unlike anything I'd ever seen before," remembers Young. "I answered detailed questions about my emotions, what times of the year and temperatures I preferred and all about my symptoms."

The lengthy and unusual questionnaire wasn't the only part of the visit that differed from Young's consultation with her gynecologist. Dr. Howard also took Young's pulse, examined her tongue and studied her eyes—routine diagnostic tools in Traditional Chinese Medicine. After a long interview, Dr. Howard prescribed a combination of herbal tinctures, which she blended just for Young. She also gave Young biweekly acupuncture treatments. Her symptoms eased in a few weeks.

Young's periods have now ended—and so have her menopausal symptoms. "I'm glad to be back to my old self again," she reports.

effects," says Christina Stemmler, M.D., a Houston physician who integrates TCM and acupuncture with Western medicine and previously headed the American Academy of Medical Acupuncture. As Dr. Stemmler explains it, hot flashes are a release of yang energy produced because your body has a yin deficiency. (For a more complete explanation of the role of yin and yang in Traditional Chinese Medicine, see page 278.)

To combat the yin deficiency, says Dr. Stemmler, each woman needs to be evaluated by her TCM practitioner, who is likely to prescribe an individualized regimen of Chinese herbs, dietary changes and acupuncture. "What's important to know is that the path through menopause is completely different for each woman, depending on the dysfunctions that she's acquired during her life as well as her diet, her love life, her parents and her lifestyle," says Dr. Stemmler.

A small Swedish study of 21 women appears to confirm the use of acupuncture for hot flashes, indicating that hot flashes could be relieved via regular acupuncture treatments. In this study, 30-minute acupuncture treatments were given twice a week for two weeks and then once a week for another six weeks. The number of hot flashes experienced by the women decreased and remained noticeably reduced for up to three months after the treatments stopped.

Homeopathy May Help

Homeopathic practitioners offer effective, highly individualized treatments for hot flashes as well as menopausal discomforts, including irregular bleeding, mood swings and insomnia (often triggered by hot flashes).

"Each woman's hot-flash experience will be different," says Joyce Frye, D.O., an osteopath who uses homeopathy in her obstetrics and gynecology practice, chairperson of the gynecology department at Presbyterian Medical Center and a clinical faculty member at Jefferson Medical College, all in Philadelphia. "Some women will get hot faces, others will have hot chests and others will wake up during the night drenched in sweat. Classical homeopathy can help make menopause a peaceful transition with treatment tailored to the individual."

EASING VAGINAL DISCOMFORT

During menopause, the lining of your vagina may become drier, thinner and less flexible, due to lessening amounts of estrogen. You probably notice it most during sex—you may find that you don't become as lubricated when you're aroused, so sex is uncomfortable (or even impossible).

Here's what healers say you can do to remedy the situation.

Have sex regularly. Regular sexual activity promotes better circulation to the vagina and can increase lubrication, says Adriane Fugh-Berman, M.D., former head of field investigations for the Office of Alternative Medicine at the National Institutes of Health in Bethesda, Maryland. So a good way to protect yourself against menopausal vaginal dryness is to have regular sex—and it doesn't have to be with a partner.

Open sesame! Not all alternatives involve preventive sex. "Some women report having great success using sesame oil to relieve vaginal dryness," says Dr. Fugh-Berman. Soak a Coets (quilted cotton cosmetic square) in sesame oil, squeeze out the excess oil, insert it into the vagina and leave it in overnight. Remove the Coets the next morning, and that night, replace it with a new one also dipped in sesame oil. Repeat every day for a week, then once a week for as long as necessary. "The sesame oil is supposed to induce an estrogen-like effect," says Dr. Fugh-Berman.

Apply vitamin E. Some women find that vitamin E oils, when used regularly, ease vaginal dryness.

Use an herbal salve. Herbal salves or ointments containing St.-John's-wort and calendula will ease a dry, irritated vagina, says herbalist Rosemary Gladstar, author of *Herbal Healing for Women*. In her book Gladstar offers this recipe for a soothing medicinal paste: Mix enough slippery elm powder with aloe vera gel to form a paste; apply inside the vaginal lips and vagina.

Try a water-based lubricant. If you aren't lubricated, drugstore remedies such as Astroglide, K-Y Jelly and Replens (which lasts for up to three days per application) can also reduce the friction and discomfort of intercourse.

LIFTING THOSE MOODY BLUES

If you're approaching menopause, mood swings may be cause for reflection. For example, say you practically burst into tears over a trivial incident at the office. Or you're stuck in traffic and start yelling at the driver in front of you. Are hormones playing havoc with your emotions, or what?

"There's no simple answer about whether menopause causes mood disorders," says Mary Morrison, M.D., assistant professor of psychiatry and medicine in the Department of Psychiatry at the University of Pennsylvania in Philadelphia. "My sense, though, is that some women are particularly sensitive to hormonal changes. To those women, being in their forties may unmask depressive symptoms, like mild depression, irritability, memory problems and sleep disturbances."

Here are some options to try.

Choose a relaxation technique that works for you. Dr. Morrison recommends relaxing exercises such as yoga and meditation to the menopausal women that she counsels. Other tactics that may be helpful, say Dr. Morrison and other experts, include deep breathing, visualization and exercise. Keep a journal of what you try and how it works, to help you select the most effective technique, she says.

Try a calming herb blend. "For women whose hot flashes combine with irritability, I have great success using a formula made of equal parts of tincture of chickweed, dandelion root, motherwort and valerian," says Kathleen Maier, a physician's assistant, herbalist and director of Dreamtime Center for Herbal Studies in Flint Hill, Virginia, and former adviser on botanical medicine to the National Institutes of Health in Bethesda, Maryland.

Get some help. Women who can't shake off their sadness at the time of menopause—as well as women who have mood impairments or memory problems—should seek expert help by talking to a qualified therapist, physician or psychologist, says Dr. Morrison.

MENSTRUAL AND PREMENSTRUAL PROBLEMS

Real Relief for Real Discomfort

It's not all in your head. You really do want to hang a do-not-disturb sign around your neck the week before your period. You really do get cramps that make you want to crawl pitifully into bed. Your cravings for chocolate are utterly overwhelming. And just where did that bag of potato chips go, anyway?

But you're resolved not to give in to menstrual or premenstrual discomfort. The job, the kids and life itself are just too demanding, and besides, you're not the type to hide under the covers for days on end. So what's a real woman, beset with the very real symptoms of premenstrual syndrome (PMS), cramps and other menstrual challenges to do? For the best advice that advocates of natural healing have to offer, read on.

PMS: HELP FOR THE SCREAMING MEANIES

PMS is so ubiquitous among women that one British doctor calls it the world's commonest disease. "Sixty to 80 percent of all women have premenstrual changes that are mildly annoying," says Kathleen Ulman, Ph.D., staff psychologist at Women's Health Associates at Massachusetts General Hospital and instructor in the Department of Psychiatry at Harvard Medical School, both in Boston. "About 3 to 5 percent of women have severely disruptive symptoms, like profound depression, flashes of rage and unremitting exhaustion."

What causes PMS? No one, not even the British physician Katharina Dalton, who coined the phrase "premenstrual syndrome" back in 1953, is entirely certain. What scientists do know, though, is that female reproductive hormones, specifically progesterone, probably play a significant role.

Dr. Dalton notes that there are more than 150 recognized symptoms of

PMS and they affect teenage girls, menopausal women and everyone in between. The good news, she says, is that nearly 100 different treatment options exist to help relieve PMS.

Medical options include daily doses of synthetic hormones or drugs such as Prozac (an antidepressant) and Xanax (an anti-anxiety drug). For women looking for a natural, nondrug route, alternative practitioners offer the following advice, from herbs to yoga.

De-stress with Relaxation and Exercise

"We know that stress-management techniques can alleviate many PMS symptoms," says Dr. Ulman, who runs PMS stress-management groups. Here are the strategies that she has found to be the most successful.

Keep a menstrual journal. In small notebook, note your mood and physical symptoms for each day of your cycle. Many women with PMS find that stresses that they would otherwise tolerate well (or ignore) at other times of the month seem to make PMS worse.

"Keeping a record is the only way that you can connect your PMS symptoms to events in your life," says Dr. Ulman. "When you learn what triggers your symptoms and what your bad days may be, you'll learn when you have to take it easy, go home a little early and save the hard stuff for next week."

Learn a calming discipline. It doesn't matter which relaxation technique you choose, as long as it helps you to relax, says Dr. Ulman. "Deep breathing, meditation and yoga are all excellent for PMS," she says. (For details on deep breathing, meditation and yoga, see pages 67, 233 and 309.)

Take a walk. "I have some very exciting news for women with PMS," reports Mary Jane DeSouza, Ph.D., an exercise physiologist with the Center for Fertility and Reproductive Endocrinology at New Britain General Hospital in New Britain, Connecticut. Dr. DeSouza conducted a study on 45 sedentary women. Her findings? Women who took easy to moderately brisk half-hour walks three or four times a week experienced significant improvement in PMS symptoms. "This is the first study to document that low to moderate levels of exercise can improve PMS problems and symptoms," she says. "I'd much prefer to tell a woman to go on a low-intensity walking program than tell her to take an antidepressant drug."

  Food and Vitamin Therapy to the Rescue

A few dietary changes can ease or even end premenstrual syndrome and other menstrual problems, says Loretta Mears, D.C., chiropractor and certified clinical nutritionist in private practice in New York City. "For many of the women that I work with, PMS problems are usually related, in one way or another, to nutritional problems."

Here's what she and other nutritional experts recommend.

Eat small meals—frequently. "I find that eating five small meals a day, with a good balance of complex carbohydrates and a moderate amount of protein, helps many women," says Dr. Ulman. (Half of a turkey sandwich on whole-wheat bread is a good example.)

The combination of carbohydrates and protein helps buffer mood swings, says Diana Taylor, R.N., Ph.D., director of the Perimenstrual Symptom Management Research Program at the University of California School of Nursing in San Francisco.

"What doesn't help is going for hours without eating and then grabbing a candy bar," she says. Simple sugars, like candy, soft drinks, juice drinks, cookies and ice cream, cause your body to release additional insulin, which can cause a low-blood-sugar rebound effect, sometimes resulting in fatigue and irritability, according to Dr. Taylor.

Focus on vitamin B_6. "I recommend that women take 500 milligrams of vitamin B_6 once a day for three days before their PMS symptoms usually start," says Dr. Mears. (Vitamin B_6 is toxic in high doses. Since this is several hundred times the daily requirement for this vitamin, you should take it for brief time periods only, and only under the supervision of your doctor.)

Other women find that far lower amounts of B_6—50 milligrams—are adequate. But even then, its use should be limited.

Nix the wake-up juice. Studies have shown that as little as one cup of coffee a day can increase the tension and anxiety symptoms of PMS. Even decaffeinated beverages can contain enough caffeine to stimulate symptoms in sensitive women.

To avoid withdrawal headaches (not unusual in coffee drinkers who try to quit), gradually replace caffeine by substituting decaffeinated versions of your favorite beverages—coffee, tea and cola—over a couple of weeks, recommends Dr. Taylor. Then, try to meet your fluid needs of 48 ounces a day with noncaffeinated beverages such as herbal teas, seltzer water or iced water with a slice of orange or lemon.

Light Therapy for Winter PMS

Do you find that your PMS symptoms seem to worsen in the winter? If so, a type of depression known as seasonal affective disorder (SAD) may be a problem for you, says Brenda Byrne, Ph.D., director of the Seasonal

Affective Disorder Clinic at Jefferson Medical College of Thomas Jefferson University in Philadelphia.

"It's been said that over one-half of all menstruating women who have SAD have PMS-type symptoms," says Dr. Byrne. "Those affected may feel that their PMS symptoms become worse during the darker, shorter days of winter. If you have seasonal affective disorder and your symptoms respond to light therapy, there's a good chance that it will improve your PMS symptoms, too."

Using light therapy for PMS may be as easy as sitting in front of a light source for a few minutes every morning. (To learn more about light therapy for seasonal affective disorder and related problems, see page 210.)

Traditional Chinese Medicine Claims Success

"Premenstrual syndrome is easily treated with Chinese herbal formulas and acupuncture," says Christina Stemmler, M.D., a Houston physician who uses acupuncture and Traditional Chinese Medicine (TCM) in her practice and previously headed the American Academy of Medical Acupuncture. In fact, PMS is one of the easiest conditions to treat with Traditional Chinese Medicine, she says.

According to Dr. Stemmler, each woman's condition needs a different approach, which might combine acupuncture, Chinese herbs, dietary changes and massage. Other practitioners say that TCM is also excellent for menstrual cramps and excessive menstrual bleeding.

"There is no standard recipe for curing PMS because PMS is a very complex problem with hundreds of subtly different nuances," says Dr. Stemmler. (For details on finding a practitioner of Traditional Chinese Medicine, see page 284.)

CRAMPS: K.O. PERIODIC PAIN

Almost half of us feel some kind of monthly pain, and 5 to 10 percent of us have pain that downs us for anywhere from an hour to three days. "What happens during a painful period is like a mini–heart attack of the uterus, where blood to the uterine muscle gets cut off," says Veronica A. Ravnikar, M.D., director of the Reproductive, Endocrine and Infertility Unit and professor of obstetrics and gynecology in the Department of Obstetrics and Gynecology at the University of Massachusetts Medical Center in Worcester.

When hormones called prostaglandins are released during your period, the uterine blood vessels constrict and cause decreased blood flow to the area. As a result, the uterine muscle clenches tightly and is felt as a cramp. Happily, cramps may lessen after you're 30, and motherhood sometimes ends them, too.

Many of the world's natural-healing systems treat cramps successfully. Read on.

Hydrotherapy: Made-to-Order for Cramps

Therapeutic use of water is a simple time-tested treatment that works especially well for menstrual cramps. "The soothing effect of lying in a tub of hot water helps relax tense uterine muscles, so that's why it helps your cramps," says Irene von Estorff, M.D., assistant professor of rehabilitation medicine at New York Hospital–Cornell University Medical Center in New York City.

Make your own heating pad. "Instead of a nice hot tub, however, you could use another, more portable variation on hydrotherapy when you have cramps—a moist hot pack."

Making your own moist heating pad is simple, explains Dr. von Estorff: Dampen a terry cloth towel in hot (not boiling) water. Wring out the towel so that it's not dripping and place it over your crampy lower abdomen. Then lie still, relax and let the towel cool naturally. Repeat as necessary.

Chiropractic: An Eclectic Approach That Works

Some chiropractors find that spinal manipulation can help relieve menstrual cramps in much the same way that chiropractic relieves back pain. "Because the spinal nerves that go to the uterus and ovaries come from the lumbar spine, any untreated back problems can exacerbate cramping," says Dr. Mears.

Dr. Mears offers additional clues and solutions.

Keep a food diary. When a woman comes into Dr. Mears's office complaining of menstrual difficulties, she will probably be advised to start keeping a food diary.

"Menstrual difficulties are complex and can be associated with food allergies," asserts Dr. Mears. "I ask women to keep track of what they eat, the timing, frequency and social situation and how they feel after they've eaten. I also ask them to keep track of their bowel movements because constipation can contribute to cramps."

Stretch, walk, massage. One woman who consulted Dr. Mears complained of severe menstrual cramps that had not responded to heavier-than-recommended doses of ibuprofen, which the woman had been taking on her own.

"I gave her a new daily regimen consisting of daily stretching exercises and a brisk 20-minute walk in the park every day, and I started her on a special soup that I use to relieve constipation," says Dr. Mears. "I also saw her twice a week for chiropractic manipulations for her lower-back pain, and I taught her how to do self-massage for her abdomen and thigh muscles. It wasn't long before she was cramp-free for the first time in her life."

For the thigh, stroke along the inner thigh muscle for a few minutes. Do not press the muscle. Use your left hand to stroke your left thigh and your right hand to stroke your right thigh.

For the abdomen, lie on your back. Beginning on your right side, in the lower groin area, press in with the fingertips of both hands. Hold for two seconds and release. Follow this pressing and releasing pattern up your right side, across the top of your abdomen under the ribs and down your left side into the lower groin area. You are pressing in the form of an upside-down letter U. Continue this U pattern spiraling into smaller and smaller U's until you reach the center.

According to Dr. Mears, if you drink plenty of water and engage in physical activity, you'll banish your constipation—and your cramps.

Exercise to Exorcise Cramps

Add menstrual cramps to the long list of ailments alleviated by exercise. "If you can relax the pelvic area and increase the blood flow to the muscles, you'll decrease pain and cramping," says Dr. Ravnikar.

And, since exercise boosts endorphins, your body's natural painkillers, working out (or just walking) might ease your cramps, suggests Christine Wells, Ph.D., professor of exercise science and physical education at Arizona State University in Tempe and author of *Women, Sport and Performance*.

Start out easy. For the first 15 minutes of your workout, take it easy, says Dr. Wells. Then, if you're up to it, pick up the pace. When you're crampy, don't add unfamiliar exercises or heavier-than-normal weights to your routine and avoid heavy lifting that stresses your abs, she says. Save crunches and other belly-buster activities till later in the week.

Stretch Like a Yogi

Your lower back and thighs may ache when cramps stimulate nerves that supply these areas, says Dr. Ravnikar. Stretching yoga-style can help.

Sit up straight with both of your legs touching and stretched out in front of you. Bend your right leg, bringing your foot to your inner left thigh. Place a folded blanket on top of your extended leg. Inhale. Push into the floor with your hands to lift your chest and lengthen your spine upward as you twist your torso so that your breastbone comes directly over your extended leg. As you exhale, bend forward from the hips, keeping your back straight. Do not hunch your spine. Rest your chest forward on the blanket. Stay stretched like this for two to three minutes. Repeat the stretch on the other side.

 ## Herbal Remedies for Cramps

According to herbalists, Mother Nature's own remedies are ideally suited to easing the pain of menstrual cramps. Herbalists often recommend the following three herbs.

Raspberry leaves. "Raspberry leaves contain fragrine, a specific constituent that tones the uterus and helps ease cramping," says Kathleen

Super Soup for Cramps

This unique soup may not win any awards from the French Culinary Institute, but it's effective for menstrual cramps aggravated by constipation, according to New York City chiropractor and certified clinical nutritionist Loretta Mears, D.C. You can find oat bran or wheat bran and flaxseed at any health food store.

1 cup fat-free and salt-free vegetable broth
    (preferably homemade)
2 tablespoons oat bran or wheat bran
1 tablespoon whole flaxseed

Heat the broth on the stove in the evening. Turn off the heat and add the bran and flaxseed to the broth. Let it stand on the stove until morning. When you get up in the morning, reheat the broth until it's warm. Don't overcook, to maintain consistency and avoid sliminess. Pour the broth into a bowl or mug. Put a tablespoon into your mouth and swish it around to mix well with your saliva. Then swallow, but don't chew the flaxseed.

Yield: 1 cup

Maier, a physician's assistant, herbalist and director of Dreamtime Center for Herbal Studies in Flint Hill, Virginia, and former adviser on botanical medicine to the National Institutes of Health in Bethesda, Maryland. Maier recommends brewing a strong cup or two of raspberry-leaf tea (*Rubus idaeus*), available at most health food stores, for cramp relief.

Motherwort. "When you want a good mother herb, motherwort's wonderful," says Maier. "I use 10 to 15 drops of motherwort (*Leonurus cardiaca*) tincture for menstrual cramps at midcycle, or ovulation time, taken daily till bleeding starts. Some women may notice that their periods are heavier during the first month they use it because motherwort relaxes the uterine muscle and thereby releases more of the uterine lining. But with consistent use, bleeding levels off. Most women see a noticeable improvement in their cramps after one month, but I'd say that, generally, it takes three to four cycles to establish a difference."

How I Healed Myself **Naturally**

Acupuncture Cured Her Cramps

Martha Peters, a 49-year-old nurse in Media, Pennsylvania, found that acupuncture relieved menstrual pain when all else failed.

"For years, I'd been seeing gynecologists for my painful menstrual cramps," says Peters (who asked us not to use her real name). "The first doctor that I saw said, 'Have a baby—that'll help your cramps.' But since I wasn't planning on having children, the advice wasn't helpful. In fact, none of the advice that I'd received from any of the doctors I'd ever seen was particularly helpful."

By the time Peters was in her thirties and working as a nurse, she'd been suffering from severe cramps for 14 years. She missed time from work every month because of the incapacitating pain, nausea, occasional migraines, weakness and dizziness that she experienced.

"Occasionally, the pain was absolutely crippling," she says. "Finally, ibuprofen came on the market. At first, it was like a godsend. I could work." Unfortunately, ibuprofen eventually caused severe stomach damage, and Peters was no longer able to take it.

Some time later, during a visit to the West coast, Peters went to an acupuncturist. "My mother-in-law's arthritis had responded to acupuncture, and she convinced me to go," says Peters. "As a nurse, I was extremely skeptical and thought that it was all in her head. But I was desperate enough to try anything."

Black cohosh. "Black cohosh is an antispasmodic—it quells muscle spasms, especially in the uterus," says Maier. "It relaxes the uterus and decreases cramps. But I use it in general relaxation formulas when there's also shoulder tension." The botanical name is *Cimicifuga racemosa*.

HEAVY BLEEDING: VITAMINS THAT HELP

An occasional change in your monthly flow is perfectly normal, say experts, and may be due to a lifestyle change. If you're bleeding more heavily than normal, ask yourself what's new or different: Have you started a new exercise program? Taken a new job? Moved into a new home?

Age could be a factor: Your uterus keeps growing until you're around age 35, so there's more uterine lining to bleed. Approaching menopause can

---

Peters had a total of nine appointments in three weeks with a woman obstetrician/gynecologist from Taiwan, a licensed acupuncturist with an M.D. from the University of Pennsylvania School of Medicine in Philadelphia.

"My exact thoughts were, 'Here goes good money after bad,' " remembers Peters. "I thought it was completely ridiculous. Much to my surprise, I got my next period without even being aware of it. I had nothing—no cramps, no nausea, no weakness. I was absolutely shocked."

Peters remained free of menstrual cramps for a couple of years. Then, gradually, they began again. With no acupuncturist accessible to her, Peters began taking birth control pills (sometimes offered as a medical solution for menstrual cramps). But as a consequence of taking the Pill, she suffered migraines that were even more painful than her cramps.

Finally locating an acupuncturist, Peters began weekly treatments for eight weeks, and once again acupuncture worked. "I knew that I was getting my period, but it was just like a miracle all over again," says Peters. "I continued to see the acupuncturist for 'booster' treatments once every six months, or whenever I felt a little twinge, and my cramps stopped again."

also mean having unpredictable, heavy periods. Experts say that you should pay attention to your cycle and know what's normal for you and be certain to get examined annually. Recording when your period stops and starts and whether you bleed heavily or lightly is also smart.

If bleeding or pain seem unusually heavy for you, or if you miss a period, consult your physician, advises Margaret M. Polaneczky, M.D., medical director of women's health and assistant professor of obstetrics and gynecology at New York Hospital–Cornell University Medical Center.

If your physician has ruled out possible underlying medical causes for your heavy bleeding, these suggestions may ease the problem.

Pump some iron. Inadequate iron intake may cause excessive bleeding, according to Linda Ojeda, Ph.D., author of *Menopause without Medicine*. And excessive bleeding, in turn, can lead to iron-deficiency anemia, which can cause fatigue. So Dr. Ojeda and others recommend that women with heavy periods eat iron-rich foods to prevent iron deficiency.

The most efficiently absorbed iron, called heme iron, is supplied by foods such as red meat, liver, egg yolks and fish. If you're watching your intake of fat and cholesterol, a multivitamin/ mineral supplement with iron is a sound alternative, she says. Vegetarians who get nonheme iron from grains, beans and dried fruit must also take vitamin C to enhance absorption, says Dr. Ojeda.

Bolster your bioflavonoid intake. What's a bioflavonoid? This nutrient, also called vitamin P, is found in grape skins, cherries, blackberries and blueberries as well as in citrus fruits, especially in the pulp and white rind. Both bioflavonoids and vitamin C can reduce excessive bleeding by strengthening capillary walls. Since it's not easy to get the 500 milligrams a day of bioflavonoids that experts recommend, some suggest taking supplements. You might also add 1,000 milligrams of vitamin C in divided doses, says Susan Lark, M.D., in her book *The Estrogen Decision Self-Help Book*. (Note, however, that excess vitamin C may cause diarrhea in some people.) In her book, Dr. Lark recommends both vitamin C and bioflavonoid supplements for heavy menstrual bleeding. Take the supplements at the same time. They are available at drugstores and health food stores.

 ## Look to the Garden

Your herb garden (or your health food store) has a number of options for treating irregular periods. Try these, all recommended by Susun S. Weed, herbalist and teacher from Woodstock, New York, and author of the *Wise Woman* herbal series.

Raspberry-leaf infusion. A cup a day (or more) acts as a tonic for the ovaries and the uterus, according to herbal medical lore. To make the infusion, add dried raspberry leaves to a quart of boiling water, then remove it from the heat and let it sit overnight.

Vitex tincture. Vitex (*Vitex agnus-castus*) has long been used in European herbal medicine. It is believed to inhibit the secretion of the peptide hormone prolactin by the pituitary gland. For irregular menstrual periods, take a dropperful two to three times a day in a small glass of water for six to eight weeks, after every irregular period. For heavy bleeding or flooding, take 25 drops several times daily for several months.

Lady's-mantle. In tincture form, clinical tests show that lady's-mantle (*Alchemilla vulgaris*) can control heavy menstrual bleeding or flooding in virtually all of the 300 or so women who participated in a study, says Weed. When taken after heavy bleeding began, lady's-mantle took three to five days to be effective. When taken one to two weeks before menstruation, lady's-mantle prevented heavy bleeding. Weed recommends taking five to ten drops of the fresh plant tincture three times daily for up to two weeks out of the month.

Cramp bark and valerian. "Heavy bleeding accompanied by nasty cramps responds well to a blend of two parts cramp bark tincture mixed with one part valerian tincture," says Rosemary Gladstar, herbalist and author of *Herbal Healing for Women.* The botanical name for cramp bark is *Viburnum opulus,* and for valerian, *Valeriana officinalis.*

OVERWEIGHT
New Ways to Get Rid of the Unwanted Pounds

Even if fleshy thighs and generous abdomens were suddenly as attractive as they were back in the days of the Flemish painter Rubens, being overweight still wouldn't be desirable.

Aesthetics aside, being overweight is simply not healthy. Carrying an extra 20, 30 or 50 pounds or more raises your risk of diabetes, high blood pressure, heart disease and cancer of the breast, colon and uterus, among other illnesses. Carrying extra pounds also strains your spine, muscles, joints and ligaments, contributing to chronic back and joint problems.

If you're like a lot of women, you probably know that you'd benefit by losing unneeded weight. And you've probably tried. According to the National Center for Health Statistics, more than half of all overweight people say that they've tried to lose weight within the past year.

IN SEARCH OF THE PERFECT WEIGHT-LOSS AID

In their efforts to lose weight, women have tried scores of diet gimmicks: over-the-counter appetite suppressants, diet shakes, high-protein diets, grapefruit pills, thigh wraps and more. Or they go on starvation diets. Invariably, the weight comes back.

"Ninety-five percent of all diets fail," says Diane Grabowski-Nepa, R.D., nutrition educator at the Pritikin Longevity Center in Santa Monica, California. "Women diet, they starve themselves, then they go off the diet and they binge and feel miserable, so they go back on a diet. It's a vicious cycle, and it isn't working."

Some women try teas and capsules containing ma huang, the Chinese name for the herb ephedra (*Ephedra sinica*). Ephedra contains ephedrine, a compound that raises your metabolism, so you burn more calories. It's natural, but it's far from safe: This herb can speed up your heart rate and blood pressure and trigger a heart attack. Some weight-loss products even combine ma huang with caffeine, enhancing its risk.

"These pills are harmful and shouldn't be used," says Susun S. Weed, an herbalist and teacher from Woodstock, New York, who is the author of the *Wise Woman* herbal series and who speaks widely on the topic of healing herbs at medical gatherings.

Medical doctors agree that diet gimmicks are dangerous or useless or both. At the other end of the spectrum are prescription drugs such as dexfenfluramine (Redux). This so-called miracle drug prompts your body to raise your level of serotonin (a brain chemical), which in turn dampens your appetite, so you eat less.

Though medically approved, this prescription drug is no miracle. In a year-long study of 900 severely overweight men and women, almost two-thirds of those taking dexfenfluramine lost less than a tenth of their total weight. The remaining third lost virtually no weight at all.

Questions have arisen over the safety of dexfenfluramine as well. The drug has been linked to serious brain and lung problems.

SAFE, NATURAL WEIGHT LOSS

Women who want to lose pounds have other, safer options. A vegetarian diet can help you lose weight permanently, without starving yourself. Certain foods, herbs and minerals can speed up your metabolism safely. And acupuncture can increase serotonin and regulate appetite naturally—as can listening to music. Even the way that you think can help you lose weight.

Coupled with more conventional wisdom about what works and why, safe alternative methods can and do work.

FAT-DUMPING STRATEGIES

It's no mystery that much of the unwanted fat on your body comes from fat that originates on your dinner plate. In a study conducted at Indiana University in Bloomington, of 17 lean and 15 severely overweight women, the overweight women consumed diets much higher in fat. Among the very overweight women, 36 percent of their total calories came from fat, compared to just 29 percent for the lean women. So, getting no more than 30 percent of your daily calories from fat—about 30 grams of fat a day—helps keep the fat off your body, says Michael Steelman, M.D., president of the American Society of Bariatric Physicians in Oklahoma City, Oklahoma.

Fat has three strikes against it. Strike one: Gram for gram, fat contains more calories than carbohydrates—nine calories per gram of fat versus four calories per gram of carbohydrate.

Strike two: It's easier for your body to store fat calories than calories converted from carbohydrates to fat. To digest, transport and store fat uses just 3 percent of the fat calories eaten. But carbohydrates—whole grains, fruits and vegetables—burn 24 percent of the calories that are going to be transformed and stored as fat.

Strike three: Fat is less satisfying than carbohydrates. After eating high-fat foods, you don't feel as full as you do after eating carbohydrates, so you overeat, says Ken Goodrick, Ph.D., psychologist at Baylor College of Medicine in Houston.

The study also found that the lean women consumed an average of 22.7 grams of fiber, compared with 15.7 grams consumed by the overweight women.

Together, dumping fat and adding fiber are effective first steps on the road to lasting weight control. Here's what alternative-minded practitioners suggest.

Switch to a high-fiber, natural-food vegetarian diet. Giving up animal foods is the single easiest way to cut fat and calories from your diet, says Joel Fuhrman, M.D., physician in Belle Mead, New Jersey, and author of *Fasting—And Eating—For Health.* "Three hundred calories worth of meat—about six ounces of beef—takes up very little room in your stomach. In comparison, 300 calories in fiber-rich foods such as whole grains, fruits and vegetables makes you feel full and satiated. These foods don't turn into fat in your body as rapidly. Plus, the typical serving of meat gets 50 percent of its calories from fat."

Double your fiber intake. Fiber is the part of food that doesn't break down—the skins of fruits, outer layers of beans, the bran in brown rice and oats and other components of food that simply pass through your digestive tract since your body doesn't produce the enzymes needed to digest them.

Experts say that we should consume between 20 and 30 grams of fiber a day. Yet many women consume much less. And too little fiber translates into too many pounds, says Marg Alfieri, R.D., coordinator of the bariatric clinic at the London Health Science Center in London, in Ontario, Canada. In a study at the center that examined the eating habits of 150 people (including 125 women), researchers found that moderately or severely overweight people ate significantly less fiber than those who were not overweight.

"Normal-weight individuals ate an average of 19 grams of fiber a day," says Alfieri, who conducted the study. "In contrast, overweight people consumed far less—only 13 grams."

Fiber facilitates weight loss in a couple of ways. "First, most high-fiber foods are great in volume and low in calories, so they fill you up without a lot of calories," says Edward Saltzman, M.D., medical director of the Obesity Consultation Center at the New England Medical Center at Tufts University in Boston.

"Second, foods with more fiber, especially raw vegetables like carrots and celery, take longer to chew. You spend more time chewing. People get tired of chewing, so they eat less," Dr. Saltzman says.

Eating fruits, vegetables and whole grains every day gives you the dietary fiber that you need every day to lose weight, says Dr. Saltzman. It's best not to increase your fiber through supplements, says Dr. Salzman. Adding supplements to an unhealthy diet is not a nutritionally sound way to lose weight.

How I Healed Myself **Naturally**

She Reaches Her Goal Weight—At Last

Dorothy Day, a middle-age accountant from Hillsborough, New Jersey, says that after all else failed, a vegetarian diet enabled her to lose weight permanently.

Like many women, Day began gaining weight in her late twenties. And she battled the same stubborn 30 to 40 pounds for most of her adult life.

Name a weight-loss gimmick and Day had tried it—protein drinks, fasts, skipping meals, living on nothing but salads and devouring chocolate-flavored diet shakes. Nothing really worked.

"A pattern started," she says. "I'd go on a diet and try to lose weight, but I'd never get down to where I wanted to be. Then I'd gain it all back."

At age 46, Day attended a public talk on vegetarianism by a local medical doctor. She decided to try a vegetarian diet. It succeeded where other diets had failed.

Today, Day weighs in between 120 and 127 pounds—leaner than she had ever dreamed she could be. Occasionally, she will eat turkey, dairy products and lean ground beef. Otherwise, however, her diet is comprised of whole grains, fruits, vegetables and vegetable protein.

FOODS THAT BOOST YOUR METABOLISM

You've probably known women who seemed incapable of losing weight no matter how little they ate. They probably attributed their excess weight to slow metabolism.

Some people do burn calories more slowly than others, making it harder for them to control their weight. Perhaps you're one of those women.

In about one person out of four, the problem isn't slow metabolism, per se, but a defect in the way that their bodies metabolize sugar and convert it into fat. In the normal course of consuming and burning calories and carrying on everyday functions, your body produces insulin, a hormone produced and released by your pancreas. Insulin controls the rate at which blood sugar—your body's fuel—is absorbed by cells throughout your body.

Some people, it seems, produce higher-than-normal levels of insulin—not necessarily high enough to bring on diabetes but high enough to affect their metabolisms, appetites and weights. Too-high levels of insulin trigger the body to manufacture more fat cells than normal when certain foods are consumed. The more easily foods are converted into sugar in the body, the more pronounced this effect. The overmanufacture of fat cells also slows down your metabolism. The net effect is that you gain weight.

By selecting what some doctors call low-glycemic foods—foods high in carbohydrates and fiber that don't stimulate overproduction of insulin—people who've failed to lose weight may at last succeed. Here are the do's and don'ts.

Load up on fibrous fare. Eat plenty of oatmeal, barley, sweet potatoes, whole-grain breads like rye and pumpernickel, beans, fruits and broccoli and other vegetables, recommends Dr. Steelman. These foods don't seem to stimulate insulin production easily. Yogurt, chicken and turkey also seem to be low-glycemic foods.

Skip the white stuff. In contrast, white potatoes, bread, pasta and noodles made from white flour seem to prompt an increase in blood sugar levels, says Dr. Steelman. Known as high-glycemic foods, these foods are quickly absorbed into your system, sending a signal to your pancreas to produce and release more insulin, so they're best avoided. Sugar does the same thing.

Fight fat with flaxseed. If you don't get enough omega-3 fatty acids (essential compounds found in some oils), your fat cells become insensitive to insulin, prompting your pancreas to produce too much insulin. Taking a tablespoon a day of flaxseed oil—a rich source of omega-3 fatty acids—helps improve the function of your insulin, notes Michael Murray, doctor of naturopathy in Bellevue, Washington, instructor at Bastyr University of Naturopathic Medicine in Seattle and author of *Natural Alternatives for Weight Loss*.

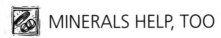

MINERALS HELP, TOO

While modifying what you eat and stepping up the number of calories that you burn are the mainstays of weight control, other factors exert smaller but significant effects on the effort.

Consider chromium. Taking 200 micrograms of chromium a day also helps regulate insulin levels, says Dr. Steelman. (Before taking this much chromium, talk to your doctor.) Chromium works closely with insulin in controlling the intake of blood sugar into your cells. Without enough chromium, the insulin's action is blocked and blood sugar levels rise, contributing to weight gain. Foods rich in chromium include whole grains, such as oatmeal and whole-wheat bread, vegetables, wheat germ, soy, brewer's yeast and chicken.

Caution: While some authorities cite studies in which people consume up to 1,000 micrograms of chromium a day with no toxic effects, it's best to consume no more than 200 micrograms a day from supplements without medical supervision.

Mind your magnesium. Dr. Steelman suggests taking 500 milligrams a day of magnesium. This mineral can help cut down on chocolate cravings, which are sometimes the downfall of women trying to lose weight. "We see magnesium levels drop in premenstrual women, which is when the cravings usually pick up," he says. "So it only makes sense that magnesium might help reduce the cravings." If you have heart or kidney problems, talk to your doctor before taking magnesium supplements.

Rely on mineral-rich herbs. Use herbal infusions that are made with herbs rich in calcium, magnesium and potassium, says Weed. Calcium may help to regulate your thyroid, an endocrine gland in your neck that regulates your metabolism, so every little bit helps. Try herbal infusions made from stinging nettle, oatstraw, red clover, peppermint or lemon balm, says Weed. To make an herbal infusion, take one ounce of a dried herb, put it in a quart jar, fill it to the top with boiling water and let it sit overnight. Then strain and drink it hot or cold. You can find these herbs in health food stores.

MOVE IT TO LOSE IT

If you aren't exercising, you may be missing out on one of nature's most valuable weight-loss aids and metabolism boosters.

Exercising will burn calories and raise your metabolic rate both during and after your workout. Researchers at the University of Vermont in

Burlington compared women who exercised regularly to women who were sedentary. The active women had significantly faster metabolic rates. More than ten hours after their workouts, they were burning calories 6 percent faster than inactive women.

Exercise is like marriage. In order for it to work, you have to be committed to it, come rain or shine. But also like marriage, commitment is a lot easier if you also enjoy it.

Experts agree that when it comes to weight loss and maintenance, the following forms of exercise are among the best when done several times a week and coupled with calorie control. Here's what they recommend.

Walk to keep it off. Walking is an effective exercise for keeping the weight off once it's gone, says Philip Ewbank, exercise physiologist and supervisor of exercise physiology at the William Beaumont Hospital Division of Preventive and Nutritional Medicine in Birmingham, Michigan. It's easy to do, convenient and a good activity to do with friends, he says.

Ewbank and fellow researchers traced a group of 45 formerly obese people who had lost an average of 62 pounds on very low calorie diets. Typically, people who go on very low calorie diets gain back all the weight that they've lost, and then some. But in this study, people who exercised regularly for two years, mainly through walking, regained just 24 percent of the weight that they'd lost (about 15 pounds). This high-activity group burned 1,575 calories a week through walking 16 miles per week. In comparison, those in the low-activity group who walked 4.8 miles a week burned about half as many calories through exercise—fewer than 850 calories. And they gained back more than twice as much weight—72 percent (roughly 45 pounds).

How much walking is enough? In the study, the exercisers who minimized weight gain were walking three miles a day, five to seven days a week. That's about an hour's worth of walking a day, nearly every day.

Pump iron. Walking alone may not be enough to reach your goal. For those last stubborn pounds, you may need to add resistance training—working out with light weights such as dumbbells, for example.

Lifting weights for about an hour three times a week may help speed up your metabolism, says Ben Hurley, Ph.D., director of the exercise science lab at the University of Maryland College of Health and Human Performance in College Park.

When you build muscle, you facilitate weight loss in two ways. Muscle burns more energy than fat does, so the more muscle you create, the more calories you'll burn, says Dr. Hurley. In contrast, fat is not as metabolically active, so it burns fewer calories.

Building muscle also increases your resting metabolism. In other words, if you lift weights every other day or so, your body burns more calories while you're sitting around or sleeping than it would if you didn't exercise. Since you spend about 16 hours or more a day at rest, the afterburn effect can give your weight loss effort an additional assist, he says.

MOZART AND MANICOTTI

Practiced regularly, mind-body therapies such as imagery, visualization and music therapy can be perfect complements to an overall weight-loss

How I Healed Myself **Naturally**

By Working Out, She Lost 85 Pounds

Kathy McCreedy, 36, a nurse in Beverly Hills, Michigan, was able to lose 85 pounds in just over a year. The key to her success? Exercise.

McCreedy is five feet four inches tall and at her heaviest weighed 235 pounds. She was divorced—and very depressed.

"I'd eaten my way through my divorce, and I remember wondering how I could be so miserable yet so unmotivated to do anything about it," she recalls. "I decided to get really serious about exercise."

McCreedy started with walking. She began with a 15-minute mile, then worked up to two miles and then moved up to four. "When I got down below 200 pounds, I finally worked up the nerve to try in-line skating. I bought a pair of in-line skates, and now I go out and skate whenever I can, as long as it's not raining.

"I also started cycling. Just the other day, I rode 60 miles," says Mc-Creedy, with pride. "It's one of the coolest things I've ever done.

"I don't count calories in food, but I do try to be careful to eat lots of vegetables, fruits and very little meat. I am rigid about keeping an exercise log and tracking the calories that I burn. I try to burn at least 2,500 calories a week and average about 3,000 calories a week." That's about an hour of exercise a day, she says.

"Over the last 14 months, I've missed maybe four days of exercise, total," says McCreedy. And it has paid off. "Now, my weight averages between 145 and 150 pounds, and I wear a size 10. I'll never be heavy ever again. I am so much happier with myself now."

program, says Peter Miller, Ph.D., clinical psychologist, executive director and founder of the Hilton Head Health Institute in Hilton Head Island, South Carolina, and author of *The New Hilton Head Metabolism Diet*.

Imagery may be as simple as picturing how you'll look thin and wearing a sleek, black cocktail dress. Music therapy may consist of listening to Mozart as you munch manicotti to make you eat more slowly.

Here are some effective mental strategies to aid your weight-loss efforts.

Munch to music. Listening to gentle music while you dine forces you to concentrate on what you're eating, which means that you'll eat more slowly and probably be more satisfied with what you've eaten, says Dr. Goodrick. "We know that if you watch TV and eat without being aware of it, you'll probably eat more, simply because the eating becomes automatic. From the very beginning of behavior modification, we've talked about focusing on the food so that you're better able to appreciate it."

See yourself reject food. Envisioning yourself avoiding the pitfalls of overeating is a creative tool in weight loss, says Dr. Miller.

Visualize a situation that makes you vulnerable to cravings. Maybe you know that you're going to find yourself home alone with half a cheesecake leftover from a party. "Imagine smelling it, looking at it, letting the craving develop and not fighting it. The next step is to see yourself destroying the food or putting it away in the refrigerator, out of sight," he notes. "Then, when the situation arises, your mental rehearsal will help you avoid devouring the food."

To keep cravings under control, practice your craving-control visualizations two or three times a day for about five minutes, recommends Dr. Miller.

Picture yourself thin. Another positive visualization is to see yourself achieving your weight-loss goal, says Dr. Murray. "You should put yourself into a relaxed state and see yourself losing weight and imagining what it would feel like. Imagine how your body would feel and what it would look like. This programs the subconscious mind to do what you want."

Ask for acupuncture. Acupuncture is best known for relieving chronic pain. But acupuncture may possibly help weight loss. Research suggests that by stimulating certain energy channels, or meridians, acupuncture can prompt the release of serotonin, the brain chemical that suppresses appetite, says Lixing Lao, M.D., Ph.D., licensed acupuncturist and assistant professor in the Department of Family Medicine at the University of Maryland in Baltimore. But unlike some medications, acupuncture has few harmful side effects. (For information on finding a practitioner qualified to provide acupuncture treatments, see page 33.)

Try cognitive therapy. Another key to losing weight and keeping it off is to figure out what drives you to overeat in the first place, says Dr. Murray. Cognitive therapy, or talk therapy, can help. "Many people want to be thin but don't believe that they can be. A therapist can help people realize that they have the power to achieve their weight-loss goals," he notes.

Visits to a health professional trained in cognitive therapy can also help you to mentally adjust to your new body once you've achieved your weight-loss goal. "When some women start to lose weight, it changes how they see themselves, and they're not prepared to deal with it." If you don't address these emotional and psychological issues, the weight will most likely return, he says. (For information on how to locate a cognitive therapist in your area, see page 81.)

PELVIC PROBLEMS
Nature's Solutions for Pesky Pain
and Devilish Discomforts

Before Victoria Homeier learned to use visualization to ease the pain, endometriosis left her down and out one week out of every four.

"The pain during my menstrual periods was debilitating," recalls Homeier, a 30-year-old undergraduate student at the University of Colorado in Greeley, who was diagnosed with endometriosis at age 18. "My doctor prescribed painkillers, but the drugs made me so drowsy that I'd end up sleeping through the week."

A condition in which pieces of the endometrium (the lining of the uterus) grows outside of the uterus, endometriosis is a fairly common problem. And a puzzling one. No one knows exactly why endometrial tissue shows up where it shouldn't. Some women have tissue attached to their ovaries, intestines and even their lungs. Though displaced, the endometrial tissue bleeds when a woman has her period, just as the lining of her uterus does. The bleeding can cause cysts and scarring that can lead to chronic pain or infertility. In extreme cases, doctors may recommend surgery to remove the stray tissue or a hysterectomy to remove the uterus.

"I didn't want to consider surgery until I'd tried everything else," says Homeier. "So when we learned about visualization in one of my classes, I decided to try it and see whether it could help. And it did."

To deal with endometrial pain, Victoria set aside 20 minutes a day for visualization. "I'd visualize the inside of my pelvic wall, imagining the endometrium tissues attached there getting smaller and smaller until they disappeared," she explains. "What a relief it is to no longer have debilitating pain."

Certain alternative therapies, like visualization, food therapy, herbal medicine, and vitamin and mineral therapy can help treat a range of gynecological problems, from endometriosis to vaginal itching, among others, says Tori Hudson, doctor of naturopathy, professor of gynecology at

National College of Naturopathic Medicine and director of A Woman's Time clinic, all in Portland, Oregon.

"Natural remedies are, by and large, nontoxic and safe, so you don't have to worry about the side effects that you might get with drugs or the complications associated with surgery," says Dr. Hudson.

Here's a problem-by-problem guide to common gynecological problems and their recommended natural therapies, followed by across-the-board strategies that can also help.

CERVICAL CHANGES: KEEP TROUBLE IN CHECK

No one likes getting a Pap test. No matter how high you register on the aplomb scale, it's hard to feel comfy lying on an exam table, waiting patiently while a doctor uses a tiny spatula to scrape cells from your cervix. But a Pap test is something that you shouldn't forgo. An annual test can save you from cervical cancer. A Pap test tells your doctor whether your cervical cells are normal or whether they are developing abnormalities that could lead to cancer. Given early warning, your physician can treat precancerous abnormalities before they become cancerous or treat early cancer before it spreads.

Since cervical changes usually come with no symptoms attached, the Pap test is absolutely essential, says Chris Meletis, doctor of naturopathy and clinic director, chief medical officer and medicinary director at the National College of Naturopathic Medicine in Portland, Oregon.

What causes cervical abnormalities? Research points the finger at the sexually transmitted human papillomavirus (HPV). Not everyone who has HPV, however, develops cervical abnormalities. A strong immune system, it seems, can help protect you from abnormalities even if you have HPV, says Dr. Hudson.

If you've been diagnosed with cervical abnormalities (cervical dysplasia), you should be under a doctor's care, says Dr. Hudson. If abnormalities are cancerous, you'll need surgery. If things haven't progressed that far, a variety of alternative treatments can help reverse abnormalities.

Fortify with folic acid. The supplemental form of the B vitamin folate, folic acid can help prevent and, in high doses, help reverse cervical abnormalities, research suggests. Population studies find that women who get little of this vitamin run a higher risk of developing cervical changes. To help fend them off, Dr. Hudson recommends 2,500 micrograms of folic acid daily for women who are at higher risks, such as smokers, women on birth control pills and women with changing sex partners. (Amounts higher than 400 micrograms can mask signs of B_{12} deficiency, so higher doses should be used with a doctor's guidance.) It is best to take folic acid with other B vitamins as found in a multivitamin/mineral or B-complex supplement, he advises.

If your doctor has determined that you have cervical abnormalities, ask her if a prescription-level dose of folic acid can help restore your cells to normal.

Add antioxidants. Vitamins such as beta-carotene and vitamins C and E, along with the mineral selenium, protect healthy cells from damage by free radicals—byproducts of oxidation that occurs in the normal course of living and breathing, in all tissues. Your body needs antioxidants to build healthy cervical tissue and keep your immune system going strong, says Dr. Meletis. In a preliminary study conducted at the University of California in Irvine, women with cervical dysplasia took 30-milligram (50,000 international units, or IU) supplements of beta-carotene daily for 19 months. When checked 6 months later, 21 of the 30 women were free of abnormalities.

To prevent and reverse cervical changes, Dr. Meletis recommends a good diet that includes dark leafy greens, 800 micrograms of folic acid, 25,000 IU of beta-carotene and 400 IU of vitamin E every day. He also recommends 500 milligrams of vitamin C two to three times daily and up to 100 micrograms of selenium. (If high doses of vitamin C give you diarrhea, cut back.)

See a naturopath. To treat cervical dysplasia, a naturopath might take a multi-pronged approach: She may prescribe supplements of immunity-boosting vitamins, plus antiviral herbs (such as echinacea), and paint your cervix with a solution made from natural ingredients like zinc chloride, among others, that encourage your body to shed abnormal cells, explains Kareen O'Brien, a naturopathic physician and academic dean at Southwest College of Naturopathic Medicine and Health Sciences in Scottsdale, Arizona.

ENDOMETRIOSIS AND UTERINE FIBROIDS: VITAMINS AND IMAGERY HELP

If your menstrual periods have progressed from minor annoyances to disabling episodes of heavy bleeding, cramps and pain, you probably don't need a book to tell you to seek medical help. But diagnosing the problem can be tricky, even for doctors.

For many women, the cause of severe pelvic pain turns out to be either endometriosis or uterine fibroids, sinewy growths that develop in the uterus.

Fibroids can compress the endometrial lining, causing excessive bleeding during and between periods. If uterine fibroids grow in such a way that they block the ureters, the tubes draining the kidneys, they can trigger kidney problems. Fibroids are noncancerous growths.

Like endometriosis, uterine fibroids are puzzling. No one knows exactly what causes them. It's clear, though, that excessive estrogen levels makes fibroids worse.

Some women have such severe uterine fibroids or endometriosis that surgery (to remove either the problem tissue or the entire uterus) is the

How I Healed Myself **Naturally**

Vegetarian Diet Shrinks Her Fibroids

Suffering from heavy menstrual bleeding, cramps and pain, Marie Jackson, a 41-year-old mother of two from Belle Mead, New Jersey, went to three doctors before she found one who gave her an accurate diagnosis and an option other than drugs or a hysterectomy.

"When I was 39 years old, I started bleeding heavily during and between my periods," says Jackson. "I had terrible pain and cramping. I went to a gynecologist who did a D and C (a dilation and curettage). In this procedure, the doctor scrapes away the uterine lining. It's supposed to cure the problem.

"Shortly after the D and C, I started bleeding again," says Jackson. "My doctors suggested a hysterectomy, but I didn't want that. So they put me on birth control pills, but I didn't like taking hormones, so I stopped after a month.

"Finally, I went to see a physician, an M.D. who advocated therapeutic fasting. An ultrasound test showed that I had a uterine fibroid that was causing the bleeding. He suggested that I fast, but I didn't want to just then, so I went to another gynecologist. He also suggested a hysterectomy. I still didn't want surgery, so he prescribed medication. When I took it, I started to develop severe headaches, so I went back to the doctor who recommended fasting.

"I decided to follow his advice and go on a complete vegetarian diet—no meat, dairy or eggs—for three months followed by a ten-day fast, supervised by the doctor," says Jackson. "Then I resumed the vegetarian diet.

"Things have improved greatly," says Jackson. "Another ultrasound showed that the fibroid has shrunk by 50 percent. I have no more bleeding, cramping or pain. The diet has really been remarkable." (To read more about the therapeutic use of fasting, see page 122.)

only effective option, says Dr. O'Brien. In less severe cases, doctors may prescribe hormones that mimic menopause and limit estrogen production, shrinking fibroids or endometrial fragments. Or doctors may prescribe oral contraceptives, which can control the bleeding from endometriosis. The catch is, birth control pills can deplete a woman's folate stores, increasing her risk of cervical dysplasia, says Dr. O'Brien.

If endometriosis or fibroids are mild enough, natural remedies for pelvic pain due to endometriosis or uterine fibroids may get equally good results, Dr. O'Brien says.

Bring on the bioflavonoids. Found in citrus fruits, garlic, onions and all vegetables, bioflavonoids are plant compounds related to vitamin C. Among other benefits, bioflavonoids seem to reduce excessive bleeding by strengthening capillary walls. They may also help lower excessively high estrogen levels. Dr. Hudson recommends supplements of 1,000 milligrams of bioflavonoids daily. They're available at health food stores.

Bolster your Bs. B vitamins help your liver rid your body of excess estrogen, notes Susan Lark, M.D., author of *The Estrogen Decision Self-Help Book*. She recommends 50 to 100 milligrams of vitamin B-complex daily and up to 300 milligrams of vitamin B_6 for women using birth control pills.

Caution: When taken over a long period of time, amounts of more than 50 milligrams of vitamin B_6 can cause unstable gait and numb feet. So don't take more without the consent of your physician.

Visualize a healthy uterus. Visualization exercises can help you manage the symptoms of endometriosis and fibroids, says Dr. Hudson. Visualize your uterus intact, free of maverick tissue and disruptive growths. You should practice this 10 to 30 minutes a day, three to five times a week.

Consult a naturopath. Naturopathic physicians may prescribe other herbs and supplements that help the liver clear excess estrogen from the body. They may also prescribe natural progesterone, a laboratory-modified herbal extract that relieves pain and reduces bleeding, says Dr. O'Brien.

Since progesterone modified in this way is essentially a drug, the only way to utilize it is via a naturopath.

INFERTILITY: THINK YOURSELF PREGNANT

When Boston's Deaconess Hospital introduced a program to help women deal with the stress of infertility, the results were both predictable and surprising. As expected, nearly all of the women who practiced stress-reduction techniques such as yoga, meditation and breath work felt less stressed-out after finishing the program. Surprisingly, almost 40 percent of them were pregnant six months later.

The high pregnancy rate among program graduates isn't proof that stress causes infertility. But it strongly suggests that stress contributes to the problem and that stress relief can help solve it, says Alice Domar, Ph.D., psychologist, program founder and author of *Healing Mind, Healthy Woman*.

Aside from stress, an array of physical problems can impair fertility. As mentioned, severe endometriosis and uterine fibroids can also contribute to infertility in women, as can aging. Fertility drops slightly between the ages of 25 and 35, then drops sharply after age 35, followed by an even more dramatic fall after age 40.

Among women, the most common causes of infertility are chlamydia and gonorrhea, which can scar the fallopian tubes, explains Adriane Fugh-Berman, M.D., former head of field investigations for the Office of Alternative Medicine at the National Institutes of Health in Bethesda, Maryland.

If you're having a hard time getting pregnant, you and your partner should see a doctor who can help you get to the heart of the matter. Some problems, like blocked fallopian tubes, require surgery. But depending on the cause, fertility can be restored with simpler measures. Here's what you can do to boost your odds of getting pregnant.

Use "reverse" birth control. Sometimes, infertility is no more than a matter of bad timing, says Joseph B. Stanford, M.D., assistant professor at the University of Utah School of Medicine in Salt Lake City. Studies find that nearly all pregnancies can result from intercourse during the time that starts five days before ovulation and ends with the day that you ovulate. If you don't have intercourse during your fertile period, you won't get pregnant.

To figure out exactly when you're fertile—and when to have intercourse—Dr. Stanford says, "Use Natural Family Planning." (For information on how to use Natural Family Planning, see page 466.)

Slip your man some supplements. Supplemental doses of vitamins E and C, selenium and folic acid can improve sperm quality and improve the odds of conception, says Dr. Fugh-Berman. She recommends 150 micrograms of selenium, 500 milligrams of vitamin C, 400 IU of vitamin E and 800 micrograms of folic acid daily. Talk to your doctor before taking more than 100 micrograms of selenium, and keep in mind that amounts higher than 400 micrograms of folic acid can mask signs of B_{12} deficiency.

Cut out caffeine. High doses of caffeine can lead to delayed pregnancy, says Dr. Meletis. A study that followed 1,400 women found that among those who downed more than 300 milligrams of caffeine daily and had unprotected intercourse, most took more than a year to get pregnant—considerably longer than those who curtailed caffeine. For the record, 300 milligrams is about what you'd get in three cups of coffee.

Say, "I can be a mother." In addition to yoga, meditation and breath work, the stress-reduction program at Deaconess Hospital teaches women cognitive therapy techniques. The basic premise behind cognitive therapy is that you can enjoy better mental and physical health if you scuttle irrational and negative beliefs.

Natural Birth Control
An Alternative to the Pill

If you're not ready to have a baby and prefer not to take oral contraceptives, Natural Family Planning is an attractive alternative. It's natural, it's side effect–free and it's as effective as the Pill in preventing unwanted pregnancy. And used in reverse, Natural Family Planning can help you get pregnant.

"If you learn Natural Family Planning from a qualified instructor and use it exactly as you're supposed to, it works as well as the Pill," says Joseph B. Stanford, M.D., assistant professor at the University of Utah School of Medicine in Salt Lake City. Studies find that among couples who consistently and correctly use Natural Family Planning, a mere 1 percent conceive during a year of use (about the same failure rate as couples who rely on the Pill). Here's how it works.

Know your mucus. Watch for changes in your cervical mucus, the discharge from your vagina, to determine when you're fertile. As you get closer to ovulation—the stage in your menstrual cycle when your ovaries release an egg—mucus secretion increases. At this stage, the mucus is usually the consistency of egg whites, is easy for sperm to swim through and actually contains nutrients that sustain them. Flow of this egg-whitish mucus peaks on the day before you ovulate. Once you've ovulated, however, the mucus changes, getting thick and rubbery and inhospitable to sperm.

Plan for sex (or avoid it). Once you know when you're fertile, use that information to either achieve conception or avoid it. To prevent conception, avoid intercourse from the day that you first see the appearance of a mucous discharge to the seventh day after flow peaks.

Women with fertility problems are often bogged down with negative thinking, repeatedly telling themselves things like, "I'll never be a mother," Dr. Domar notes. You can use the following cognitive therapy technique to disabuse yourself of such notions, she says. The next time you tell yourself that you can't have a baby, ask yourself, "Did the doctor say that I couldn't have a biological child?" The answer is probably no. In light of that, ask yourself, "Is my belief logical?" Again, the answer should be no. By repeating the exercise, you should be able to snap yourself out of illogical, negative thinking.

That's your fertile time, explains Dr. Stanford. Conversely, if you're trying to conceive, this is the optimum time to have intercourse.

Don't confuse Natural Family Planning with the highly unreliable rhythm method. Like the rhythm method, Natural Family Planning requires you to abstain from sex during your fertile period. But the similarities end there, says Dr. Stanford.

Practicing "rhythm" also involves avoiding sex midway through your cycle, when you ovulate. The problem is, the rhythm method relies on the calendar, not on changes in your body, to signal when you're ovulating. Rhythm assumes that every woman has a 28-day menstrual cycle and will be fertile—and should avoid unprotected sex—roughly 14 days after her menstrual period ends. Not so, says Dr. Stanford. Women's cycles usually range from 25 to 35 days but sometimes can be even longer or shorter. So, as a form of birth control, the rhythm method is unreliable.

Take lessons. Because recognizing changes in mucus flow demands a certain degree of expertise, you should learn Natural Family Planning from qualified instructors, says Dr. Stanford. Each group teaches a slight variation on the method for charting mucus flow, but the technique is essentially the same. Contact the American Academy of Natural Family Planning, 615 South New Ballas Road, St. Louis, MO 63141; Natural Family Planning Center, P.O. Box 30239, Bethesda, MD 20824-0239; Couple to Couple League, P.O. Box 111184, Cincinnati, OH 45211; or Northwest Family Services, 4805 Glisan NE Street, Portland, OR 97213.

VAGINAL DRYNESS: EASING PAINFUL INTERCOURSE

Sex should feel wonderful. But it can feel downright painful if your vagina loses its natural ability to self-lubricate and ease intercourse.

More often than not, dryness is the result of hormonal change or nutritional deficiency, says Dr. Meletis. Certain drugs or menopause can cause hormonal changes that contribute to dryness. When you stop menstruating, your ovaries produce less estrogen, the hormone that helps keep vaginal tissues moist, thick and flexible, says Dr. Meletis.

If your doctor has ruled out thyroid problems or other medical causes, these remedies can restore vaginal moisture.

Rebuild with supplements. To maintain delicate vaginal tissue, your body needs a variety of vitamins and minerals. To make sure that you have enough of the essentials, Dr. Meletis suggests that you take 400 IU of vitamin E, 25,000 IU of beta-carotene, 15 milligrams of zinc and 800 micrograms of folic acid daily. (If you take more than 400 micrograms of folic acid, your doctor needs to monitor your vitamin B_{12} levels.)

Take a tablespoon of flaxseed oil. If your vagina is parched, you may be deficient in essential fatty acids, oils found in plants and fish that are essential to the health of vaginal tissues, says Dr. Meletis. The remedy? Swallow a tablespoon of fatty acid-rich flaxseed oil daily. You can find the oil in the refrigerated section of health food stores.

Use a lubricant. Over-the-counter lubricants like K-Y Jelly, Replens or Astroglide work well if you're dry. (You can buy vaginal lubricants at any drugstore.)

Or try a small dollop of olive oil, applied to your vagina, says Dr. O'Brien. But don't use the olive oil if you're also using a condom, since any oil will damage the latex, she says. (For practical solutions for vaginal dryness associated with menopause, see page 436.)

VAGINAL ITCHING: A SIGN OF INFECTION

Few things are as maddening as vaginal itching or pain. Often, it's the result of an infection or an allergic reaction, says Dr. O'Brien.

If you see a doctor, she may diagnose the problem as vaginitis, a catchall term for any inflammation of the vagina, whether it's caused by an allergy or an infection.

Vaginal infections are very common. And the most common vaginal infections of all are trichomoniasis, yeast infections and bacterial vaginosis. Chlamydia, herpes and gonorrhea infections are also relatively widespread.

The trick to relieving vaginal problems is knowing what you have. Many vaginal infections have similar symptoms but varying causes and consequences, explains Dr. O'Brien.

Trichomoniasis is caused by a parasite and is usually sexually transmitted. Telltale symptoms of "trich" infections include itching, burning and soreness and a yellow-gray, foamy, foul-smelling vaginal discharge. Some women, though, don't have any symptoms.

Yeast infections, on the other hand, are almost always itchy and are often accompanied by a cottage-cheesy discharge. Bacterial vaginosis can cause itching or burning, unpleasant odor and white or gray vaginal discharge. Both yeast infections and bacterial vaginosis are often caused by overgrowths of organisms native to your vagina, explains Dr. Meletis. With yeast infections, the culprit is usually an organism called *Candida albicans*. With bacterial vaginosis, the culprits may be Gardnerella, Bacteroides or Peptostreptococcus bacteria.

Normally, yeast, Gardnerella and the like are kept in check by other beneficial organisms found in your vagina. But douches, birth control pills, hormonal changes during pregnancy and antibiotics can kill off helpful bacteria and lead to an overgrowth of yeast, Gardnerella, Bacteroides or Peptostreptococcus.

Since yeast, Gardnerella and these other irritating organisms thrive in a moist environment, wearing stockings or nylon underwear that don't allow vaginal moisture to evaporate can also lead to increased chance of infection, says Dr. Meletis.

Bacterial vaginosis may increase your risk of complications during pregnancy, including premature birth. If the infection spreads through your cervix, uterus and fallopian tubes to your pelvic cavity, it can lead to painful pelvic inflammatory disease.

Other sexually transmitted infections—such as HIV, herpes, syphilis, gonorrhea, chlamydia and human papillomavirus—can cause other complications, says Dr. O'Brien.

Syphilis, a bacterial infection that causes a painless vaginal or vulvar sore, later a rash and still later involvement of almost any organ, can be fatal if untreated. Gonorrhea, which may cause vaginal discharge and, in rare cases, pain during urination or cause no symptoms at all, can lead to pelvic inflammatory disease. Chlamydia, which is usually symptom-free, can also lead to PID. Human papillomavirus is also virtually symptom-free but may lead to cervical changes that can progress to cancer if untreated. Herpes announces itself with painful vaginal blisters. Many of these sexually transmitted diseases make it easier for HIV infection to occur.

CHECK IT OUT

You should see your doctor for a diagnosis if you have vaginal burning, pain or discharge, says Dr. Fugh-Berman. And every sexually active woman should have tests for gonorrhea and chlamydia during an annual gynecological exam. You'll need antibiotics for bacterial vaginosis, chlamydia, gonorrhea or syphilis, she says. For yeast infections, your doctor may recommend an anti-yeast cream like Monistat or Gyne-Lotrimin.

Alternative approaches can help prevent or soothe less serious infections, like yeast infections. Here's what works.

Cover up. Protect yourself from sexually transmitted infections by using condoms, says Dr. Fugh-Berman. If you're sexually active, using condoms, spermicides, diaphrams, cervical caps and female condoms can protect against some sexually transmitted diseases, but male latex condoms are the best, she says.

Shield yourself with zinc and C. If you're prone to vaginal infections, Dr. Meletis suggests 15-milligram doses of zinc daily. "Zinc makes membranes more resistant to infection," he says. Add 500 milligrams of vitamin C two to three times daily to shore up your immune system, Dr. Meletis suggests. (If you get diarrhea from high doses of vitamin C, take less.)

Meet some nice bacteria. Among the organisms that normally inhabit your vagina are lactobacillus acidophilus, good-guy bacteria that help keep potentially irritating types like yeast in check. To reinforce your lactobacillus troops—and prevent or recover faster from yeast infections—eat eight ounces of lactobacillus-fortified yogurt daily, says Dr. Meletis. (Check the label to make sure that the yogurt contains live lactobacillus.)

If you don't like yogurt or are in the throes of a stubborn yeast infection, a naturopath can write you a prescription for a concentrated dose of lactobacillus in vaginal suppository form, adds Dr. O'Brien. (So can an M.D. or osteopath.)

Or you can tap the powder out of a lactobacillus capsule, mix it into a paste with water and put it into your vagina, says Dr. Fugh-Berman.

Adjust amino acids, help herpes. People with herpes tend to have too little of the amino acid L-lysine and too much of the amino acid arginine in their bodies, says Dr. Hudson. This imbalance can trigger blister outbreaks. By correcting the imbalance, you can help keep outbreaks under control, she says.

To do that, avoid high-arginine foods like nuts and chocolate. And take 2,000 milligrams of the amino acid L-lysine daily during an acute outbreak, says Dr. O'Brien. You can find the amino acid in most health food stores.

Allow breathing room. You can lower the odds that you'll get repeat yeast infections if you wear cotton underpants and pantyhose with cotton crotches, says Dr. Meletis. That's because yeast like moisture. And cotton, unlike nylon, lets excess moisture evaporate.

Ban all chemicals. Steering clear of scented tampons, sanitary napkins, toilet paper, douches and vaginal deodorants will help you steer clear of vaginal itching and pain due to chemical irritation, says Dr. Meletis.

WHOLE-BODY STRATEGIES FOR GYNECOLOGICAL HEALTH

Here's a rundown on other important approaches that can help prevent and treat more than one gynecological problem.

Adopt a low-fat, high-fiber diet. A diet sparse in meat and fat, devoid of all dairy products and abundant in complex carbohydrates such as vegetables and fruit may help ease endometriosis and symptoms of uterine fibroids. Why? A high-fat diet prompts your body to produce an excess of the female hormone estrogen. And high estrogen levels exacerbate conditions like uterine fibroids.

Since meat is relatively high in fat, some women find that symptoms of both conditions improve when they switch to mostly vegetarian diets, says Christiane Northrup, M.D., in her book *Women's Bodies, Women's Wisdom*. Dr. Northrup is a practitioner of obstetrics and gynecology in Yarmouth, Maine, and assistant clinical professor of obstetrics and gynecology at the University of Vermont College of Medicine in Burlington.

Eat your share of fruits and vegetables. Filling up on brightly colored fruits and vegetables, instead of fat, is a good bet because bright yellow, red and green produce is rich in vitamin C and beta-carotene, nutrients that fortify your immune system and help you fight off infections, including vaginal infections, says Dr. O'Brien. Research suggests that adequate levels of folate (400 micrograms), a B vitamin abundant in leafy greens, may help prevent the human papillomavirus from causing cervical dysplasia.

Sweat it out three times a week. Exercise benefits reproductive health indirectly: Exercise boosts immunity by raising levels of natural killer cells and T cells that kill viruses, fungi and bacteria. And it increases the activity of immunoglobulins, key factors in the defense against invaders, so that you're better able to resist and fight infections.

Regular exercise also helps you burn calories and control your weight, which is important because research finds that both overweight and underweight women have a harder time conceiving than normal-weight women do.

Dr. O'Brien recommends an hour of aerobic exercise, such as running, walking, swimming and the like, three times a week. If you're running marathons, however, cutting back on exercise may help you conceive. Intense exercise can lead to an absence of menstrual periods, a sign that exercise has interfered with ovulation.

Reserve 15 minutes for stress reduction. Feeling overwhelmed? If so, your gynecological health can suffer. Studies indicate that stress may stimulate hormones that suppress the function of immune cells, leaving you more vulnerable to infections. Stress can also contribute to vaginal dryness, making intercourse painful. "If you're stressed-out, your body isn't going to lubricate easily," says Dr. O'Brien. And research suggests that stress contributes to infertility, too.

For good gynecological health all around, Dr. O'Brien recommends 15 minutes of stress management daily. Yoga, visualization, breath work, exercise, meditation and music therapy are all good choices, she says. "Do something that you enjoy. No one method is right for everyone."

Quit smoking. Snuffing the cigs may also help you conceive. Research finds that women who smoke have higher levels of nicotine, which is toxic to sperm, in the mucus lining their cervixes. Quitting may also lower your risk of developing precancerous and cancerous cervical changes, and it can help reverse those changes if they've already occurred, says Dr. Meletis.

Bid farewell to booze. Alcohol may contribute to endometriosis and uterine fibroids by putting undue strain on your liver, the organ responsible for clearing alcohol from your system, says Dr. O'Brien. Your liver is also responsible for ridding your body of excess hormones like estrogen. So if your liver is expending a lot of effort detoxifying the alcohol, Dr. O'Brien explains, it isn't as efficient at clearing out the excess estrogen. Since excess estrogen contributes to endometriosis and uterine fibroids, drinking can make both problems worse, she says.

Drinking can also make conceiving tougher. Studies show that women who drink have more difficulty conceiving than teetotalers do, says Jacob Teitelbaum, M.D., clinician and researcher on the treatment of chronic fatigue syndrome at Anne Arundel Medical Center in Annapolis, Maryland, and author of *From Fatigued to Fantastic!* (Drinking affects men's fertility, too.)

PREGNANCY PROBLEMS
Comfort Strategies for Moms-to-Be

Trembling with anticipation, you head to the drugstore and buy an at-home pregnancy test. You race home. You read the instructions. You follow them to the letter. You wait the appointed time. You watch, hardly daring to breathe. And, finally, there it is before your eyes, the irrefutable proof that you are, indeed, pregnant. At long last, your body's wondrous design meets its greatest challenge.

As soon as that test turns color, your mind starts to wonder, wander and churn. And, if you're like most women, more than a few worries are likely to mingle with the wonderment and joy.

What changes will the next few months bring? What kind of prenatal care will you opt for? What will childbirth be like? How much will it hurt? What if something goes wrong? And, of course, will your baby be healthy?

Perhaps you've heard that high-tech medicine (ultrasonic fetal monitoring, for example) is great for high-risk pregnancies. But what about your pregnancy? Do you want the high-tech procedures for insurance, or do you want to trust the birth methods that were used long before the word sonic ever entered the human vocabulary?

Some advocates of natural childbirth are just plain opposed to the high-tech route. "I've been delivering babies in the mountains of western North Carolina for 21 years, and I worry about some of these high-tech birthing procedures," says Lisa Goldstein, R.N., a midwife practicing in Burnsville, North Carolina. "In some hospitals, for example, you're hooked up to a fetal monitor from the minute that you arrive in labor. You can't move around naturally. The beeping of the monitor is distracting and scares some women. Fear then causes adrenaline to surge through your system. This lessens the blood supply to the baby, slows labor and amplifies the perception of pain, which then increases fear. It's a cycle."

Beyond Midwifery

So, you're pregnant.

If your goal is a comfortable, uncomplicated delivery, go out and get yourself a doula. A what?

A doula (from the Greek word meaning "woman who helps other women") provides continuous physical, emotional and informational support to mothers before, during and after childbirth.

Unlike a doctor, nurse or midwife (medically trained to assist in childbirth), a doula makes no medical decisions or interventions during labor or delivery. What she does do, however, is facilitate your birthing plans, explain medical procedures to you as they happen, stroke, massage and tend to you and in general see to it that you and your partner have the most comfortable possible labor and delivery. A doula's main role is to provide continuous emotional support, comfort, reassurance and praise to the woman during labor and to support both parents, according to authors Phyllis and Marshall Klaus, M.D., and John H. Kennell, M.D., in their book *Mothering the Mother*.

"Women attended by midwives or doulas during childbirth are calmer because they feel safer," says Lisa Goldstein, R.N., a midwife practicing in Burnsville, North Carolina. "That calmness produces endorphins and other brain chemicals that help reduce pain and help labor progress."

According to researchers at Jefferson Davis Hospital in Houston, women who have doulas to help them are 55 percent less likely to have a cesarean delivery and 40 percent less likely to have their baby delivered by forceps, the tool that doctors sometimes use to coax babies down the birth canal. They spend significantly fewer hours in labor, and the labor can be less painful, which lessens the need for pain medication.

And the benefits of a doula don't necessarily end in the delivery room. Some doulas will accompany you home after childbirth to help with the baby, the housework and your older children. In fact, some doulas work only postpartum, helping you at home but not during labor.

If you would like to locate a doula in your area, contact Doulas of North America (DONA), 1100 East Twenty-third Avenue, Seattle, WA 98112.

BUILDING BLOCKS OF A NATURAL PREGNANCY

Rest assured, though. If you're pregnant, high-tech delivery isn't your only option. Many alternative health practitioners offer more natural approaches to childbirth—safe, time-tested ways to help keep you comfortable and healthy. The process begins with competent prenatal care, sees you right through the birth and continues after your baby is born, explains Goldstein.

To relax and help condition your body and mind for delivery, you can choose from yoga, the Alexander Technique, exercise, visualization and meditation.

 ## What Naturopathy Has to Offer a Mom-to-Be

Because naturopathic medicine draws on the medical wisdom of ancient cultures, it's been called the oldest medicine known to humankind. Yet a naturopath's medical education is similar to that of a conventional medical doctor's, and today's naturopaths blend the healing arts of the past with modern medical science.

During your pregnancy, a naturopath would work with you to optimize the way that your body functions.

"Naturopathic prenatal care starts, ideally, even before a woman becomes pregnant," says Lisa Alschuler, naturopathic physician and chairwoman of the Department of Botanical Medicine at Bastyr University of Naturopathic Medicine in Seattle.

Beyond the basic advice to avoid alcohol, cigarettes and refined sugar, a naturopath may recommend a detoxification program including herbs and nutrients to increase liver and gastrointestinal functioning before you conceive, says Dr. Alschuler. And as delivery time approaches, a naturopath may also prescribe certain herbal tonics depending upon your individual needs. "Exactly when and which herbs are used varies from woman to woman," she notes.

Some naturopaths are also midwives who'll take care of you from your first prenatal visit through delivery. In most states, however, a naturopath needs special midwifery training and a license in order to deliver babies.

 ## Traditional Chinese Medicine: East Meets Mom

"There's no reason to choose between your obstetrician and practitioner of Traditional Chinese Medicine (TCM)—they complement each other,"

says Harriet Beinfield, licensed acupuncturist and co-author of *Between Heaven and Earth: A Guide to Chinese Medicine.*

"Each system has its advantages. For example, the morning sickness that can accompany pregnancy can be easily treated with Traditional Chinese Medicine instead of drugs, which can potentially damage the fetus. Acupressure, for example, has no side effects," says Christina Stemmler, M.D., a Houston physician who integrates TCM and acupuncture with Western medicine and who previously headed the American Academy of Medical Acupuncture.

Traditional Chinese Medicine can also help women who have certain types of infertility not caused by anatomical problems, says Dr. Stemmler. And she notes that "there are some women for whom acupuncture helped induce labor and provided pain relief with no need for a local or general anesthetic and no adverse affects on the fetus."

Diet for a Healthy Baby

Once you're pregnant, eating for two doesn't mean eating twice as much food—it means eating foods that are twice as healthy, says Andrew Weil, M.D., professor of herbalism, director of the Program of Integrative Medicine at the University of Arizona College of Medicine, near Tucson, and author of *Spontaneous Healing.*

Bag the junk food and go organic. Moms-to-be should eat a diet that includes a wide variety of organically grown vegetables, grains and cereals, according to Dr. Alschuler. Like many naturopaths, she says that pregnant women need to avoid the pesticides, preservatives and chemicals in processed, nonorganic foods.

Add a little fish to your diet. Essential fatty acids, also known as omega-3 fatty acids, are food substances essential for the normal growth and development of your baby. Omega-3's also improve the health of the placenta, which carries the nutrients that nourish a child in the womb. Studies show that these fatty acids are largely responsible for the health of your baby's nervous system and for her eyesight.

Fish and flaxseed, among other foods, are rich in omega-3 fatty acids. If you're planning to become pregnant, now's the time to start supplementing your diet with them. An adequate intake before conception sets the stage during pregnancy for the way that your body transfers fatty acids to your developing baby.

"To make sure that you get an adequate amount of omega-3 fatty acids, eat a four-ounce serving of salmon or sardines three times a week, or take a tablespoon of ground flaxseed daily," says Dr. Weil. Other good sources are nuts, seeds and whole grains.

VITAL VITAMINS FOR BABY'S HEALTH

Conventional doctors and alternative healers alike seem to unanimously agree that taking vitamins before and during your pregnancy is critical. Here are some guidelines.

Go the prescription route. If you're pregnant, it's better to take special prenatal vitamins prescribed by your doctor or midwife than to rely on over-the-counter vitamins, says Joyce Frye, D.O., an obstetrician/gynecologist and chairperson of the gynecology department at Presbyterian Medical Center and a clinical faculty member at Jefferson Medical College, both in Philadelphia.

This will ensure that you get protective amounts of folic acid, an essential B vitamin that helps prevent neural tube defects—severe problems that can affect the baby's spinal column and brain development.

Medical experts and alternative healers recommend that pregnant women get at least 400 micrograms of folic acid to prevent neural tube defects. If the woman has a family history of neural tube defects, her doctor may advise significantly larger amounts. Standard over-the-counter vitamins usually supply no more than 8 micrograms of folic acid, as compared with prescription prenatal vitamins, which contain one milligram of folic acid. One milligram, Dr. Frye says, is the appropriate amount for pregnant women as well as for women who are planning a pregnancy.

Vitamins prescribed by your doctor or midwife also contain other vitamins and minerals, including calcium, which is necessary for both mother and baby. In the prescription dose, you'll get more of the calcium and other minerals in the proportions that you need, says Dr. Frye. Ask your doctor if you might need additional calcium and other supplements, she adds.

Protect your pearly whites. "If your water isn't fluoridated, take a fluoride supplement during the last three months of pregnancy and continue taking it as long you're breastfeeding," advises Dr. Weil.

Dr. Fugh-Berman goes one step further, advising pregnant women to take fluoride right from the start. Fluoride helps prevent tooth decay. Since breast milk is low in fluoride, the American Academy of Pediatrics recommends that nursing moms take a daily 0.25-milligram fluoride supplement.

Exercise: It's Only Natural . . .

"One of the best gifts that you can give yourself during your pregnancy is the gift of fitness," says Lisa Stone, American Council on Exercise certified prenatal and postnatal fitness instructor and founder of Fit for 2, a prenatal and postnatal fitness program in Atlanta.

One study shows that women who continue to exercise during pregnancy are better able to control excessive weight gain during pregnancy. If you haven't been exercising regularly before your pregnancy, check with your doctor before you begin, recommends Stone. Ask your doctor about joining a prenatal exercise class. She's likely to be familiar with good ones in your area.

But whether or not you take a class, here are some guidelines to follow once you have your doctor's okay.

How I Healed Myself **Naturally**

Natural Tactics for a Heavenly Pregnancy and an Angelic Baby

Karen Wingenroth turned to massage, chiropractic care and exercise to "train" for childbirth and ease delivery. The 36-year-old marketing executive from Ephrata, Pennsylvania, glows when she describes her experience.

"I gave birth to a calm, happy and healthy little angel who slept through the night when she was eight weeks old," says Wingenroth. "I think that prenatal massage, my chiropractor and the running program that I maintained up until a day or two before she was born were key."

Despite her regular running schedule, Wingenroth gained 38 pounds during pregnancy. "I had an amazing recovery, though," she says. "In just four weeks after delivery, I lost all the weight. I think that running contributed to my rapid weight loss. And running gave me the endurance that I needed to get through a long, arduous labor and delivery."

Wingenroth's pregnancy was normal, but began, as do so many pregnancies, with morning sickness that lasted for three months.

"Not only did I have morning sickness, but early in my pregnancy, I had to take several business trips," Wingenroth recalls. "I typically get queasy when I fly, so it was a real double whammy. I was afraid that I'd have to spend most of the flight time in the restroom."

But she didn't. "I got ginger capsules from the health food store and used acupressure on a spot just above my wrist that's said to control nausea and vomiting," Wingenroth reports. Together, ginger and acupressure took enough of an edge off her nausea to make flying bearable. "It wasn't a perfect remedy because I still felt a little queasy, but I'm sure that I felt a lot better than if I'd done nothing at all."

Seeing her chiropractor twice a year had always kept her back on

Take your body and your baby for a walk. If you already exercise, you're ahead of the game. If not, says Dr. Alschuler, consider walking: It's easy and convenient, even when your body gains girth.

Take baby steps. Start your exercise program slowly with a moderately brisk walk of 15 to 20 minutes about every other day, says Adriane Fugh-Berman, M.D., former head of field investigations for the Office of Alternative Medicine at the National Institutes of Health in Bethesda, Maryland. Standard advice says to walk at a rate at which you can carry

the right track, but when she became pregnant, she increased the frequency of her visits. "I got adjustments every month till my eighth month and then weekly adjustments to ease the serious back and neck pain that I started feeling," says Wingenroth. "My doctor would take just five to ten minutes to readjust things, and that made me feel so much better.

"My chiropractor knew how to work with pregnant women. The adjustments he used when I was pregnant were different than what he'd used before, and they alleviated the pain."

In addition to seeing a chiropractor, Wingenroth also put herself in the skilled hands of a massage therapist. "I don't know how I would have lived without massage during my pregnancy," she notes. "At first I had a massage every three weeks or so. Later I saw her every week. My therapist gave me the tender-loving care that my slowly swelling body needed."

Wingenroth's massage therapist used a variation of classic Swedish massage, specially adapted for use during pregnancy. Therapists get specific training and learn which techniques are best for moms-to-be.

"My pregnancy massages were a little gentler than normal ones, and I'd turn on my side rather than my stomach so she could do my back," says Wingenroth. "There was only one area that my therapist said was taboo for massage purposes: my ankles. My therapist said that ankle massage late in pregnancy can induce labor.

"In fact, my therapist told me to call her if I was slow to go into labor. She said that she'd help me along with a brisk ankle massage. Happily, that wasn't necessary," Wingenroth says with a smile.

on a conversation. If you're out of breath, slow down.

Make exercise routine. Consistent exercise is most effective. Aim to walk daily or at least three times a week, says Dr. Fugh-Berman.

Get off your back. After the first three months of pregnancy, avoid exercises that are done while lying on your back, such as sit-ups.

Take water breaks. Drink water before, during and after your workout. That helps to regulate your body temperature and also your baby's.

If you hurt, stop. When you exercise, listen to your body, says Dr. Fugh-Berman. If you feel dizzy, get light-headed or feel any kind of cramp or pain, stop immediately.

MORNING SICKNESS: BANE OF THOSE EARLY MONTHS

Morning sickness, the infamous hallmark of early pregnancy, is experienced by about half of all pregnant women. Happily, it generally disappears by the end of the first trimester.

Morning sickness can be as mild as a faintly nauseated feeling when you wake up or as severe as nausea and vomiting that lead to dehydration and weight loss. Despite its name, morning sickness can occur any time of day.

What causes morning sickness? "When you're pregnant, increased hormonal activity slows down your digestion, and that can cause nausea above and constipation below," says Dr. Fugh-Berman.

Fortunately, natural medicine offers safe remedies for your queasy feelings. Here are some of the best.

 ## Acupressure Eases Morning Sickness

"Acupressure can lessen both the nausea and the vomiting of morning sickness," says Dr. Fugh-Berman. Studies show that pregnant women who applied acupressure to the point just above their wrists for ten minutes, four times a day, significantly reduced their nausea, she adds. (To locate the P6 point, see the diagram in the acupressure chapter on page 14.)

 ## Herbal Medicine: Ancient Medicine for Modern Morning Sickness

Herbal medicine offers safe remedies for morning sickness, according to Susun S. Weed, an herbalist and teacher from Woodstock, New York, and author of the *Wise Woman* herbal series.

But you should use only herbs deemed safe and effective for use during pregnancy. Herbs normally used during cooking are fine, but pregnant women should not consider using more potent medicinal herbs without advice from an expert herbalist, says Dr. Fugh-Berman. The following mild herbs are fine, according to herbalists. (But be sure to examine packages carefully—some ginger tea, for example, may contain licorice root, which can raise blood pressure if consumed daily in large doses.)

Try ginger candy. Crystallized gingerroot candy, available in health food stores, can ease morning sickness, says Rosemary Gladstar, herbalist and author of *Herbal Healing for Women*. Keep it on your nightstand for first-thing-in-the-morning use.

Sip raspberry-leaf tea. Try some raspberry tea as soon as you get out of bed. Weed says that the tea—or sucking on ice cubes made from the tea—helps relieve early-morning digestive distress.

Try some morning mint tea. Peppermint or spearmint infusions, sipped first thing in the morning, are effective against nausea, says Weed. To make an infusion, pour one quart boiling water over one ounce dried mint leaves in a quart glass jar. Cover tightly and allow the mint leaves to steep overnight, or for at least four hours. Refrigerate. If kept refrigerated, the tea will last for up to a week. If you wish, you can strain the leaves out or reheat the tea before drinking it. Many women keep the infusion by their bedside at room temperature and sip it as needed.

Banish Morning Sickness with Homeopathy

"I have had excellent results using homeopathy for morning sickness, even when no other type of remedy has worked," says Goldstein.

Homeopathic remedies are available in different potencies (concentrations), expressed by a number and commonly followed by the letter "c". Goldstein and other homeopaths suggest that beginners start by choosing remedies labeled 6c. Take these every two to eight hours as needed. If the remedy hasn't helped ease discomfort after the third dose, it's probably the wrong remedy. Here are a few of the many effective remedies for morning sickness.

Pulsatilla. If nausea hits later in the day or evening, accompanied by intolerance to heat and perhaps a dry mouth (but not thirst), and you also feel teary or crave sympathy, Goldstein and other homeopaths suggest pulsatilla. This is a homeopathic remedy derived from the windflower, a plant native to Europe.

Ipecac. If nausea and vomiting are constant or persistent and you're salivating excessively, feeling a noticeable lack of thirst, and your tongue feels clean rather than coated, homeopaths recommend a homeopathic version of ipecac, derived from the dried root of a South American plant. Signs of mucus in your vomit also calls for ipecac, says Goldstein.

Practitioners emphasize that in addition to pulsatilla and ipecac, there are several other homeopathic treatments for morning sickness worth trying. Ask your practitioner for additional recommendations, suggests Dr. Alschuler.

PRENATAL ACHES AND PAINS: PAMPER YOUR BODY

As your baby grows, so will your girth, and your posture will change to accommodate your altered center of gravity. Your new swaybacked stance is likely to cause pain in your lower back. In addition, you may feel discomfort in your pelvic area as your hip joints loosen a bit in preparation for birth.

Here are some safe, natural remedies to ease pregnancy-induced aches.

 ### Alexander Technique: Taking a Stand against Pain

The Alexander Technique is a form of movement therapy which stresses improved coordination and enhanced mind-body functioning. According to proponents of this technique, women who learn it early in their pregnancies can avoid backaches, varicose veins and other problems. (For details on learning the Alexander Technique, see page 40.)

 ### Get Thee to a Masseuse

"Massage therapy can ease cramps, lower-back pain, chronic tension and hip pain," says Carole Osborne-Sheets, a licensed massage therapist with expertise in prenatal massage.

"One of the benefits of massage therapy during pregnancy is that it reduces stress and activates the parasympathetic branch of the nervous system, which lowers blood pressure, deepens breathing and facilitates blood flow to internal organs," says Dr. Fugh-Berman.

Many women have back pain during their pregnancies, notes Osborne-Sheets. One-third to one-half of all pregnant women will have back pain in late pregnancy, and of those, one-third will have pain that's debilitating enough to keep them from working or performing everyday chores, she adds.

Massage is also useful for discomfort related to fluid retention throughout the body during pregnancy. "Massage can reduce the swelling and discomfort that some pregnant women experience," says Dr. Fugh-Berman. But certain areas, like the ankles, shouldn't be massaged during pregnancy.

Find a certified massage therapist who has received special training in pregnancy massage, recommends Robert A. Edwards, licensed massage therapist and director of the Somerset School of Massage in Somerset, New Jersey.

BREAST CHANGES: PREPARING FOR BABY

One of the earliest signs of pregnancy is breast tenderness. Because your breasts increase in size early in pregnancy and continue to grow and change throughout your pregnancy in preparation for breastfeeding, feelings of heaviness or discomfort are common.

Your breasts will look different, too: The nipples and surrounding skin may darken and the veins may become more prominent. Toward the end of your pregnancy, your nipples may leak a yellow, watery fluid. This is colostrum, a rich first food that protects your baby against infections.

To minimize breast tenderness that you may encounter during pregnancy, try these tactics.

Shop for a supportive bra. Sports bras provide the extra support that pregnant women need, says Stone. Look for a bra with extra-wide straps. You may even be able to find sports bras with nursing features for use after delivery, she says.

Wear two for comfort. "The women in my exercise classes taught me another trick for easing breast tenderness, especially while you're exercising: Wear two sports bras, one atop the other, for extra support," says Stone.

Warm up a compress. As with breast tenderness associated with premenstrual changes, some women whose breasts grow tender during pregnancy find that warm compresses help, says Dr. Weil. Hold a comfortably hot towel or hot-water bottle against your breasts for 10 to 15 minutes.

SLEEPING PROBLEMS: WHEN YOU JUST CAN'T GET COMFY

When you're pregnant, sleeping isn't what it used to be. Many women find that sleeping is a cinch early in pregnancy: Anytime, any place, you can catch a nap just like that. But when your belly gets bigger and your baby starts moving, you may find that getting a good night's sleep is hard work.

Relaxation techniques, including visualization, breathing exercises and meditation are just a few safe exercises that aid sleep.

Water Births: No More Wailing

Imagine a delivery so calm, so peaceful, that your precious little one arrives blissfully asleep.

Going through labor, even delivery, in water can achieve an unusual level of relaxation for mother and baby, say proponents of water birth.

"Seeing a baby born asleep is an incredible experience, and it takes a while before you realize that a baby born this way isn't in trouble—she's just sound asleep," says Barbara Harper, R.N., author of *Gentle Birth Choices* and president of the Global Maternal/Child Health Association, a nonprofit corporation that promotes water births and midwifery.

In a water birth, the woman sits in a tub of warm water at various stages of labor, including delivery. The baby is born completely submerged and begins breathing when lifted into the mother's arms, seconds later.

In the United States, water birth is catching on slowly but steadily: About 1,000 water births are reported each year and about 60 hospitals and birthing centers have installed special tubs for the purpose. Water birth is more popular in England, where more than 200 hospitals have birthing tubs.

Only a small percentage of women offered water birth choose it as an option. "But so far, the women who choose it are very pleased," says Elizabeth K. Dickson, a certified nurse-midwife and founder and director of the Carolina Birth Center in High Point, North Carolina.

The advantages of laboring in water include complete relaxation for mother and baby and non-narcotic, all-natural pain relief, says Harper. The water also softens the perineum so that it can stretch, minimizing the need for episiotomy. "In a fluid environment, a woman can remain in control of her labor and follow her instincts much better. Women seem to melt into the warmth of the water and actually enter almost an altered state of consciousness," she says.

Water births should be attempted under proper supervision only, not on your own. For more information about water births, contact the Global Maternal/Child Health Association, P.O. Box 1400, Wilsonville, OR 97070.

Breathe yourself to sleep. Deep-breathing exercises are often all that you need to nod off, suggests Jeff Migdow, M.D., a holistic medical doctor, director of yoga teacher-training at the Kripalu Center for Yoga and Health in Lenox, Massachusetts, and co-author of *Take a Deep Breath*. Here's how.

Lie on your back and breathe rhythmically—four counts in, eight counts out. As you breathe, picture a light wind moving in and out of your body and enveloping your entire body. As you become sleepy, you may wish to shift to your favorite sleeping position and continue breathing to the rhythm that you've established.

Wide-awake at 3:00 A.M.? Meditate. "Meditation has definitely been found to be effective in helping pregnant women get a good night's sleep," says Mark Epstein, M.D., psychiatrist in New York City and author of *Thoughts without a Thinker: Psychotherapy from a Buddhist Perspective.*

Meditation can help you get to sleep by letting you focus on, and then release, what's keeping you awake, no matter whether it's emotional or physical discomfort, suggests Dr. Epstein.

And you don't need meditation experience to meditate yourself back to sleep. Just follow Dr. Epstein's suggestions whenever you have insomnia.

Rouse yourself to full awareness, then sit up in a comfortable position and use your breathing (or an object) as a focus point. Fully experience all that's keeping you awake, whether it's disturbing thoughts or discomfort. Focus on your disturbance or discomfort and then release your disturbance or discomfort. Lie back and go to sleep.

RAYNAUD'S SYNDROME
Natural Ways to Warm Up

Mary Kildare (not her real name) lived in Alaska and, like other 26-year-olds, she loved to ski and snowmobile. Then she developed Raynaud's disease, a circulatory problem that periodically triggers spasms in the blood vessels of the fingers and toes. At relatively mild temperatures of 50°F or so, Kildare experienced the kind of tingling and severe pain that most people feel in subzero temperatures. Her fingertips turned white, her toes turned blue and the pain was excruciating. She had to wear gloves to take food out of the refrigerator.

Having Raynaud's meant that skiing and snowmobiling were now out of the question. In fact, Kildare's symptoms were so severe that she couldn't even drive a car in winter. By the time that she got to the car and got it warmed up, the agony was incapacitating.

HYDROTHERAPY WITH A TWIST

Kildare's doctors tried the usual treatments for Raynaud's. First, they prescribed calcium channel blockers, medications customarily used to relax coronary blood vessels and treat the heart-related chest pain angina. But the drugs caused unpleasant side effects. Her doctors also tried rauwolfia alkaloids (Reserpine)—a drug normally used to treat high blood pressure, it controls nerve impulses along certain nerve pathways. The drug worked for four months, but Kildare's symptoms recurred.

Doctors know that Raynaud's disease sets in when tiny arteries in the fingertips constrict. With blood flow cut off, people get painfully cold sensations in their fingers and toes. Surgery can sometimes correct the condition, and Kildare's doctors considered it at first. But before going ahead, they sent her to the U.S. Army Research Institute of Environmental Medicine in Natick, Massachusetts. There, medical researchers taught Kildare an innovative cold-reconditioning technique that holds promise for men and women with Raynaud's disease.

Standing in a cold room, Kildare dipped her hands in 105°F water four times a day, every other day, for eight minutes. After just one week, she started to improve. She found that she could tolerate colder and colder temperatures without pain, and the constrictions were fewer and less severe.

Kildare practiced the cold-reconditioning technique at home on her porch. Every year, before the onset of winter, she repeated the reconditioning sessions. After seven years, she was still controlling Raynaud's without medication—and was once again able to ski and snowmobile.

Researchers who developed the cold-reconditioning technique, also called the submersion technique, say it works by training your blood vessels to relax (dilate) rather than constrict when exposed to cold.

The submersion technique may be somewhat time-consuming, but the results are worth it, says Murray Hamlet, director of research, plans and operations at the U.S. Army Research Institute of Environmental Medicine. For best results, he advises doing it in winter when you can use a cold outside area as well as a warm inside area. Then follow this procedure.

- Fill two buckets or Styrofoam coolers with water of about 100°F. Place one container in a cold area such as an outdoor patio and the other in a warm room.
- Dressed lightly, in the warm room, immerse both your hands in the water for two to five minutes.
- Wrap your hands in a towel and go to the cold area. Again put your hands in the 100°F water—this time for ten minutes.
- Return indoors and put both hands in the 100°F water for two to five more minutes.
- Repeat the procedure three to six times a day, every other day.

Many people who try the submersion technique experience remission of Raynaud's after only a few repetitions, notes Dr. Hamlet. Some people, however, may need to repeat the procedure as often as 40 to 50 times over the course of several days.

Brain-Train Your Body with Biofeedback and Visualization

When combined, biofeedback and visualization can help women with Raynaud's to warm up their fingers and toes without drugs, says Richard Surwit, Ph.D., professor and vice-chairman of the Department of Psychiatry and Behavioral Sciences at Duke University in Durham, North Carolina.

"Raynaud's occurs when body temperature drops and blood flow slows," explains Dr. Surwit. "So if you learn to raise finger temperature and increase blood flow voluntarily, you'll be able to prevent the spasms." And biofeedback uses special equipment, in an office setting, to help you control body sensations.

To get set for biofeedback, you wrap a monitor around one finger, then watch a liquid-crystal display change color. The colors change as your hand gets warmer. "Each square of color on the band represents a different temperature," says Dr. Surwit. So you learn how to concentrate on making your hand warmer while watching the results. (To locate a biofeedback instructor who can teach you this technique, see page 65.)

Once you begin using biofeedback, you'll be able to treat Raynaud's yourself using self-statements and visualization. Here's how.

Find a warm spot. Set aside a few minutes of quiet time in a warm room, with no distractions.

Concentrate on hand-warming images. Visualize yourself holding a warm rock or immersing your hands in warm water.

Talk your hands warm. Say to yourself, "My hands are getting warmer" or "My hands are getting heavier."

If you practice this routine regularly at home, you should be able to follow the same sequence to warm your hands when you're actually exposed to cold. If your Raynaud's acts up when you get into your car on a cold winter morning, for instance, begin the self-statements and visualization as soon as you head for the car. Or start doing it whenever you have to take your gloves off, suggests Dr. Surwit.

He says this technique has two advantages for women with Raynaud's. First, you don't have to rely on vasodilating drugs. These drugs relax the blood vessels but can lower blood pressure—which is especially problematic for women, who tend to have lower blood pressure than men, says Dr. Surwit. "Second, you can use this technique only when needed, instead of taking a drug daily for a problem that occurs occasionally."

 ## Vitamins for Warmer Hands

Taking vitamins can end the deep freeze for some women with Raynaud's, says Alan Gaby, M.D., professor of therapeutic nutrition at Bastyr University of Naturopathic Medicine in Seattle. Here's how.

Start with a little E. To help circulation, Dr. Gaby recommends taking between 400 and 1,200 international units of vitamin E a day. Talk with your doctor before taking amounts of more than 600 international units.

Go easy with niacin. Dr. Gaby also recommends up to 2,000 milligrams a day of niacin, a B-complex vitamin known for its ability to dilate blood vessels. But don't take doses higher than 100 milligrams without medical supervision, since niacin can cause liver damage in high doses.

  ## The Hydrotherapy-Aromatherapy Rescue

A warm bath spiked with essential oils can warm your heart and hands, says Paul Petit, D.C., certified chiropractic sports physician, aromatherapist and naturopath in Poway, California. Sitting in a warm (not hot) bath helps increase circulation to the extremities, he says.

To maximize the healing power of a bath, put essential oils such as birch, cypress, rosemary and savory into the mix, suggests Dr. Petit. But you need to dilute the oils in milk, stirring well, or the oils will simply float on top of the water and irritate your skin. He suggests mixing one-sixth ounce of combined essential oils with one cup milk.

RESPIRATORY PROBLEMS

Wheeze Whackers and Decongestants for Breathing Woes

You've probably heard that taking vitamin C can prevent colds, that steam can loosen nasal congestion and that gargling with saltwater will soothe a sore throat. But did you know that acupuncture can ease wheezing triggered by asthma? Or that a special herb used in Europe can cut short a bout with the flu?

From nagging coughs to annoying cases of the flu, alternative medicine has a wealth of natural options to offer, including ways to stop a scary asthma attack short.

ASTHMA: AN ARSENAL OF NATURAL WEAPONS

Imagine trying to suck an orange through a straw. Sure, you'd get bits and pieces of fruit and some trickles of juice now and then, but for the most part, it would be an exercise in frustration, especially if you were hungry. Well, that's not far from what someone with asthma goes through every time she has an attack.

During an asthma attack, the smaller bronchi and bronchioles—tubes through which oxygen passes into the lungs—constrict and then swell. At the same time, these passages produce excess mucus, which congests the airways even further, making each gasp more difficult. Difficulty breathing along with wheezing or coughing and a "tight" chest are symptoms of asthma.

In some people, asthma is triggered by the body's reaction to exposure to cold, respiratory infections or allergens such as pollen, dust, mold and animal hair and dander that inflame the lungs. In many, the tendency toward asthma is inherited.

Asthma should never be ignored. Bronchodilating drugs are a vital part of most treatments. These are medications that instantly relax constricted breathing passages, and for some people, they're essential. Inhaled steroids, which reduce inflammation, are now an important foundation of treatment. While you should never stop taking your asthma medication unless you have your doctor's approval, there's plenty that you can do to lessen your dependence on asthma medication and help yourself breathe easier, says Adriane Fugh-Berman, M.D., former head of field investigations for the Office of Alternative Medicine at the National Institutes of Health in Bethesda, Maryland.

See yourself breathe. Regularly picturing clear bronchial openings in your lungs can help relax you and help your body to breathe a bit easier, says Judith Green, Ph.D., professor of psychology and biofeedback in the Department of Behavioral Sciences at Aims Community College in Greeley, Colorado, and author of *The Dynamics of Health and Wellness.*

Bronchi, which branch off into the lungs, resemble the limbs of an upside-down tree and branch off into even smaller tubes called bronchioles. Dr. Green suggests visualizing all the little bronchial tubes in your lungs as being open, relaxed and elastic and breathing perfectly. At the same time, picture your antibodies (substances in the body that fight infection) looking the other way, since allergic asthma is often an overreaction to antigens (substances that trigger the production of antibodies). Do this for a few minutes several times a day whenever you have time, she suggests.

Get your feedback. Learning to relax with biofeedback can help ease the severity of an asthma attack, says Angele McGrady, Ph.D., professor of psychiatry and physiology at the Medical College of Ohio in Toledo and past president of the Association for Applied Psychophysiology and Biofeedback based in Wheatridge, Colorado. A technique for monitoring muscle tension, biofeedback can help you learn to relax when you feel the familiar chest tightness that precedes a bout of asthma, she notes. "You still need asthma medicine, but biofeedback helps you deal with the panic you might feel when you have trouble breathing."

Fight back with fatty acids. Essential fatty acids, natural substances present in certain dietary fats, can help cut down on inflammation, says Andrea Sullivan, Ph.D., a naturopathic and homeopathic physician in Washington, D.C., and author of *Naturopathic Medicine for African Americans.* "Flaxseed oil and cod liver oil contain omega-3 fatty acids, which are helpful for any condition associated with the release of prostaglandins (body chemicals that cause inflammation)."

Dr. Sullivan suggests taking one or two tablespoons of flaxseed oil twice a day or 1,000 milligrams of cod liver oil once a day. Refrigerate flaxseed oil and keep cod liver oil in a cool, dark place. She also notes that salmon and halibut contain ample quantities of omega-3 fatty acids and recommends eating a half-pound of the fish two to four times a week.

Consider vitamin C. "There's good evidence that vitamin C deficiency combined with air pollution can increase the incidence of asthma, especially in children," says Gary Hatch, Ph.D., health effects researcher for the Environmental Protection Agency in Research Triangle Park, North Carolina. "Vitamin C protects against exposure to nitrogen oxides, pollutants that are present in car exhaust, smoke and both indoor and outdoor air."

In two studies of men and women, those with asthma had 50 percent less vitamin C in their blood than those who didn't have asthma. Apparently, people with asthma have overactive inflammation cells that produce substances that oxidize vitamin C. The key is to get vitamin C in the form of foods, which supply a mix of antioxidants, says Dr. Hatch. Eating plenty of vitamin C–rich foods such as spinach, broccoli, turnip greens, tomatoes and citrus fruits will supply a balance of nutrients, which is hard to duplicate by taking individual supplements.

If you do opt for supplements, keep in mind that a vitamin C deficiency can't be cured overnight. It takes weeks for levels of vitamin C to build up again, notes Dr. Hatch.

Leaf your woes behind. Magnesium, a mineral that's abundant in green, leafy vegetables like broccoli and spinach, could help reduce the severity of wheezing, says Scott Weiss, M.D., physician and professor of medicine at Harvard Medical School's Brigham and Women's Hospital in Boston. "Magnesium relaxes muscles, including the muscles that surround the bronchial tubes in the lungs." In a study at the University of Nottingham City Hospital in Nottingham, United Kingdom, and at Brigham and Women's Hospital, Dr. Weiss and other physicians looked at the health and diets of 2,633 people ages 18 to 70 and found that those who consumed the Daily Value of 400 milligrams of magnesium a day had better lung function and less reactive airways.

Dr. Weiss recommends eating magnesium-rich foods rather than taking magnesium supplements. "The more fresh green vegetables you eat, the more magnesium and the more vitamin C you'll get," he notes.

Walk away the wheeze. Some women have asthma that is induced by exercise. But over the long haul, regular exercise can gradually increase your lung capacity, helping you to breathe more efficiently and to lessen the severity of the condition, says Wade Lillegard, M.D., a sports medicine physician in Duluth, Minnesota.

Prep your lungs. To prepare your lungs for longer, more strenuous workouts, says Dr. Lillegard, do 5 to 10 minutes' worth of shorter, intense exercise, like cycling, about 15 to 30 minutes before a longer exercise session, like a tennis game. That way, your airways won't start to constrict when you exert yourself more continuously.

Note: If your physician has prescribed cromolyn sodium, a drug commonly used as a preventive measure against exercise-induced asthma, consult your physician before incorporating this lung-prepping technique into your asthma-control program. At the very least, she has probably advised you to keep your inhaler handy at all times, especially when exercising.

Exercise indoors. If you get allergic asthma and it's allergy season, you might have to work out indoors. Indoor aerobic exercises, such as riding a stationary bike, are a good way to improve asthma by opening up your airways, says Garrison Ayars, M.D., allergist and clinical associate professor of medicine at the University of Washington in Seattle. He recommends doing some form of indoor exercise three to five times a week.

Rub it out. Massage is a soothing way to promote relaxation and stress reduction, says Mary Malinski, R.N., licensed massage therapist and staff clinical nurse at Allergy, Asthma and Dermatology Associates in Portland, Oregon. "Stress is often a factor in asthma attacks, and when people are massaged, they have a chance to experience the positive effect of relaxation, improving both their stress levels and their overall quality of life."

In a pilot study of 19 people with chronic asthma, 17 women and 2 men received 15-minute upper-body massages once a week for 12 weeks. At the conclusion of the study, 89 percent of the men and women reported improvements in their energy levels, mental health, physical activities and their ability to handle emotional problems. They also reported decreased levels of chest tightness, wheezing, physical pain and fatigue. (If you'd like to try self-massage, a head-to-toe routine appears on page 227.)

Work the kinks out with Hellerwork. A few sessions with a Hellerwork practitioner can be a boon to your breathing, says Sandra Sullivan, a certified Hellerworker and director of practitioner relations at Hellerwork International in Mount Shasta, California. "During the first few sessions, the Hellerwork practitioner hones in on how you breathe and teaches you to relax your body at the neck, shoulders and abdomen in order to help you be able to take deeper, fuller breaths."

A Hellerworker also shows you how to use your body in ways that don't restrict breathing, she notes. You'll learn how to breathe normally, rather than holding your breath, when you're under stress. And you'll learn to avoid tensing your muscles unconsciously. (If you want to try Hellerwork on your own, see page 166.)

COLDS: THE ROUTE TO FAST RELIEF

Getting a chill can stress your immunity and give a cold virus free reign. But you don't just get colds when it's cold outside. Anyone who's ever had a miserable summer cold can attest to that. Colds deserve their name, though, because they *can* stop you cold. When you get struck by a common cold, aches, a stuffy or runny nose, coughing, sneezing and a sore throat, you can end up feeling out of sorts for seven days or more.

More than 100 different viruses cause colds. Cold medicines treat symptoms only, and many leave you drowsy or fog your thinking. Here are some nondrug approaches to ease the misery of a cold.

How I Healed Myself **Naturally**

Fasting Cleared Her Asthma

Judy Sutterley, 36, a housewife in Glen Gardner, New Jersey, helped ease her asthma by fasting, then by following a vegetarian diet.

"I've had asthma since I was a kid," says Sutterley. "At first, I got attacks only in the winter when I went from the outdoors, where it was cold, to the indoors, where it was warm. When I went to college, asthma hit me a bit more often, and by the time I got married, I was taking over-the-counter medicine to try to control my daily asthma attacks.

"It got to the point where I was admitted to the emergency room three times in one year," says Sutterley. She also took steroids intermittently over an eight-year period, but even those powerful drugs never fully controlled her asthma symptoms. When her asthma was at its worst, she needed to use a nebulizer every three to four hours to dispense bronchodilating drugs to open up her airways.

"Then I heard that fasting could help asthma, and I had to try it—nothing else was working," says Sutterley. "I quit my job and fasted under medical supervision for 21 days. About a week into the fast, my asthma symptoms started to dissipate."

By the end of the fast, Sutterley no longer needed medications and was breathing freely. "I was completely off medication for about two years," she says. "Also during this time, I was eating no meat, dairy or fish—mostly just pasta, veggies and rice. I ate beans and soy products for protein. When I began to veer from this diet, I started having symptoms again, and I ended up doing a 14-day fast.

"I exercise three times a week, either doing aerobics or walking, and I don't need an inhaler," says Sutterley.

"Fasting was the jump start that I needed, and vegetarianism is what's kept me asthma-free," she adds. (For information on how to fast and when it's recommended, see page 122.)

Sink it with zinc. Taking a zinc supplement as soon as you sniff that first sniffle is an effective way to sideline a cold, says Sherif Mossad, M.D., clinical doctor in the Department of Infectious Diseases at the Cleveland Clinic. "The key is to start taking it within 24 hours of the first cold symptoms."

To study the effectiveness of zinc, Dr. Mossad prescribed zinc gluconate lozenges for 50 of a group of 100 employees of the Cleveland Clinic who had early cold symptoms. The other 50 took a mock look-alike drug. The employees who received the zinc gluconate lozenges, who were mostly women, took 13.3 milligrams every two hours during waking hours for as long as they had the symptoms. Among those who took zinc, most symptoms lasted about 4½ days, compared with about 7½ days for the other 50 people not taking zinc. And, in fact, many people find sucking on zinc lozenges to be an effective way to fight off colds. You can buy zinc lozenges at health food stores and drugstores. Follow the package directions.

Zinc may help to prevent the attachment of common cold germs inside of the nose, says Dr. Mossad. He recommends that you take a daily dose of up to 150 milligrams of zinc gluconate when you start to feel a cold coming on. Talk to your doctor before taking supplements higher than 15 milligrams for more than a few days.

Stock up on C. Another effective standby in the battle against the common cold is vitamin C, says Dr. Sullivan. "Take extra vitamin C when you're under stress or in the winter, both of which leave you more susceptible to a cold. I recommend taking 1,000 milligrams of vitamin C three times a day when you have a cold, to help shorten the duration." Large amounts of vitamin C may cause diarrhea in some people, so cut back if you start experiencing problems.

Pick up some echinacea. The herb echinacea is a natural cold-killer, says Dr. Sullivan. "It stimulates the immune system, specifically the white blood cells, to fight infection." Most of the time, echinacea is taken in liquid form—no more than 20 drops three times a day when you start feeling the symptoms of a cold. Or take two standardized capsules three times a day, says Dr. Sullivan.

Whip up a batch of pesto. Because it's a potent antibiotic and antiviral herb, crushed or mashed garlic can help prevent colds and reduce symptoms, says Dr. Fugh-Berman. As an alternative to garlic-laden food, she suggests enteric-coated garlic capsules, available at most health food stores. Typically, garlic is taken in 300-milligram dosages, three times a day, for as long as cold symptoms last. Or you can take half a clove of the real thing three times a day.

Hurry to homeopathy. Homeopathy offers a variety of cold remedies, depending on your particular symptoms, says Linda Johnston,

M.D., diplomate in homeopathic therapeutics, founder of the Academy of Classical Homeopathy in Van Nuys, California, and author of *Everyday Miracles: Homeopathy in Action.* For example, if your left ear aches, the left side of your throat hurts and you feel worse at night, you might benefit from taking 200c (which means it's been diluted 200 times) of lachesis, a homeopathic remedy that, among other effects, fights infections, she says. For other cold symptoms, select a homeopathic remedy based on the descriptions noted on the packages.

Needle that cold. Acupuncture can cut short a cold's stay, notes Joseph S. Acquah, licensed acupuncturist and doctor of oriental medicine in Los Angeles. "Stimulating with acupuncture of the lung, colon and liver meridians enhances the body's innate healing ability to clear phlegm from the nose and lungs, detoxify the liver and eliminate excess waste through the colon. All of these things are part of the common cold," he says.

CONGESTION: BREATHE EASY RIGHT NOW

Whether due to a cold or allergies, the stuffy, clogged-up discomfort of congested nasal passages is still a major pain in the . . . head.

Over-the-counter nasal sprays and decongestants can help, but sprays can't be used for longer than three days, and decongestants, for more than seven. Overuse can result in a rebound effect—that is, your nose gets stuffed up all over again. And some people find that over-the-counter drugs tend to make them jumpy.

Before nasal congestion drains all of your patience, try these safe, non-drug remedies.

Spice up your menu. Eating any kind of spicy food can temporarily help loosen congestion by thinning out your mucus and making your nose run, says Dr. Fugh-Berman. Eating cayenne (ground red pepper), green chilies or jalapeño peppers can increase secretions in your nose and throat, she notes. Or add some hot-pepper sauce (like Tabasco) to soup, salad or pasta sauce. If you can't stomach spicy foods, try taking two cayenne capsules four times a day, she suggests.

Unclog the cause. Spending about five minutes in a hot shower also allows steam to loosen mucus-clogged sinuses, says Irene von Estorff, M.D., assistant professor of rehabilitation medicine at New York Hospital–Cornell University Medical Center in New York City. This can also be done leaning over a pot of steaming water with a towel over your head.

Rub on an aromatic oil. The essential oils of camphor (from camphor trees), menthol (derived from peppermint) and the herb eucalyptus are natural decongestants, says Dr. Fugh-Berman. When applied to the skin, these essential oils cause a cooling sensation, which seems to enhance their decongestant properties. Put some on your neck, under your nose, on your temples or anywhere that you can smell it. Essential oils should never be applied straight. They should always be mixed with a neutral oil such as grapeseed or corn oil.

Many commercial rubs contain those three essential oils, notes Dr. Fugh-Berman. You can also make your own rub by adding a couple drops of eucalyptus, camphor or menthol to a handful of corn oil and rubbing it on your chest and neck, she says.

COUGHS: SOOTHING RELIEF

Coughs seem to have a knack for perversity. They'll happen during your best friend's wedding, in the middle of a boring speech and at 3:00 A.M. with sleep nowhere in sight.

No matter how hard you fight back a cough, that hacking, choking sound has to come out eventually. That's because coughing is a natural reflex—many times it's your body's way of trying to get rid of mucus in your lungs.

How I Healed Myself **Naturally**

Echinacea Killed Her Colds

Barbara Moore, 45, owner of a real estate company in Rehoboth Beach, Delaware, credits the herb echinacea for helping her cut down on frequent colds.

"I used to get a cold every summer and every fall with the change of seasons, and they'd last for two weeks," says Moore. "I read an article that said Native Americans discovered that echinacea fought off colds. So I tried it. That was two years ago, and I haven't had a cold since.

"I take echinacea when I first feel the symptoms of a cold coming on, and now I just swear by it."

Interestingly, echinacea was the plant most commonly used by Native Americans in times past. Now, it's enjoying a renaissance—at the start of every cold and flu season, echinacea flies off drugstore shelves.

If you've been coughing for more than two weeks and it doesn't seem to go away or you're coughing up discolored phlegm (anything other than clear or white), see your doctor. Otherwise, try nature's cures for silencing your cough.

Try nature's cough drops. Cough drops containing eucalyptus or horehound take the edge off your hack, says Dr. Fugh-Berman. Found in drugstores and health food stores, these lozenges help thin excretions of bronchial mucus that can make you cough.

Mind your vitamins. Drink plenty of juices made from vitamin-packed veggies like carrots and beets and greens like kale or collards, suggests Dr. Sullivan. These vegetable juices, available at health food stores or prepared in a juicer, help you fight germs that cause coughs, thanks to generous amounts of immune-boosting nutrients like vitamins A and C, she says. A deficiency of vitamin A damages the natural protective mucous membrane barrier of the respiratory tract, leaving your throat and lungs vulnerable to bacteria and viruses. Vitamin C boosts immunity by enabling white blood cells to fight infection.

"Drink one glass of vegetable juice a couple of times a day," notes Dr. Sullivan. "If you make the juice yourself in a blender, add a little water because the vegetables need to be diluted."

EMPHYSEMA: BETTER BREATHING WITH YOGA

Emphysema slowly robs you of your ability to breathe effectively. Your lungs are less and less able to transfer the oxygen from each breath into your bloodstream. Typically, you'll start to notice that vigorous activities leave you out of breath, and eventually, ordinary efforts like climbing stairs or walking a few blocks leave you gasping for air. This disease—often the outcome of smoking—damages the air sacs of the lungs. Some sacs lose their elasticity and others are destroyed, making breathing increasingly difficult.

With emphysema, the damage is irreversible. Since it's often the outcome of smoking, one "must" is to stop smoking, if you haven't already. To further ease your breathing, take the following steps.

Stretch to better breath. People with emphysema often hunch their shoulders and jut their heads forward, says Mary Schatz, M.D., physician and author of *Back Care Basics*. "In order for your chest and lungs to be able to expand, you need to position your body so that your head isn't sticking out in front of your chest."

When you do yoga, you improve your breathing by correcting your posture. Yoga also relaxes tight neck, shoulder and chest muscles—the muscles that help you breathe, says Dr. Schatz. "The stretching and strengthening of yoga helps balance the muscles and allows the bones of your neck and shoulders to loosen into a better position to help with breathing."

Work out your lungs. When you regularly get short of breath, you'll probably tend to decrease your activities. Yet cutting back on activity causes you to become breathless from even less effort, so you decrease your activity level further. It's a vicious cycle, says François Haas, Ph.D., director of the Pulmonary Function Laboratory at New York University Medical Center in New York City and co-author of *The Chronic Bronchitis and Emphysema Handbook.*

Exercise actually helps. If you have emphysema, the best workout is walking at least three times a week. "I've had patients who were unable to walk one block, but after two months of exercise, they could walk a mile or more. And they were much less out of breath." They were considerably more fit, lots more confident and no longer frightened when they occasionally did run out of breath, he adds.

When you walk, try to walk indoors during extreme temperatures, because hot and cold weather make walking much more of an effort. A mall is ideal, says Dr. Haas. Before you exercise, though, talk to a rehabilitation professional who specializes in working with people living with chronic lung disease. Call your state chapter of the American Lung Association for a recommendation.

Walk to the music. An enjoyable distraction, like walking with a friend or walking to music, will help you be less aware of feeling breathless and get you farther than you probably would otherwise, says Dr. Haas. That's the message behind a study that Dr. Haas conducted on 36 people who have chronic obstructive pulmonary disease, which includes both emphysema and chronic bronchitis. The participants walked on a treadmill while listening to music. Then they listened to gray noise (a machine-produced sound similar to static on a radio) and then silence. When they listened to music, they regularly exerted their greatest efforts and felt the least breathless.

Pucker up and breathe. One thing that you can do to help you breathe more effectively is pucker up when you breathe out, says Dr. Haas. Pursed-lip breathing helps move stale air out of your lungs.

First, breathe in through your nose. Then purse your lips as if you were going to kiss someone and exhale, says Dr. Haas. "Pursing your lips enables you to maintain adequate pressure inside your airways, which helps to keep them open."

Strengthen your breath. To help you get the most out of each breath, Dr. Schatz recommends doing a simple exercise whenever you have a few free minutes. Purse your lips if you find it helpful—it may make breathing easier.

- Inhale through your nose or mouth.
- Exhale through your nose or mouth.
- Pause and count, "one-thousand one, one-thousand two," before taking the next breath.

Repeat the steps and continue to breathe this way for several minutes.

FLU: FIGHT BACK WITH HERBS

The flu bug is the most sadistic of germs. At its worst, you'll feel body chills that make you pile on the wool blankets while at the same time, you're coping with a fever. Add to those miseries a headache, achy joints and a general feeling that you'll never get out of bed again and it all spells misery.

So what can you do about this highly contagious respiratory infection? If you drink plenty of fluids, get plenty of rest and take acetaminophen to help with muscle and joint pains and reduce fever, you should be better in about a week. But if you'd like to rid yourself of the flu a few days earlier—and who wouldn't?—try these tactics.

Grab some echinacea. If you're just starting to feel that tired-all-over general malaise of the flu, try echinacea. This immune system–boosting herb fights colds and flu, and it could shorten the virus' stay, says Dr. Fugh-Berman. Take two capsules three or four times a day, or take 20 to 40 drops (40 drops equals about one dropperful) of tincture three or four times a day, she says.

"It's very important to take echinacea every few hours instead of just once a day because it doesn't stay in your system for very long," adds Dr. Fugh-Berman. Continue to take echinacea until you feel better, but no longer. If used long-term (for more than a few weeks) echinacea loses its effectiveness, she notes.

To prevent colds, Dr. Fugh-Berman recommends taking echinacea before a long airplane trip. Because the air in planes is drier and continually recirculated, you're exposed to more viruses, and you're more vulnerable, she explains. "A lot of people pick up viruses on airplanes. So I suggest that you take echinacea the day before and the day of your trip."

SINUS PROBLEMS: RELIEF FOR CLOGGING

If you have a cold or have allergies, your sinuses may clog up with mucus. Tiny openings in the sinuses are obstructed, so mucus can't drain.

With nowhere to go, fluids build up, causing pressure and pain. Worse, bacteria can set up camp in the pools of mucus and infect your sinuses, causing fever, headaches and facial pain.

If you have a fever, which is a key indicator of infection, see your doctor. If you have pain but no fever, however, you can take the following steps to help drain your sinuses, says Dr. Fugh-Berman.

Create a sinus-soothing steam. As with ordinary nasal congestion, breathing menthol, camphor or eucalyptus oil can help clear congested sinuses and relieve pain, says Dr. Fugh-Berman.

"Heat up some water on the stove until it's boiling, then pour it in a bowl and add a couple of drops of essential oil," she notes. "Drape a towel over your head and, keeping a comfortable distance away, breathe in the steam from the bowl for about five minutes." Both the humidity of the steam and the action of the essential oil work to loosen mucus.

Sleep with a vaporizer. You can relieve stuffy sinuses as you sleep at night by putting a few drops of the essential oil of eucalyptus, camphor or menthol into a steam humidifier set up by your bed, Dr. Fugh-Berman says.

Clear your head with yoga. A legs-against-the-wall yoga pose can help clear your sinuses, says Larry Payne, Ph.D., director of the Samata Yoga Center in Los Angeles and chairman of the International Association of Yoga Therapists.

Lie on your back with your buttocks pushed against the base of the wall. Raise your legs and hold them against the wall for 7 to 15 minutes, says Dr. Payne. "This changes blood flow within the body and changes the flow of your body's lymphatic fluids—the fluids that flow from the space between the body cells into the bloodstream. For the first few minutes, pressure in your sinuses will increase. But after awhile the mucus in your sinuses starts loosening."

Caution: If you have high blood pressure, stroke risk or glaucoma, you should not do this exercise, notes Dr. Payne.

SKIN PROBLEMS
On-the-Spot Remedies for Minor Vexations

Wise women know that true beauty isn't reflected in a mirror. But it's hard for even the wisest of us to remember that fact when we're hit with an outbreak of adult acne or some other, equally unattractive eruption.

"In a culture that puts so much emphasis on youth and beauty, it's easy to panic when you get any kind of blemish or flaw, especially when it shows up on your face," says Deb Soule, an herbalist in Rockport, Maine, and author of *The Roots of Healing: A Woman's Book of Herbs*.

Skin problems ruin more than your appearance, though. A bad sunburn, outbreak of hives or fresh batch of mosquito bites can make you miserable. Unless treated correctly, burns or cuts can heal slowly or get infected. Ongoing or frequent episodes of eczema, psoriasis or shingles beg for effective treatment.

You don't have to suffer through skin problems. Here's what you can do.

ACNE: CURES FROM NATURE

You thought that you and your acne broke up after high school but, sadly, it's back, worse than ever. The scourge of your teen years has reared its ugly whiteheads and blackheads for all the world to see, smack dab on your 30-, 40- or even 50-something face.

What causes midlife acne? The quick answer is that acne is the result of too much sebum, an oily substance secreted by your skin. Sebum can collect dirt and bacteria, plugging hair follicles in skin pores. If plugs lodge near the pore's surface, blackheads or whiteheads form. If a blockage ruptures, it becomes an inflamed pimple, infected bump or pustule or sometimes a larger, fluid-filled bump or cyst, which can leave serious scars.

Various triggers can shift sebum production into high gear. Common triggers are hormonal fluctuations, stress, diet, irritating ingredients in cosmetics or a combination of these factors. Many women, for example, tend to sprout blemishes just before their menstrual periods or as they approach menopause.

If acne should revisit you, here's what alternative medicine has to offer.

 ## Herbal Relief for Spots and Pimples

Herbalists offer these tactics for erasing acne.

Reach for a weed. An infusion of yarrow is a tried-and-true remedy for acne, says Susun S. Weed, an herbalist and teacher from Woodstock, New York, and author of the *Wise Woman* herbal series. "To make an infusion of yarrow, put one ounce of dried yarrow flowers into a quart jar. Fill the jar with boiling water and cover. Steep overnight. Strain out the plant material and store the infusion in a plastic bottle. Dampen a washcloth in the liquid and gently pat it on your face every morning, evening and as needed in between."

Discard and prepare a fresh batch every three to seven days, or sooner if it becomes cloudy, advises Lisa Meserole, doctor of naturopathy, research consultant and faculty member in the botanical medicine department at Bastyr University of Naturopathic Medicine in Seattle.

Yarrow is a powerful herbal antiseptic that can kill bacteria that contribute to acne, says Weed. You can buy yarrow (*Achillea millefolium*) in herbal or health food stores.

Brew up burdock. "Burdock is a safe, effective way to clear up the skin," says Weed. For adult acne, make a very strong tea out of dried burdock root. Brew overnight and drink a cup or two a day.

Acne rosacea, a chronic form of acne that occurs on the cheeks, nose, chin and forehead, also responds well to burdock, says Weed. "For acne rosacea, take 10 to 20 drops of burdock seed or root tincture three times daily, which will usually bring slow but steady improvement," says Weed. Burdock tinctures are available at health food stores. Look for *Arctium Lappa*.

Treat your face to an herbal steam bath. "Herbal steaming is really good for women with acne because it helps remove the pus, blackheads and dirt that become embedded in your pores," says Soule. She recommends a steam bath using a combination of elder flowers, yarrow and chamomile in particular. Put a handful each of the dried herbs into a large pot, cover with a quart or two of cool water and bring to a very slow, gentle simmer. Continue simmering, and cover the pot and your head with a towel so that the steam touches your face. Keep your eyes closed, and don't get so close that you burn your skin or the towel. Steam for up to 15 minutes.

BURNS, BRUISES, CUTS AND SCRAPES:
NATURAL FIRST-AID

As a kid, you probably suffered your share of burns, bruises, bumps and cuts. As an adult, you probably still get your share of minor wounds. You flip a fritter a little too fast and splash your skin with hot oil. Or you're taken by surprise on a cloudy day that suddenly morphed into sunlight, stranding you without your sunblock—and with a sunburn. Or you walk into the coffee table and scrape your skin.

You can usually handle most minor burns, bruises and cuts on your own, if you know what to do. Next time you nick or burn your skin, turn to these natural remedies to soothe the pain and speed healing.

Smear on some aloe. Healers have used the aloe vera plant, with its long, spiky, cactuslike leaves, since ancient times.

To soothe a minor burn (including sunburn), scrape or other skin irritation, just snap off an aloe leaf from a mature plant, cut it down its length and apply the transparent gel from inside the leaf to your skin, advises Michael Murray, doctor of naturopathy in Bellevue, Washington, in his book *The Healing Power of Herbs*. Dr. Murray is also an instructor at Bastyr University of Naturopathic Medicine.

Aloe contains vitamins C and E and zinc—nutrients that speed wound healing. In fact, research shows that fresh aloe gel reduces inflammation and appears to promote wound repair when applied to cuts and burns. In a controlled clinical study of 27 people, for example, burns treated with aloe vera gel healed in just 12 days, which was significantly faster than the 18 days it took to heal burns merely covered with petroleum jelly–coated gauze.

Turn to aloe for frostbite. Aloe has also been used as a first-aid for frostbite, possibly because it acts against thromboxanes, substances that constrict blood vessels. When aloe is applied, the blood vessels relax, helping to heal frostbitten skin. In one study, 56 men and women treated with standard first-aid—including rewarming, pain medication and antibiotics—*plus* aloe healed faster than others treated with standard first-aid alone.

Grow your own. Fresh aloe gel works better than aloe-containing products, according to Dr. Meserole. Most plant stores and greenhouses sell aloe plants, and they're easy to grow at home. "Every household should have an aloe plant for an easy, inexpensive, ready and pure first-aid remedy."

Soothing relief. For minor cuts and scrapes, mix 15 drops of lavender essential oil with one ounce of aloe vera juice (both are available at health food stores). Place the mixture in a spray bottle and store in the refrigerator for a soothing, cooling mist that you can spray on the hurt, says Mindy

Green, instructor at the Rocky Mountain Center for Botanical Studies in Boulder, Colorado, and co-author of *Aromatherapy: A Complete Guide to the Healing Art*.

Plant on some plantain. This common weed found in lawns and along driveways soothes pain, binds together torn tissue and strengthens the skin's surface, says Weed. Plantain can be used fresh. Crush a thin leaf or two and apply to minor cuts and scrapes. Rub the leaves briskly between your palms or chop them with a knife. Hold the crushed or chopped leaves in place with an adhesive strip. Leave this on for 12 to 24 hours. It's okay if it gets wet. You can also use a plantain salve, found in health food stores, to ease itching and promote healing, she adds.

Take homeopathic arnica. *Arnica montana*, available in health food stores and drugstores, is an amazing remedy for bumps and bruises that are apt to leave you black and blue, says Richard J. Weintraub, M.D., consulting psychiatrist at the Spaulding Rehabilitation Hospital and assistant clinical professor of psychiatry at Tufts University School of Medicine, both in Boston. For best results, take the dosage recommended on the package immediately after an injury.

Caution: Never ingest nonhomeopathic arnica, such as arnica tincture or arnica essential oil, as it is highly poisonous.

DANDRUFF:
AN HERBAL END TO A FLAKY SCALP

Nothing nixes the sex appeal of that little black dress faster than little white flakes on your shoulders.

The familiar flaking and uncomfortable itching are signs of dandruff, or seborrheic dermatitis, an inflammation of the scalp. Dandruff can also show up on your eyebrows, the sides of your nose, your chest and behind your ears.

To de-flake yourself, try these remedies.

Rinse away with herbs. To make a dandy antidandruff herbal rinse, combine a handful each of dried nettle tops (*Urtica dioica*), dried rosemary (*Rosmarinus officinalis*) and dried calendula flowers (*Calendula officinalis*), says Soule.

Place the herbs in a two-quart glass jar and cover with a quart of organic apple cider vinegar. Let the herbal rinse sit for one month, then strain it. If you like, scent the rinse with a few drops of your favorite essential oil, such as lavender oil. (You can use the rinse after two weeks, but it's more potent after one month. So the best strategy is to always have a batch or two in the works.)

Use a cup or so to rinse your hair after every shampoo, and leave it in, says Soule. If you find that it's too strong, you can use one to two tablespoons in one cup of water, she says.

Soule also recommends using a tea brewed from the herbs if you can't wait two to four weeks. Pour a cup of boiling water over one to two tablespoons of dried chopped herbs, cover and steep for 10 to 15 minutes, then strain. Rinse your hair with this room-temperature tea. You can rinse it out twice if you wish.

ECZEMA: SOOTHE THE ITCH, HEAL THE RASH

"Eczema isn't just any nasty skin rash—it typically refers to a pink, scaly rash that itches intensely," says Jeffrey Thompson, D.O., a dermatologist in private practice in Murrysville, Pennsylvania.

Eczema, or atopic dermatitis, is hereditary. But stress, allergies or extremes in temperature can trigger the rash. Many people who have eczema also have hay fever or asthma.

When eczema is severe, your skin can thicken and crack, especially around folds near your neck, knees and elbows. That's painful.

So far, no one has discovered a permanent cure for eczema, but you can take steps to soothe the rash and minimize discomfort.

Avoid food culprits. "The first thing that you should do if you have eczema is to rule out food allergies," notes Dr. Murray. Milk is the number one culprit, but it's not the only trigger. (To find out if you have food allergies that could be aggravating your skin, see page 338.)

Follow the three-minute moisture rule. "If you have eczema, moisturizing your skin thoroughly and regularly is vital," says Dr. Thompson. "Choose a thick moisturizing lotion and put it on within three minutes of taking your shower or bath, while your skin is still damp. The goal is to seal in the moisture." He recommends plain old solid vegetable shortening, such as Crisco. If you find shortening to be too greasy and messy, Dr. Thompson suggests skin lotions like Aquaphor and Eucerin.

Baby your skin. Above all, don't irritate skin that's already irritated, advises Dr. Murray. Avoid itchy fabrics like wool. Launder your clothes, towels and bedding with mild, fragrance-free detergents, and rinse them well. Also, avoid getting sweaty. Hot, moist skin aggravates dermatitis. If you do work up a sweat, shower off as soon as possible.

 The Vitamin-and-Mineral Rescue

Taking a combination of vitamins and minerals can significantly ease the rash of eczema, say experts. Here's what they suggest.

Zinc. Take 50 milligrams a day. Research shows that zinc speeds wound healing, making it particularly valuable in treating eczema, says Dr. Murray. (Doses of zinc above 15 milligrams per day should be taken only under medical supervision.)

Quercetin. Quercetin is a flavonoid, a plant compound related to fruit and vegetable pigment, found in lemons, asparagus and other plants. Studies show that flavonoids block the flood of histamines, substances that the skin releases when exposed to allergy triggers.

Take two capsules of quercetin daily, recommends Willard Dean, M.D., medical director of the Center for Self Healing in Santa Fe, New Mexico, and author of "The Immune System," one in a series of booklets titled *The Holistic Health Series*. The capsules combine quercetin with vitamin C, notes Dr. Dean.

Evening primrose oil. Take two to four capsules of 500 milligrams each, three times a day. Evening primrose oil contains essential fatty acids, substances that help reduce inflammation. If you find that it is too expensive, Dr. Murray suggests that you switch to flaxseed oil as your eczema improves. Flaxseed oil delivers essential fatty acids less efficiently, but it's not as expensive as evening primrose oil. (Some people experience nausea, diarrhea or headaches when taking evening primrose oil. If you experience side effects, discontinue its use.)

HIVES:
COOL THE ITCHING AND SWELLING

Allergies are notorious for making your skin or eyes itch, your nose run and your throat scratchy—symptoms caused by the release of histamines during an allergic reaction to something that you've breathed in or touched. But some allergies can also trigger hives.

Hot or cold weather and certain foods can also cause hives, even if you don't have allergies. And hives can be caused or aggravated by stress. If you break out in hives, act fast. Here's what to do.

Apply a cold compress. Dip a washcloth in cold water and apply it to the welts to shrink blood vessels and block the further release of histamines into your skin, says Leonard Grayson, M.D., a retired clinical associate allergist and dermatologist at Southern Illinois University School of Medicine in Springfield.

Two caveats: Don't use a cold compress if you break out in hives or experience other allergic reactions when exposed to the cold. And if you get hives in your mouth or throat, get emergency medical help immediately.

Try vitamin C and quercetin. If the hives linger or return, Dr. Murray recommends supplementing your diet with 1,000 milligrams of vitamin C three times a day. Or, if you suspect that the hives are triggered by food, take 250 milligrams of quercetin (often combined with vitamin C in capsules) 20 minutes before each meal. Its antihistamine action may help reduce the hives.

Identify the source. If you get hives frequently, you need to take preventive action, advises Dr. Murray. He suggests that you try an elimination diet to test for food allergies or see a naturopath experienced in treating food allergies. (For guidelines on following an elimination diet, see page 339. For details on locating a naturopath, see page 251.)

INSECT BITES: BATTLE NATURE WITH NATURE

Bring on the sounds of summer . . . the buzzing, the swatting, the slapping, the moaning. When mosquitoes and other invaders dive in, outdoor fun takes flight.

Spraying yourself with a powerful chemical insect repellent containing DEET (N,N-diethyl-meta-toluamide) will keep bugs away. But DEET is a nervous system toxin—it can make you sick. The safety of powerful chemical repellents is in question, especially for use on children.

If you'd rather not resort to chemical warfare against biting bugs, try these safe, all-natural homemade repellents.

Make a mosquito mister. "Fill a pocket-size four-ounce mister with warm water and add two to four drops of essential oil of cedar or citronella. Shake well and mist yourself as needed," says Weed. "This recipe keeps everyone bite-free, even during my summer outdoor herb workshops. It works great against mosquitoes and no-see-ums, and here's the best part: You can't smell it, but the bugs can."

Concoct a bug oil. "I make a bug repellent using half a cup of olive oil, to which I add five or six drops each of essential oils of citronella, eucalyptus, rosemary and lavender and two drops of pennyroyal," says Soule. "Avoid using the pennyroyal if you are pregnant or if you are giving the mixture to children under age eight. Dab the mixture on as needed, with your fingers. Be sure to avoid contact with your eyes and wash your hands after applying the mixture."

A good smell for bad bugs. If you don't care for the smell of citronella, Green offers a bug banisher made from other equally effective essential oils. Combine five drops eucalyptus, two drops rosemary, four drops lavender, two drops juniper, eight drops cedar, one drop peppermint, one drop clove, one drop cinnamon and two ounces vegetable oil. Mix together in a glass bottle and apply liberally.

You could also use two simpler versions of the formula. Combine ten drops each of lavender and rosemary, or combine ten drops each of lavender, rosemary and cedar. (Look for pure essential oils in aromatherapy shops and some health food stores.)

POISON IVY:
FIGHTING THE PLANT WARRIORS

"Three leaves, leave it be." You heed Grandma's poison-plant warning whenever you venture outdoors. So how come you're covered with poison ivy?

Most likely, your dog or cat or kids or husband brought it home. And you got the itchy rash because you're allergic to the plant's oil.

"The substance in poison ivy that makes you break out transfers easily from other people's clothing or your pet's fur to your skin," says William Epstein, M.D., professor of dermatology at the University of California at San Francisco.

"If you put poison ivy oil on a patch of cloth, you can transfer enough oil to cause a reaction 2,000 rubbings later," says Dr. Epstein. "Your pet can just brush against poison ivy, come inside and hop in your lap or be petted. If you're sensitive, that's all it takes to give you the rash." (Four out of five people are allergic to poison ivy or other related plants such as poison oak or sumac.)

Quarantining yourself and your family indoors is a sure way to prevent a brush with poison ivy, oak or sumac. Short of that, here's what you can do.

Reach for the alcohol. No, not the chardonnay. "Rubbing alcohol is the safest and best solvent that you can use to get poison plant oil off your skin," says Dr. Epstein.

Even if you just think that you've come in contact with poison ivy, oak or sumac, slosh yourself down, head to toe, with rubbing alcohol. Liberally splash it on your hands, face, arms, legs and any other exposed skin, but keep it out of your eyes. As you are doing this out in your yard, rinse the alcohol off with a garden hose. Do this before going in the house. The alcohol extracts the oil, and the water washes it away.

Act quickly: You have four to six hours before the oil penetrates your skin, says Dr. Epstein. If you're camping or hiking and can't use the alcohol until long after exposure, at least rinse yourself off with water as soon as you can, he adds.

Lather down. An alternative to rubbing alcohol is Fels Naptha soap, says Green. Just jump in the shower and lather. You can find naptha soap at your local hardware or grocery store.

Quarantine your clothes. Make sure that clothes contaminated by poison plants don't touch anything except the inside of your washing machine. Wash them separately so that they can't contaminate clothes not exposed to poison plants.

Make a plantain poultice. All varieties of plantain, a common lawn and roadside weed, contain a mucilaginous substance that contains healing properties. If this weed grows in your yard, you're in luck. Soule suggests bruising some fresh plantain leaves, placing them between thin sheets of cotton gauze and placing the poultice directly on your poison ivy.

Wear jewelweed. You might call jewelweed, also known as pale touch-me-not, nature's cortisone. Applied directly to poison ivy, jewelweed can reduce the inflammation as well as cortisone creams customarily used for the rash, says Dr. Dean. In one study, 108 of 115 men and women with poison ivy responded most dramatically to jewelweed cream applied directly to their rashes. Their symptoms disappeared within two to three days.

Jewelweed (*Impatiens biflora*) grows wild along roadsides. It is a tall annual with succulent stems and yellow or red-brown orchidlike hanging blossoms that appear in summer. Apply the sap from the stem directly onto the affected area. Or, for convenience, you can buy jewelweed cream in health food stores.

PSORIASIS:
GET BACK IN CONTROL

Psoriasis is a cinch to diagnose: Skin cells grow abnormally, triggering itchy, uncomfortable and unsightly red patches and silvery scales anywhere on your body but usually on your scalp, the backs of the ears, your elbows or behind your knees. It's not contagious, but comes and goes.

When it comes to treating psoriasis naturally, doctors face a challenge. "I call psoriasis the great humbler because it's the greatest treatment challenge that dermatology has to offer," says Alan M. Dattner, M.D., a dermatologist in private practice in Putnam, Connecticut. Doctors can't cure psoriasis, says Dr. Dattner, who uses alternative treatments in his practice. But some treatments can control it pretty well. Here are some of the most promising tactics.

Catch some rays. Getting out in the sun for about an hour a day helps four out of five people with psoriasis, according to the National Psoriasis Foundation. According to Dr. Murray, exposure to ultraviolet light slows down the abnormal growth of cells that causes the problem.

Because sunshine therapy can be such valuable therapy for psoriasis, Dr. Murray says that this is one time when you can modify the usual rules about sun exposure. You can sunbathe any time of the day, but limit your exposure to what won't produce a sunburn on you (which may be less than five minutes if you're very fair). Be sure to cover or use sunblock on areas that are free of psoriasis.

And don't make the mistake of thinking that tanning salons offer light-therapy benefits, says Dr. Thompson. "They don't, and they're dangerous."

Just say ohm. Dealing with stress can help you combat psoriasis, not because stress causes psoriasis, but because stress can make it worse in some people, says Dr. Dattner. "Learning how to meditate can help put psoriasis in perspective and help deal with the severe life stresses that can make it flare up in some people."

Look to the East. The National Psoriasis Foundation reports that acupuncture and Chinese herbs have helped some people with psoriasis. Both are part of Traditional Chinese Medicine, a system of diagnosis and treatment using a number of healing methods customarily applied in China. (The foundation recommends that you work with a qualified medical professional trained in these techniques. To locate a doctor of Traditional Chinese Medicine in your area, see page 284.)

PUFFY EYES:
GET RID OF THE BAGS

For many people, baggy pouches under the eyes result from a run-in with pollen or other allergens. For them, dealing with the allergies can solve the problem. (For information on how to handle allergies, see page 333.) And in some people, puffy eyes are genetic, like brown hair or freckles. More often, though, puffy eyes are an unwelcome legacy from a late-night soiree.

"Undereye puffiness can often be traced to a night on the town," says Adriane Fugh-Berman, M.D., former head of field investigations for the Office of Alternative Medicine at the National Institutes of Health in Bethesda, Maryland. "Bags under the eyes usually are a matter of too little sleep or too much alcohol, or both. Though fluid retention causes the puffiness, we don't know exactly what causes the fluid retention. Doctors consider puffy eyes more of a cosmetic annoyance than a health problem." (If eye puffiness extends around the whole eyes, you should see a doctor.)

Even so, before you reach for a cosmetic cover-up, try these tried-and-true, good-for-you herbal remedies.

Make yourself a cup of dandelion-leaf tea. "Help de-bag your eyes with this tonic tea," says Soule. Drink a cup of dandelion-leaf tea, or take half a teaspoon of dandelion-leaf tincture three times a day, recommends Soule. Dandelion is a mild diuretic, which helps your body get rid of excess fluid. You can buy herbal tinctures at health food stores.

Brew an herbal infusion. Combine 1½ tablespoons each of dried calendula flowers, eyebright (*Euphrasia*, all varieties), borage flowers (*Borago officinalis*) and raspberry leaf (*Rubus idaeus*). Place the herbal mixture in a glass quart jar, fill with boiling water and cover. Let the mixture steep at room temperature for two to eight hours. Once the infusion has cooled, soak a washcloth with the liquid, lie down and rest with the cloth over your closed eyes, says Soule. Store any leftover infusion in the refrigerator for two to three days, then bring to room temperature before soaking the washcloth and using again.

Slice a cucumber. For years, women have used cucumbers to relieve puffy eyes. This modern folk remedy works because cucumbers contain a natural substance that reduces swelling and eliminates puffiness, says Shawne Bryant, M.D., who incorporates healing herbs and massage therapy into her gynecology practice in Virginia Beach, Virginia. Slice one-fourth-inch rounds off the cucumber. Gently press the rounds over your puffy eyes and lie down for a bit.

SHINGLES:
NATURAL RELIEF FOR A SERIOUS PAIN

The same virus (herpes zoster) that may have given you childhood chickenpox can strike again in adulthood to give you this painful, blistery rash.

"The classic shingles outbreak looks like a straight-sided patch of little red-edged blisters," says Dr. Dean. "The virus travels along spinal nerves and comes out on either the left or the right side of your body, resulting in a rash."

Shingles pain can sometimes last weeks or months after the rash has healed, especially for the elderly or chronically ill. Fortunately, natural medicine offers soothing solutions for shingles. Here are some of the best.

Go soak in vinegar. Soak a soft dish towel in slightly chilled apple cider vinegar and drape it over the affected area for 10 to 15 minutes, suggests Dr. Dean. It's soothing.

Try a tincture. I take 30 to 50 drops of St.-John's-wort tincture in one to two ounces of water, three to six times a day, says Weed. I also use the oil on dry, itchy rashes hourly if needed. It even helps relieve lingering pain from shingles and burns, she notes. I especially like to use the oil on exposed skin to prevent sunburns. Whether using the oil or the tincture, use caution when going out in the sun. Both can cause photosensitivity.

Save yourself with gel. Aloe vera gel can often provide soothing relief for shingles, suggests Dr. Dean. "The plant gets pretty high marks for reducing inflammation and promoting healing." You can use the fresh gel or purchase some at health food stores.

URINARY TRACT PROBLEMS

What Works for Bladder Trouble

When it comes to urinating, each gender has its own advantages. Isn't it great that we don't have to relieve ourselves just a bent-elbow away from the guy at the next urinal?

Well, sure. But men have the option of being able to walk behind any tree and efficiently take care of their business in a fully upright, standing position.

Obvious differences.

But the biggest drawback for women is perhaps not so obvious. In fact, it's medical. Women are more susceptible than men to three kinds of urinary problems. First, we have more stress and urge incontinence, which means unintentional leakage of urine. We're also more prone to interstitial cystitis, a painful disease of the bladder that causes you to urinate many times throughout the day and night. And we're at greater risk of urinary tract infections, a bacterial invasion that triggers a burning sensation when you urinate.

WHY THE PROBLEM?

For two out of these three conditions, doctors have an idea why women seem more vulnerable in matters of urinary health. In the case of urinary incontinence, childbirth plays a role. Having babies weakens a woman's pelvic-floor muscles. Those are the sling-shaped muscles holding the bladder and urethra in place. And when those muscles start to go, controlling urine flow is simply more difficult.

On the other hand, doctors aren't sure why women are more prone to interstitial cystitis than men. We just are, it seems.

As for urinary tract infections, the difference has to do with the urethra, the tube that empties urine from the bladder. The urethra is shorter in women than in men, and that means it's easier for bacteria from outside sources like the rectum to work its way up to the bladder and cause an infection.

In every case, you can do something to improve, treat or prevent urinary conditions, says Denise Webster, R.N., Ph.D., professor in the School of Nursing at the University of Colorado Health Sciences Center in Denver. "There's something powerful and healing and positive about taking control of a disease and being active in your own treatment," she adds.

INCONTINENCE: NO MORE ACCIDENTS

Even in your teens and twenties, you accidentally let loose a little dribble once in a blue moon. That's normal.

But as you head into your thirties and forties—and especially if you've had children—those dribbles could become regular little "accidents" that you cannot ignore. The most common kind of urinary incontinence, stress incontinence, is usually triggered by sneezing, coughing or lifting. When you have pelvic-floor muscles already weakened by childbirth, the extra strain eases up the muscles that surround and close the urethra, allowing some urine to leak out.

With urge incontinence, the second most prevalent type of urinary incontinence, your bladder muscles contract uncontrollably and you feel an urgent need to urinate. Urge incontinence may be caused by a urinary tract infection. For some women, leaking becomes worse after menopause. Before menopause, the female hormone estrogen keeps muscles surrounding the bladder limber. When estrogen production wanes, bladder muscles dry out.

Many women suffer from a combination of stress incontinence and urge incontinence, says Guy Fried, M.D., physiatrist at Magee Rehabilitation Hospital and an instructor at Thomas Jefferson University Hospital, both in Philadelphia. Sometimes the incontinence is so uncontrollable that some doctors may suggest surgery to restore pelvic-muscle function.

Usually, though, surgery isn't necessary. About 85 percent of women with urinary incontinence can either be cured, or much improved, with nonsurgical options. To stay dry, try these strategies.

Give your bladder muscles the squeeze. Learn to isolate and strengthen the pelvic-floor muscles by exercising them, advises Dr. Fried. "While urinating, you should stop your urine stream and squeeze so that you feel where those muscles are."

Once you're familiar with the muscles at the neck of the bladder that control urine flow, you can exercise them. These exercises are called

Kegels, named after the doctor who invented them. Squeeze these muscles and hold them tight several times a day—while driving or sitting at your desk or watching TV, for example. Hold each squeeze for about ten seconds, then relax for ten and repeat. After you've learned Kegels, you shouldn't do them with a full bladder. Otherwise, you can increase your chance of getting an infection, says Adriane Fugh-Berman, M.D., former head of field investigations for the Office of Alternative Medicine at the National Institutes of Health in Bethesda, Maryland.

The goal is to do six to ten at a time, about half a dozen times a day, says Dr. Fried. "The beauty is that no one has a clue that you're doing Kegels. You could be sitting in a meeting doing Kegels and no one could tell."

Learn biofeedback. If you're having trouble isolating your pelvic-floor muscles, making it difficult to do Kegels effectively, biofeedback can help show you where your pelvic-floor muscles are and make it easier to get them in shape, says Dr. Fried.

During the first session, a probe is inserted inside your vagina or rectum to measure the amount of muscular tension you exert when bearing down on the pelvic-floor muscles. A video screen shows you a printout that registers the tension level of your muscles as you're exerting pressure.

Your goal when using biofeedback for urinary incontinence is to identify the muscles involved. After a few sessions of training, you should be able to control the muscles on your own, says Dr. Fried.

While biofeedback for urinary incontinence is certainly more invasive than biofeedback for headaches, it's a far cry from surgery. And it works: In one study of 43 women who used biofeedback for incontinence associated with a disability, the procedure proved very effective. Before using biofeedback, the women averaged three or four incidents of urinary leakage a day. After six sessions of biofeedback, where the women learned to isolate their pelvic-floor muscles, the women averaged one incident or less per day.

Give acupuncture a try. Sometimes, not completely emptying the bladder every time you urinate can cause problems. When that happens, you may leak urine at a later time, notes Patrick Lariccia, M.D., director of the Acupuncture and Pain Clinic at the University of Pennsylvania in Philadelphia. "You might have a bladder that's not contracting forcefully enough, so you retain some urine every time," he explains.

In his clinical practice, Dr. Lariccia has found acupuncture to be helpful at times for this type of problem. Acupuncture sessions can help you to empty your bladder every time you go to the bathroom, he says. However, you should first have your problems diagnosed by a medical doctor, he advises. (For information on locating an acupuncturist, see page 33.)

INTERSTITIAL CYSTITIS: GET BACK IN CONTROL

Imagine, if you can bear to, having to run from your office to the bathroom every half-hour. Even worse, imagine having to go some 30 times a day and then being awakened with the urge 20 times during the night. Those nightmare scenarios are reality for many of the 450,000 women who have interstitial cystitis (IC), a mysterious bladder inflammation that affects women ten times more often than men.

"During an acute attack, a woman could end up almost living in the bathroom," explains Dr. Webster.

Besides an urgent need to urinate frequently, IC is accompanied by frequent abdominal pain above the pubic area. Doctors aren't sure what causes the problem. Some explanations point to a possible defect in the bladder's lining, a virus or even an autoimmune disease that affects many women of childbearing age. Rheumatoid arthritis and lupus erythematosus, for instance, are conditions in which the immune system doesn't function the way it should, and they may be associated with interstitial cystitis.

You can try out a whole gamut of powerful anti-inflammatory and pain medications if your doctor prescribes them for IC. But other natural, easy-to-do remedies are available. Here are the nondrug tactics that work best.

Avoid acid in foods. Cutting back on acids in your diet is one of the most helpful ways of reducing the frequency of interstitial cystitis attacks, says Dr. Webster. Foods such as tomatoes, strawberries, citrus fruit and curry or other spices contain acids that irritate the bladder, she notes.

Reach for the baking soda. To further help reduce acidity in urine, Dr. Webster recommends drinking sodium bicarbonate: Mix one-half teaspoon of baking soda with eight ounces of water and stir to dissolve the soda. Drink it three or four times a day, at no less than four-hour intervals. Do not use for more than a few days, though. Long-term daily use of baking soda is not recommended, she says.

Nix the caffeine. Dr. Webster also tells women with interstitial cystitis to avoid coffee, since it's a diuretic that makes you urinate more.

Visualize cool zones around the pain. One way to control the misery of interstitial cystitis is to use imagery to take your mind off the pain, says Dr. Webster. "You don't forget about the pain, but instead you redefine it as another sensation. For example, try concentrating on the pain being cool, a sensation often associated with comfort, rather than hot, a sensation often associated with discomfort.

"Also, try to focus on areas of comfort in your body, like your arms or shoulders, instead of concentrating on where the pain is," Dr. Webster suggests. In a survey of how 300 women with IC deal with attacks, very few

How I Healed Myself **Naturally**

Acupuncture Eased Her Cystitis Pain

Desperate for relief from interstitial cystitis, Kirsten Kurtz, 57, a nurse in St. Louis Park, Minnesota, turned to the Eastern practice of acupuncture— with good results.

"The pain started when I was pregnant with my daughter 20 years ago," Kurtz says. "I had a gnawing discomfort, I thought, in my intestinal area. It just hurt all over.

"I'd go the bathroom every hour, and I was losing sleep," she says. "I was pretty irritable about the whole thing. The doctors offered me tranquilizers, which I turned down."

Kurtz was referred to a physician who said that she had an autoimmune problem of some kind, which means the immune system overreacts and turns on itself. "I was referred to a urologist who finally told me, 11 years after the first symptoms, that I had interstitial cystitis."

A year after her diagnosis and now desperate for help, Kurtz started acupuncture. "I noticed a marked relief in the discomfort within the first couple of treatments. I no longer needed to take ibuprofen every four to five hours. And I can go up to three hours without having to get up and urinate at night," she adds.

Acupuncture enabled Kurtz to do things she'd always wanted to do, like going to her son's cross-country running and cross-country skiing meets. Before she started acupuncture, Kurtz says that she couldn't even watch a whole meet. "I'd have to time it so that I would get there and be gone within an hour. And I was lucky if I could wait that long," she says. But with the new therapy, things are different. "Last winter, I was able to stay for a couple of hours."

Kurtz also took a three-week trip to Russia. "Fortunately, bathrooms were readily available. But before acupuncture, I would never have had the courage to go."

Kurtz now goes for acupuncture treatments every four to six weeks. She also credits a low-acid diet (no citrus fruit, for example), drinking a lot of water, exercise and prayer for reducing her pain. "The quality of my life has been improved sensationally," she says.

of them reported using imagery. But those who did found it to be very effective, she adds.

Do meditative breathing. Deep breathing can help relax you so that interstitial cystitis won't seem to cause as much discomfort, says Steven Brena, M.D., former chairman of the Board of Pain Control and Rehabilitation of Georgia in Atlanta. Tense muscles can make IC pain feel that much more intense, he notes. When you shift your attention away from pain and toward your breathing, you'll be more relaxed.

First sit comfortably, with your back straight. Then focus on your muscles and relax them in sequence. "When I do this, I start with my feet and lower extremities—first tensing them, then relaxing them, working all the way up to the shoulders," he says. At the same time, he concentrates on his breathing. "I feel how my muscles relax when I breathe very slowly. I say, 'One in,' as I breathe in and, 'One out,' as I breathe out." Dr. Brena suggests doing a form of "meditating breathing" like this for at least twice a day for 15 minutes.

Walk away from pain. If you have IC, enjoying a daily walk could be a vital way of keeping up your spirits and maintaining overall good health, says Dr. Webster. "But most women with interstitial cystitis have to avoid any exercise that jiggles the bladder, such as running or aerobics. Walking is gentle, yet strenuous enough to keep your energy level up. Theoretically, it may also increase the flow of endorphins, which are natural painkillers in your body," she notes.

URINARY TRACT INFECTION: FIGHT FUTURE ATTACKS

When you gotta go, you gotta go. But sometimes, you just *think* you gotta go because when you go, you don't gotta go nearly as badly as you thought you had to.

With a urinary tract infection (UTI), your bladder may seem confused. But if you have a frequent, urgent need to urinate and you get a burning or pain in your urethra when you go the bathroom, you probably have a UTI. A doctor's visit is definitely in order, especially if you see blood in your urine, since you might have a more serious bladder or kidney disorder. Your doctor will most likely give you a short course of antibiotics to kill the bacteria that enters the bladder and causes the problem in the first place. But whether or not you're on antibiotics, you'll want to try these healing helpers to reduce immediate discomfort and prevent future infections.

 Go with a flow. Drinking plenty of fluids will help your bladder get rid of accumulated bacteria in the urine, notes Richard J. Macchia,

M.D., professor and chairman of the Department of Urology at the State University of New York Health Science Center in New York City. "When you have a urinary tract infection, you need to flush the bacteria out. If the urine stays in the bladder, the bugs keep doubling their population rapidly. Constantly flushing keeps their numbers down." You should drink enough to keep your urine colorless. Colorless urine is a good sign that you're drinking enough fluids, he notes.

Get juiced. Drinking cranberry juice cocktail can both prevent and treat urinary tract infections, notes Dr. Macchia. "In several published studies, just drinking three eight-ounce glasses of cranberry juice cocktail a day significantly reduced the incidence of urinary tract infections in elderly women." So while you're drinking lots of fluids, be sure to include some glasses of cranberry juice cocktail.

Cranberry juice cocktail is effective because it has an unidentified ingredient that prevents the bacteria in the urine from sticking to the lining of the bladder, Dr. Macchia notes. It proved its antibacterial properties

---

How I Healed Myself **Naturally**

Cranberry Juice Cured Her Urinary Tract Infections

Plagued by frequent urinary tract infections, Rhonda Hershey, a 34-year-old bankruptcy representative in Manhattan Beach, California, heard that cranberry juice might help. She gave it a try—with good results.

"I've been getting urinary tract infections since I was about six years old," says Hershey. "For some reason, I seem to be susceptible. Maybe it's because I don't drink enough water."

When a urinary tract infection strikes, Hershey is miserable. "I'd be doubled over in pain, with a burning pressure that's horrible. You can't do anything."

Hershey's mother told her about the benefits of drinking cranberry juice, citing evidence that it curbs infections by making the bacteria less adherent to the bladder.

"We have a cafeteria at work, so I can easily get cranberry juice, even on the job," she says. "And I love the taste. So whenever I start feeling the symptoms of a urinary tract infection coming on, I drink two large glasses of cranberry juice cocktail. It really helps. I almost never get full-blown infections anymore."

when a group of 153 women drank either three glasses a day of cranberry juice cocktail or had a drink that looked and tasted like it but wasn't actually cranberry juice cocktail. Only 15 percent of the urine samples of the women who drank cranberry juice cocktail contained bacteria that could potentially cause a UTI, while 28 percent of the other urine samples had the bacteria.

Sip blueberry juice. Another good fruit for fighting urinary tract bacteria is the blueberry, says Dr. Fugh-Berman. "Cranberries and blueberries are related, so, like cranberries, blueberries have the qualities that make bacteria less adhesive." She suggests eating about a pint of blueberries a day or putting them in a blender with enough water to make a tasty blueberry juice. You can also try alternating the blueberry and cranberry juice cocktails if you want variety, she notes.

Try nature's blend. The herbs buchu and uva ursi, combined with juniper berries, have the power to remove bacteria from the urine and make you urinate, says Andrea Sullivan, Ph.D., a naturopathic and homeopathic physician in Washington, D.C. "Mix equal amounts of each tincture—buchu, uva ursi and juniper berry—together. Put 30 drops in warm water and drink it three or four times a day," she says. "They work as renal antiseptics, which help clean out the kidneys and bladder." Stop using the tincture if you don't see an improvement within seven days since uva ursi shouldn't be used for more than a week, cautions Dr. Fugh-Berman.

Have an essential soak. Sitting in a bath half-filled with warm or tepid water and a few drops of essential oils can ease the external burning of a UTI, says Valerie Cooksley, R.N., holistic nurse and aroma practitioner in the Seattle area and author of *Aromatherapy: A Lifetime Guide to Healing with Essential Oils.*

To concoct this soothing bath, you need three drops of essential oil of sandalwood (*Santalum album*), two drops of tea tree (*Melaleuca alternifolia*) essential oil, one drop of essential oil of chamomile (*Anthemis nobilis*), two tablespoons of honey and two tablespoons of apple cider vinegar, according to Cooksley. In a small dish, combine the essential oils and honey. Add the cider vinegar to the bath and then the honey mixture, which helps hold the oils together so they don't just float to the top of the water. Soak for 15 to 20 minutes, she suggests.

"Sandalwood is antibacterial, tea tree is a wide-spectrum antiseptic and chamomile is anti-inflammatory. When you sit in the bath, the whole combination of oils is very cooling and healing," she says.

Note: If you find you're allergic to any of the essential oils, omit it from the blend. To test for an allergy to an essential oil, place one drop of any essential oil on a cotton swab and wipe it on your inner forearm. If the area appears red or feels itchy within 30 minutes, don't use the oil.

Keep in mind that while an essential-oil soak will temporarily soothe your symptoms and complement medical treatment, it's not a substitute for antibiotics.

Get vital vitamins with a good multivitamin. Vitamins A and C and beta-carotene (the plant form of vitamin A), along with the mineral zinc, can strengthen your immune system. And the stronger your immune system, the better it will fight a urinary tract infection, notes Dr. Sullivan. She recommends 10,000 international units of vitamin A, 25,000 to 50,000 international units of beta-carotene and 30 to 50 milligrams of zinc a day. (Check with your doctor before taking amounts of zinc over 15 milligrams a day.)

Caution: Women who are pregnant should never take daily supplements of 10,000 international units or more of vitamin A and other women of childbearing age should check with their doctors before taking that much.

If you have a UTI (as opposed to an irritated bladder), Dr. Sullivan recommends taking 1,000 milligrams of vitamin C, which can help make the urine more acidic and less hospitable to bacteria. You can take that amount of vitamin C up to four times a day—but no more than that. More than 1,200 milligrams of vitamin C a day can cause diarrhea in some people.

Check your contraception. Some birth control methods may contribute to recurring urinary tract infections, says Dr. Fugh-Berman. Diaphragms may kink the urethra, causing urine to back up into the bladder, preventing the bladder from emptying completely. Also, spermicides may change the vaginal flora, causing an overgrowth of the bacteria E. coli, the most common cause of urinary tract infections, she explains.

VARICOSE VEINS AND SPIDER VEINS
Feel-Good Therapies for Pain and Splotches

Every year, Yvonne Williams dreaded summer. As warm weather approached, the 35-year-old wedding consultant from New York City worried about hiding her unsightly varicose veins.

"I would never wear shorts or skirts. Absolutely never," says Williams (who asked us not to use her real name). "I always wore pants, no matter how hot it was." Even dark-colored tights didn't help: The bulging veins in her calves were still noticeable, even through navy or jet-black tights.

For ten years, Williams lived with varicose veins—knotty, protruding, blue or purple veins that run along the lower legs, usually on the calves and behind the knees. Veins become varicose, or swollen, when valves along the vein's walls fail to do their job adequately. Normally these valves prevent blood from flowing back down when it's making a return trip to the heart. But when those valves start to weaken and gravity pulls blood toward the feet, the blood-vessel walls bulge like water-filled balloons. Blood pools in the lower legs, resulting in dull pain, heaviness and slight swelling of the ankles.

When Williams started to experience swelling, pain and night cramps in her legs, she decided to do something about her veins. First, she went the medical route. Her doctor performed sclerotherapy, in which an irritating fluid is injected into the troublesome veins. In response, the veins close, then shrivel and disappear. Her troubles were over—but only temporarily. For a more permanent and satisfactory solution, she still had miles to go.

A LEGACY YOU CAN AVOID

Varicose veins are hereditary—Williams's mother had them, and she, too, had undergone sclerotherapy. Williams's doctor told her that other veins in her legs could very likely become varicose since she was born with a predisposition to weak valves.

To prevent her healthy veins from giving her trouble, Williams's doctor prescribed calf raises and other exercises. Standing on a stack of books with her heels extended over the edge, Williams alternately raised herself on her toes and lowered her heels, repeating the exercise 50 to 100 times, once a day. She also made it a habit to raise up on her toes from time to time throughout the day, when she was standing. And she started walking 1½ miles a day, rain or shine.

Together, doing calf raises and walking improved Williams's blood circulation, pushing blood back toward her heart and preventing it from pooling in her legs. "The swelling in my legs never returned, and I don't get cramps at night," says Williams. "I finally started to wear shorts and skirts."

WHY GOOD VEINS GO BAD

The veins in your legs are some of the longest in the human body, where blood has to travel quite a distance on its way back to the heart. In most people, this is no problem. The veins in your legs are equipped with a series of 10 to 20 tiny valves that act like locks in a canal, allowing blood returning to the heart to collect at various points and then move on. In some people, however, these valves become faulty, so blood that was making its way up to your heart trickles back down. Over time, sections of your veins swell as the excess blood starts to collect.

Most people who get varicose veins are women. Evidently, the female hormone estrogen is partly to blame.

With the increased production of female hormones during pregnancy, the amount of blood coursing through your veins increases by a full 20 percent, overworking the valves. So having a baby—or several—is probably one of the biggest causes of varicose veins, says Luis Navarro, M.D., founder and director of the Vein Treatment Center and senior clinical instructor of surgery at Mount Sinai School of Medicine, both in New York City.

The weight of a growing fetus increases the resistence on blood that is traveling back to the heart; thus, blood is more likely to accumulate in the legs.

Or, you may reach the big 5-0 with nary a varicose vein in sight, only to experience problems later. No one is sure why, but as you get older, your blood vessels seem to lose elasticity. And if you work as a waitress, hairstylist, retail salesperson or in other occupations that keep you on your feet for hours, gravity will force blood to pool in your legs. This, together with a genetic predisposition to weak valves, can contribute to varicose veins, says Dr. Navarro.

TAKING ON THE PROTRUDING INTRUDERS

The key to relieving varicose veins is to take action early. "Once you have varicose veins, medical treatment is the only way to get rid of them," says Dr. Navarro. "But you can relieve symptoms and prevent them from getting worse."

Stock up on stockings. Elastic support hose not only hide varicose veins, they help some people's legs feel better by compressing the veins, says Dr. Navarro. The constant pressure of the stockings keeps blood from collecting in distended areas of the varicose veins and helps prevent aching and swelling.

The most effective support stockings are sold at medical supply stores and are available by prescription only. The amount of pressure the garment applies to your legs is rated numerically in millimeters of mercury (mm/Hg). The higher the number, the greater the pressure. Your doctor will prescribe what's right for you.

Put your calf muscles to work. Support hose feel great, but they only work while you're wearing them. For round-the-clock relief and prevention of varicose veins, exercise is easy and effective, says Dr. Navarro. Walking, running and cycling all help push stagnant blood from the bottom of the legs back to the heart.

"When you exercise your calf muscles, they act as a pump, taking over for weak valves," Dr. Navarro explains. "So the stronger your calf muscles, and the more you move them, the better."

Many women find that exercising on a regular basis helps to ease the pain and discomfort associated with varicose veins and can help prevent the condition from worsening.

Exercise while you sit. If you find yourself unable to get up and walk around at your office or in an airplane, for example, you can do simple exercises to help keep the blood in your legs pumping, says Dr. Navarro. Try this exercise once an hour: Flex your feet, lifting your toes while keeping your heels down, as though you're pumping a piano pedal. Repeat for a minute or two.

Invert your legs with yoga. Yoga poses that position your legs above your head can temporarily reverse the pooling of blood associated with varicose veins, says Carrie Angus, M.D., medical director for the Center for Health and Healing at the Himalayan International Institute of Yoga Science and Philosophy in Honesdale, Pennsylvania.

"Lie on the floor on your back, with your legs and feet raised up against a wall, for about five minutes," suggests Dr. Angus. "With this pose, gravity helps to push the blood back to the heart." To make this pose more comfortable, Dr. Angus suggests putting a pillow under your hips. Repeat once or twice a day. (If you have a history of back trouble, you may want to check with your doctor before trying this pose.)

Have some horse chestnut. The herb aescin, the extract from the dried seeds of the horse-chestnut plant, strengthens blood vessel walls, helping to prevent veins from softening and bulging, says Joseph Pizzorno, Jr., doctor of naturopathy and founding president of Bastyr University of Naturopathic Medicine in Seattle. "Horse-chestnut seed extract also reduces inflammation associated with varicose veins and stimulates regeneration of damaged veins," he notes. In a study of 240 people with varicose veins (194 of them women), taking 50 milligrams of aescin twice a day for 12 weeks reduced swelling in the lower legs by 25 percent.

Concentrate on fiber. Eating a high-fiber diet can take some of the pressure off varicose veins, notes Dr. Navarro. If you're constipated, you tend to push too much and too frequently when you have a bowel movement, which puts extra pressure on the valves of your legs. Chronic constipation can be one of the accelerating factors leading to varicose veins. "To relieve constipation, try a high-roughage diet with whole grains, like oats, barley, beans, peas, lentils, baked potato with the skin, brown rice and whole wheat, and plenty of vegetables and fruits," he says. Make sure that you increase your intake of water when you add fiber to your diet. Without water, adding fiber can make your constipation worse.

Seize your C. "To keep your veins healthy, you need to be sure that you're getting enough vitamin C, which is essential to strong blood vessels," says Dr. Angus. "I recommend 1,000 to 2,000 milligrams of vitamin C everyday to strengthen blood vessel walls and prevent bulging when they become distended with blood." Be careful though: Excess vitamin C may cause diarrhea in some people. If you get diarrhea, she says, cut back to between 500 to 1,000 milligrams per day.

Try an aromatic compress. Applying a cold compress soaked with witch hazel and essential oils to your legs helps soothe varicose veins, says Valerie Cooksley, R.N., holistic nurse and aroma practitioner in the Seattle area and author of *Aromatherapy: A Lifetime Guide to Healing with Essential Oils.*

To prepare the solution, put one-half cup to one cup of distilled witch-hazel lotion in a bowl and refrigerate it for at least one hour. Then add six drops of cypress (*Cupressus sempervirens*) essential oil, one drop of lemon (*Citrus limonum*) essential oil and one drop of bergamot (*Citrus bergamia*) essential oil. These oils and the cold witch hazel have an astringent effect—they shrink small blood vessels near the surface of the skin, temporarily reducing minor swelling, explains Cooksley.

To make the compress, soak a cloth in the bowl, then apply it to the affected area on your legs for 15 minutes. Elevate your feet on a few pillows as you apply the compress: That position helps the blood leave the legs and return to the heart. "The compress is very effective. You feel immediate relief as the swelling in the area goes down," she says.

Give homeopathy a try. Pulsatilla, a homeopathic remedy taken from the windflower plant, boosts circulation of stagnant blood, says Andrea Sullivan, Ph.D, a naturopathic and homeopathic physician in Washington, D.C. Recommended dosages vary from woman to woman. To determine how much you should take of this remedy, consult a homeopath or a naturopath, suggests Dr. Sullivan. Pulsatilla may not work for everyone with varicose veins, she says.

NATURAL STRATEGIES AGAINST SPIDER VEINS

At least 40 percent of women develop spider veins—networks of tiny red, blue or purple blood vessels that appear on the upper thighs, behind the knees and on the feet.

Spider veins appear when tiny blood vessels dilate near the surface of the skin, says David Green, M.D., a dermatologist at the Varicose Vein Center in Bethesda, Maryland. Most women would prefer to avoid them, if possible, since they are very unsightly.

As with varicose veins, one cause of spider veins could be the effect that the female hormone estrogen has on blood vessels. During pregnancy, nearly two-thirds of women will develop spider veins. About six weeks after delivery, pregnancy-caused spider veins usually disappear in most women.

Heredity also plays a role, says Dr. Green. "Ask a woman who has spider veins if her mom had them, and chances are that she says 'yes.'"

Spider veins may be a unsightly, but they rarely cause the pain and swelling of varicose veins, says Dr. Green.

Foods and Herbs to Try

Doctors treat the majority of spider veins the same way they do varicose veins—with sclerotherapy. But spider veins are like gray hairs—you can pluck them out as they appear, but that won't stop new ones from cropping up, says Dr. Green.

Alternative practitioners suggest a few strategies to help reduce the appearance of spider veins.

Put blueberries on your cereal. Eating foods like blueberries and raspberries provides bioflavonoids—natural compounds that help strengthen your blood vessels, says Dr. Pizzorno. "Bioflavonoids work with vitamin C and other nutrients in the body to help make capillaries less fragile." The darker the color of the fruit, like blackberries and cherries, the more bioflavonoids they have.

Eat all your grapefruit. The white membranes of citrus fruit such as oranges and grapefruit are also a rich source of bioflavonoids, says Dr. Pizzorno.

Go for ginkgo. Taking the herb ginkgo (*Ginkgo biloba*), which comes from the leaf of the ginkgo tree, also helps to strengthen the tissues that make up your vein walls, says Dr. Pizzorno. "Ginkgo is also high in bioflavonoids." Dr. Pizzorno recommends taking 40 milligrams of ginkgo three times a day for spider veins. These supplements are readily available in health food stores.

WHOLE-BODY CONDITIONS

Top Techniques for Head-to-Toe Complaints

Like many women who experience baffling medical conditions, 49-year-old massage and polarity therapist Kathy Johnson didn't know what to make of the bone-crushing tiredness that started to creep over her. It affected her whole body, making her feel perpetually achy and tired. And when it lingered for more than two weeks, she went to see her doctor.

According to her doctor, Johnson displayed many symptoms of the condition known as chronic fatigue syndrome (CFS). Most tellingly, she had headaches, a sore throat, short-term memory loss, muscle and joint pain and extreme tiredness.

"All the doctor told me to do was go home and rest," she recalls. "For the first year, I could barely move or do anything. I couldn't stand for longer than five minutes."

Johnson recalls how she felt, after a year of nearly total inactivity, when she found a new doctor who said he could help her. "I just sat in the doctor's office and cried tears of relief. I thought that I'd never work, never play and never read again. It was like being in a living coma," she says.

The doctor's next step was to put her on Cortef, a prescription anti-inflammatory supplement to ease her symptoms. To complement the medication, he also began giving her weekly vitamin B_{12} shots and started what Johnson describes as a "huge mega–vitamin and mineral regime" that included magnesium, iron, manganese and copper. On her doctor's recommendation, she drank at least eight glasses of water a day.

"Getting sick was like piling bricks on a wheelbarrow. You pile them on and on until one tumbles you over into illness," she says. "Getting back to health was like pulling one brick off at a time and figuring out what I needed. I had to look at my whole system to get better. I re-evaluated my mental, emotional and spiritual life and reorganized my life priorities."

Today, Johnson continues her regime, except for the B_{12} shots. She rates herself a "number seven on a scale of one to ten, with ten being great." The week that she found herself whitewater rafting and hiking in Colorado, Johnson knew that she'd won a major victory in her battle with CFS.

UNRAVELING THE SECRETS OF WELLNESS

Johnson was actually lucky to be diagnosed in the first place, says Arthur Brownstein, M.D., medical director of the Princeville Medical Clinic in Princeville, Hawaii. Conditions like chronic fatigue, body aches, chronic pain, insomnia and fatigue are often puzzling because they affect the whole body and it's difficult to pinpoint specific problems.

"Unfortunately, conventional doctors today aren't too familiar with how the body works as a whole," observes Dr. Brownstein. "Healing systems in other cultures have more of an awareness of the interconnectedness of everything in the body." Because of specialization, that's far less likely to be true in Western medicine, he notes. "Here, someone like a cardiologist may know everything there is to know about the heart but very little about what's going on in the rest of the body."

Here's a typical sequence, as Dr. Brownstein describes it: "A doctor will say, 'Well, it's not a kidney problem, so we'll send you to a neurologist.' The neurologist says, 'I can't find anything wrong with your brain, so I'll send you to a psychiatrist.' And you end up on industrial-strength tranquilizers. It suppresses your symptoms but crushes your spirit."

Chronic fatigue is a hard-to-diagnose medical puzzle. Other whole-body problems, such as insomnia, general aches and pains and nicotine addiction, are easy to diagnose but difficult to treat.

But where patent prescriptions and conventional therapy might not address such problems effectively, natural therapies can step in to help relieve whole-body problems. (Or, in many cases, work in concert with mainstream medicine to optimize recovery.) Acupuncture, for instance, triggers the release of brain chemicals such as endorphins and serotonin, which can help relieve chronic pain and even counteract nicotine addiction that comes from smoking. Meditation and visualization both help calm your nervous system to reduce pain as well as stress and tension. And yoga, which relaxes, stretches and tones your body, helps ease body aches while easing fatigue.

"In alternative therapies, practitioners realize that the last expression of disease is the body. It started somewhere else, maybe with stress or anxiety or sadness, and is finally expressing itself physically," says Dr. Brownstein. "You need to look at the whole person—lifestyle, diet, family relationships and everything that affects her life—before you can begin to cure what's ailing her."

ACHES: EASY STEPS TO RELIEF

Sometimes it feels like someone stole the spring out of your step and replaced it with a rusty hinge. Soon the aching has clipped your knees and snagged your shoulders, and at its worst, the feeling of affliction just won't go away.

What causes these body aches? Aging is certainly a factor, but there are other explanations as well. The biggest cause for the avalanche of aches as we age is inactivity rather than the passage of time, says Dr. Brownstein. "We've discovered that 98 percent of the pain of arthritis comes from the muscles around the joints being rigid, stiff and tight from lack of movement and stretching."

And even if you don't have arthritis, you're just asking for aches if you stay inactive. The health of the knees, hips, shoulders and back is determined by the condition of the muscles around them, says Dr. Brownstein. "If you stretch the muscles around the joint, you increase the joint's range of motion, which improves the flow of the synovial fluid in the joints that lubricates and nourishes them, reducing aches and promoting healing."

If you both work your body and baby it afterward, you can make body aches a part of your past. Here's what works.

Stretch with yoga. Doing yoga stretches can help ease or even prevent most body aches, says Richard C. Miller, Ph.D., yoga instructor and psychologist in San Rafael, California, co-founder of the International Association of Yoga Therapists and founder of the Marin School of Yoga. You should do yoga stretches for the back, legs, shoulders and hips—the major areas of the body, he recommends. Here are the stretches that he suggests.

- Stand with your arms over your head, feet shoulder-width apart. Then bend to the left, exhaling as you move. Hold this pose for three seconds and inhale as you return to an upright position. Repeat the stretch, bending to the right. Repeat three or four times, alternately bending left, then right.
- Place your hands on your lower back and lift your chest, gently bending backward, inhaling as you go. Hold for a few seconds, then come upright again, exhaling on your way back up. Repeat three times.
- With hands still on your lower back and your legs shoulder-width apart, bend your knees slightly and lean forward, as far as is comfortable. Exhale as you bend forward. Remain in the pose for three seconds, then straighten up, inhaling as you come up. Repeat three times.

Move your body. Get out and walk briskly for 30 minutes or more at least three times a week, suggests Adriane Fugh-Berman, M.D., former head of field investigations for the Office of Alternative Medicine at the National Institutes of Health in Bethesda, Maryland. She recommends walking instead of driving whenever possible and climbing the stairs at work instead of taking the elevator. Regular walking and climbing help prevent aches.

"About 90 percent of all your aches are a result of not moving your body," agrees Dr. Brownstein. "People store tension in their shoulders and upper backs, which over time results in aches. Movement and stretching help to release that tension."

Spice up your baths. Want a quick relief from aches? Sprinkle powdered ginger into a tub of warm water and climb in for a good, long soak, suggests Mary Muryn, aromatherapist and certified teacher of polarity and reflexology in Westport, Connecticut. She recommends an ounce of powdered ginger (available in supermarkets) sprinkled into your bath, for a 20-minute soak.

"For some reason, when ginger is combined with water, it gives the feeling of heat, which warms up your body and your bones and eases aches," Muryn notes.

Epsom-ize your bath. Here's a way to bathe away aches and pains accompanied by minor swelling: Pour six cups of Epsom salts into a tub filled with warm water, dissolve it well, then soak for 20 minutes and rinse with cool water, suggests Charles Thomas, Ph.D., administrator of the Desert Hot Springs Therapy Center in Desert Hot Springs, California.

For general aches, this treatment should be done no more than three times a week, always allowing one day of rest in between. (According to Dr. Thomas, Epsom salts lowers blood pressure, so after a series of three or four treatments, you may feel fatigued. If this occurs, do not repeat the treatment, he advises.) Epsom salts, chemically known as magnesium sulfate, helps to draw out carbon—one of the waste products of your body—through your pores. When the waste is removed from your muscles, your aches feel better, says Dr. Thomas.

Massage it. Getting your muscles massaged is a relaxing way of overcoming aches, notes Vincent Iuppo, doctor of naturopathy and director of the Morris Institute of Natural Therapeutics in Denville, New Jersey. Massage helps release lactic acids—substances produced during the processing of fat and glucose (a simple sugar in the body). When lactic acids build up in muscles due to overuse, they cause soreness, says Dr. Iuppo. "Massage releases the lactic acids and lets them be carried throughout your system." Eventually, the lactic acids are carried out in your urine. So massage helps your body rid itself of lactic acids faster.

ALCOHOL OVERUSE: NO MORE HANGOVERS—EVER

If you reach for a glass of wine every time you're stressed, are you an alcoholic? If you have to drink before every social gathering to "get your courage up," does that mean you're an alcoholic? Not necessarily, but it could mean that you have a drinking problem, says Jean Kirkpatrick, Ph.D., director and founder of Women for Sobriety, an organization of support groups for women alcoholics, headquartered in Quakertown, Pennsylvania.

A problem drinker, according to Dr. Kirkpatrick, is anyone who has come to rely on alcohol to deal with her problems, such as stress or social shyness, but who can still quit. The need to drink hasn't yet become overwhelming and compulsive, the way that it has for an alcoholic, she says. "Good advice for problem drinkers is to check for patterns, like needing to drink every night to unwind when you get home from work. Those are the patterns that can turn into alcoholism if not brought into check."

It's nearly impossible to track figures on how many women are problem drinkers because they're usually in denial about it in the first place, says Dr. Kirkpatrick. But more women than men seem to have a problem with negative self-image, says Dr. Kirkpatrick. And she links that to problem drinking, noting that a lot of women start drinking to feel less shy, to lose their inhibitions and to gain confidence.

One thing is certain: Even moderate drinkers—women who consume two glasses of alcohol a day—are at increased risk of developing such health problems as esophageal and liver cancer, high blood pressure and cardiomyopathy (disease of the heart muscle).

If you would like to get some help before your drinking spins out of control, you have many support groups and cutting-edge therapies to choose from. If you've become compulsive about drinking or your need for alcohol is overwhelming, you should seek professional treatment. Here are some experts' recommendations, which work well as an adjunct to therapy for problem drinkers.

Build that self-esteem. Cognitive therapy sessions with a counselor can help change the negative way that you think about yourself so you won't be as compelled to drink, says Judith Beck, Ph.D., director of the Beck Institute for Cognitive Therapy and Research and clinical assistant professor of psychology in psychiatry at the University of Pennsylvania in Philadelphia.

"At the bottom of alcoholism is a terrible self-concept or sense of helplessness that makes people want to drink to change who they are or their reactions to life circumstances," Dr. Beck observes. (To find out how cognitive therapy can help you develop a more positive self-image, see page 79.)

Mix in some acupuncture. You can curb cravings for alcohol with acupuncture, according to Lixing Lao, M.D., Ph.D., licensed acupuncturist and assistant professor in the Department of Family Medicine at the University of Maryland in Baltimore.

"Acupuncture causes the brain to release chemicals such as dopamine, which acts as a transmitter for the body's nervous system, and endorphins (the body's natural painkillers), which may help squash the desire for alcohol," he says. These soothing chemicals also ease symptoms, such as anxiety, irritability and insomnia, that heavy drinkers often experience when they stop consuming alcohol. Acupuncture helps you through these withdrawal symptoms by helping you to relax.

Handy Hints for Healing Hangovers

Welcome to Hangover Hell. It's a place where the sound of a newspaper rustling can make your head throb, a plain saltine cracker is too rich for your nauseated stomach and your bed is the only place that offers comfort.

Hopefully, you rarely visit this land of headaches, upset stomachs and general shakiness. But on occasion, one too many glasses of champagne can leave you with severe regrets—and symptoms—the morning after.

Hangovers sound harmless, but they're actually caused by toxins, says Paul Mittman, doctor of naturopathy in private practice in Enfield, Connecticut. When your liver breaks down the alcohol that you've ingested, toxins are released into your blood that contribute to the headaches and stomachaches, he notes.

Just how much alcohol is too much? "Some people drink just two drinks and get a hangover," says Alan Rapoport, M.D., director of the New England Center for Headache in Stamford, Connecticut, and assistant clinical professor of neurology at Yale University School of Medicine. "For others, tolerance is much higher. It has to do with how much you're used to drinking."

And people who weigh less tend to get worse hangovers, says Dr. Rapoport. In a smaller person, the alcohol is more concentrated and not as diluted by bodily fluids, he explains. That could explain why a woman who weighs, say, 125 pounds, may feel worse after a night on the town than her buddy, a 200-pound guy.

The best way to avoid a hangover is not to overindulge in the first place—or to have fewer drinks spaced over a long period of time. But if you're heading out for a night on the town where champagne is

Activate your alpha waves. Biofeedback can curb your alcohol craving by altering your brain waves, says Dale Walters, Ph.D., former director of education in the Applied Psychophysiology and Biofeedback Center at the Menninger Clinic in Topeka, Kansas. When you're in the first stages of relaxation, alpha waves are dominant, but once you're extremely still and drowsy, theta waves become dominant, he notes. Beta brain waves, however, dominate your brain when you're actively thinking and doing things, just as delta waves dominate when you're sleeping.

For some reason, alcoholics' brains tend to give off the activity-oriented beta waves more often than the relaxing alpha or theta waves, Dr. Walters notes. "If alcoholics want to really let go and relax, they often don't have

flowing freely, or any alcohol for that matter, Dr. Rapoport recommends keeping overall alcohol content low by diluting your drinks with water. Make sure that you drink at least 12 ounces of water an hour while you're drinking alcohol, he says. "Also, before you go to bed on a night that you've been drinking, you should drink as much water as possible."

It's also wise to eat cheese or drink milk before you start drinking. These foods give your stomach a protective coating against alcohol, says Dr. Rapoport. And you'll be better off if you consume fructose, a natural sugar found in fruits and vegetables, before you start drinking, he adds. Fructose may break down the alcohol in your bloodstream faster so it won't be as strong. He recommends eating apples, grapes and tomatoes or drinking apple, grape and tomato juice.

But what if you do get a hangover, despite all your precautions? Here's what experts advise.

Take time for tea. Spearmint or peppermint tea soothes a case of hangover nausea, says Willard Dean, M.D., medical director of the Center for Self Healing in Santa Fe, New Mexico, and author of "The Immune System," one in a series of booklets titled *The Holistic Health Series*. These mint teas soothe and settle the stomach, he notes. "Plus, you're taking in fluid, which flushes the residue of alcohol out of your bloodstream and body."

Press the point. Pressing on an acupressure point on your wrist can momentarily control the nausea of a hangover, says Dr. Dean. "Find the midway point on the inside of your wrist and press on it with your thumb for 20 to 30 seconds. That acupressure point on the wrist is the meridian that corresponds with your stomach."

the relaxing brain waves to do it. So what do they do for relief and comfort? They drink."

Research suggests that low doses of alcohol intake are related to increases in alpha rhythms and that moderate to high amounts increase delta and theta rhythms.

Biofeedback helps teach alcoholics to increase alpha and theta waves through relaxation instead of drinking, says Dr. Walters. With electrodes attached to your scalp, you hear a high-pitched tone when alpha waves are present. As you practice relaxation—by repeating phrases like, "My mind is quiet," or focusing on slow breathing—you learn to increase the presence of that brain wave more often as indicated by the tone, he explains.

It usually takes an average of thirty 30-minute brain-wave training ses-

For Women Only
An Alternative to AA

Though Jean Kirkpatrick, Ph.D., had been to Alcoholics Anonymous (AA) meetings, she felt that they always lacked something. As a woman surrounded by men, she never felt comfortable talking about problems involving deeply personal issues.

So in 1976, she founded Women for Sobriety, based in Quakertown, Pennsylvania. It's an all-woman support group, so women can seek help with their drinking problems and feel secure in the knowledge that they're surrounded by other women.

"It became clear to me that women need something different for recovery than men do. I'd say 50 to 60 percent of women alcoholics have problems with sexual abuse and incest—not something you'd talk about in a mixed group," she says.

Today, you can find some 300 Women for Sobriety programs around the world, including Australia and Ireland, with membership totaling about 5,000 women. Groups meet once a week for 60 to 90 minutes, says Dr. Kirkpatrick.

Women for Sobriety has a 13-statement program that's the philosophical opposite of Alcoholics Anonymous' 12-step program, explains Dr. Kirkpatrick. "In AA you stand up and tell your story about how you first started to drink. That just brings back guilt. Our statement is that the past is gone forever—you need to start now to rebuild your life." Another difference is that Women for Sobriety doesn't require lifetime attendance, the way that AA does.

"Our program's basis is teaching women to be empowered and to realize their strengths," says Dr. Kirkpatrick.

sions (five a week for six weeks) to produce a nearly normal brain-wave function as indicated by increased alpha waves, says Dr. Walters.

A study compared ten alcoholics who had brain-wave biofeedback for two weeks with ten who did individual and group therapy for one month, notes Dr. Walters. After 13 months, 80 percent of the biofeedback group was still sober. In the other group, 80 percent had gone back to drinking.

Seek a support group. Support groups such as Alcoholics Anonymous and Women for Sobriety have chapters in nearly every city in the United States, Dr. Kirkpatrick points out. "Support groups are like a surrogate family. You spend time with people who have the same problem, with whom you can discuss the most intimate details of your life, without being judged."

Picture yourself alcohol-free. Visualizing yourself rejecting a drink can teach you how to avoid alcohol, says Dr. Walters. "We teach people to picture a scene where they're ready to buy alcohol at the store, then turn around, take a deep breath and walk away. We also have them visualize being confident and at ease in a social setting, since many people drink to overcome social shyness." This imagery can be done for a minute whenever the craving for a drink pops into your head, he says.

Write an alcohol-free anthem. Songwriting can help you to understand yourself and your drinking problem, says Barbara J. Crowe, a registered music therapist and director and professor of music therapy at Arizona State University in Tempe. "You can write songs about feelings of anxiety and fear, which may have led you to start drinking."

Play a sobriety sonata. Music itself can be a drink substitute, says Crowe. "We show people that there are ways of getting a high other than drinking." From a music therapist you can easily learn to play such instruments as hand drums or conga drums. Sometimes people with drinking problems meet in a music therapy group session to play the drums. That helps give them the sense of community that going out to bars may have provided, she notes.

CHRONIC PAIN: TAME THE ENDLESS HURT

Pain is bad enough, but what if you suffer from frequent or constant pain that makes it difficult to do your job or to do things with your family or to sleep at night? That's called chronic pain, says Stanley Krippner, Ph.D., professor of psychology at the Saybrook Institute in San Francisco.

Some of the most common causes of chronic pain are migraines, back pain, injuries from auto accidents, falls or sports injuries, joint pain, temporomandibular disorder (a severe pain in the jaw joint), endometriosis (a painful condition in which bits of the uterus grow outside the uterus), interstitial cystitis (a chronic, severe inflammation of the bladder) and irritable bowel syndrome.

Chronic pain is depressing and frustrating, says Ann Berger, M.D., assistant professor of oncology and anesthesiology at the Cooper Hospital Pain Management Clinic in Camden, New Jersey. The psychological toll can be great. Loneliness, social isolation and possible loss of job and financial support can all make chronic pain that much more intolerable, she notes.

Natural therapies help calm the body's nervous system, which feels pain more intensely when its overly aroused, says Dr. Krippner. When you're in pain, your body releases hormones from the endocrine system, such as adrenaline from the adrenal gland and other pain-intensifying hormones from the pituitary, thyroid and parathyroid glands, notes Dr. Krippner. These hormones stay in the system for a long time, essentially "reminding" your body of ongoing pain. For reasons that doctors don't quite understand, these hormones hang around if you're tense or agitated but leave your system if you're in a relaxed state. That means that the sensation of pain will fade away more quickly if you're relaxed, he explains.

And that's where biofeedback can help, training your body to relax. It's an especially effective therapy for tension or migraine headaches, temporomandibular disorder and irritable bowel syndrome, according to practitioners.

The other effective therapies are visualization and meditation. Visualization can help reduce the pain of endometriosis. Meditation can help women deal with the pain of irritable bowel syndrome or vascular disorders such as Raynaud's Syndrome or migraine headaches.

A panel from the National Institutes of Health explained the calming effect that relaxation techniques have on the body. Therapies like meditation and biofeedback calm the sympathetic nervous system, which regulates heart rate and pulse. The result is lowered oxygen consumption and blood pressure and a slower breathing rate and heart rate, the panel's report concluded.

The panel also found that natural therapies can create more of the relaxing alpha and theta brain waves that help calm the nervous system. So if you're in the throes of chronic pain, you do have options apart from or in addition to painkilling medications. Here are some of your choices.

Meditate your pain away. Daily meditation can be the key to transforming your perception of and attitudes toward physical pain, says David Nichol, M.D., a psychiatrist in private practice in Topeka, Kansas. "As little as a minute, or preferably five to ten minutes, of meditation throughout the day can bring substantial improvements." (For more information on how to meditate, see page 233.)

Escape with music. Listening to music can also distract you from pain, says Crowe. "If you let your mind focus on the music, it can take your thoughts away from the pain, even if only briefly." You want to choose music with interesting lyrics or melodies so you can focus your attention on them. Listening to any music that relaxes you or puts you in a good mood should help ease your pain.

Breathe out. Since stress overly arouses your nervous system by increasing heart rate and speeding up breathing and pulse, learning to relax with deep-breathing exercises can tame your pain, says Thomas Rudy, Ph.D., director of the Pain Evaluation and Treatment Institute at the University of Pittsburgh Medical Center. Practice deep breathing for a couple of minutes at least three times a day and in advance of when you know you're apt to hurt the most, he says. For example, if you know that migraine headaches usually come on right after work, find a quiet place about five minutes before the end of your workday, sit down and do your deep breathing. (For more information on deep breathing, see page 67.)

Imagine away pain. Before your body gets too tensed up with pain, you can relax considerably by using imagery, says Dr. Rudy. When your pain begins, spend a few minutes in a quiet place with your eyes closed and mentally picture a relaxing scene, like a walk in the woods or a picnic in a meadow, or create your own relaxing image of a favorite place.

Exercise your right to comfort. Getting plenty of activity is important in releasing endorphins—your body's natural painkillers, says Dr. Krippner. The endorphins raise your pain threshold, which is the level at which you first become aware of the feeling of pain. Endorphins also calm you. "They produce a sense of well-being that temporarily overrides the pain for a while after you've exercised," adds Dr. Krippner. For this reason he recommends scheduling 20 to 30 minutes of exercise six days a week. If pain increases, stop and call your doctor, he says.

A study in Norway involving 16 women with chronic pain of the muscles, bones and joints shows that exercise does lessen pain. When the women did indoor physical aerobic exercise to music twice a week, they reported feeling less pain after 12 weeks of exercise than they did when they started.

Ask for acupuncture. Acupuncture increases the body's production of pain-suppressing brain chemicals like serotonin and endorphins, says Dr. Lao. "It's very hard to explain in Western terms, but in acupuncture, you stimulate various points on the body with needles, and the body responds by sending signals to the brain, which releases the chemicals."

FATIGUE AND CHRONIC FATIGUE: BEAT THE BLAHS

Poll any group of women about their health and chances are, eight out of ten will say that they're tired. Ask them why and they'll tell you that they have too much to do and too little time to do it. Or maybe they're not getting enough sleep at night. Or maybe the cause is anemia, which is a lack of red blood cells in the blood. Other possible causes are depression or problems of the thyroid, a gland that regulates how your body uses its fuel.

But a frequent cause of fatigue is the stress that you get when you have job problems or family conflicts, says Reed Moskowitz, M.D., founder and medical director of Stress Disorders Services at New York University Medical Center in New York City.

You can attribute your reactions to stress to the fight-or-flight response, a built-in reflex in which your body produces excess adrenaline and other hormones. The sudden release of these hormones is in response to a situation that makes you tense or fearful. Your heart beats faster and these hormones momentarily energize your body, explains Dr. Moskowitz.

"This biological response was only designed to be a short-term reaction to stress. These days, we're chronically running on adrenaline, with deadlines, long workdays and traffic jams," notes Dr. Moskowitz. "We get fatigued because our bodies are not designed to run long-term on the fight-or-flight response. The expenditure of energy over time can burn you out."

If you go to an alternative practitioner complaining of fatigue, chances are, she'll know all about the stress connection. Once traditional medical causes are ruled out, she'll emphasize that learning to relax, unwind and energize yourself are the best cures for a simple case of fatigue. Here are some experts' suggestions.

Breathe out stress. Relax your body with a quick abdominal exhalation of breath (one or two every second), says Dr. Miller. (With each exhalation, the abdomen should contract.) "Relax on each inhale." Because you're breathing with your abdomen and diaphragm, you're calming the sympathetic nervous system that regulates your blood pressure and pulse. With a regulated heart rate and pulse, your body will feel more relaxed and energized.

Take a whiff. Inhaling the scent of peppermint is a quick temporary pick-me-up, says Muryn. "Peppermint is a positive stimulant oil, which means that it gives you a temporary lift when you inhale it. You can use a diffuser, an air pump that blows out particles of the essential oils into the air." Put the diffuser at your desk in the office or in your living room at home—wherever you feel tired most often.

  Take a blah-beating bath. If you wake up feeling like you've hardly rested, try climbing into a bath that's been scented with lemon and lavender oil. "The invigorating scents of lavender and lemon are a real rejuvenator," says Muyrn. Add ten drops of lavender and ten of lemon to very warm (but not hot) water, and soak for 20 minutes.

Press your reflexology points. Just pressing on the sole of your foot for a few seconds can temporarily ease fatigue, says Muryn. When you're stressed at work, slip off your shoe and press in the very center of the arch of your foot with your knuckles. Repeat on the other side. According to Muryn, the pressure on the sole of your foot momentarily stimulates your adrenal gland into releasing the adrenaline that increases heartbeat and blood pressure. "That wakes you up." If you don't want to take your shoes off at work, the same technique can be used on the hand. Apply pressure to the center of the palm or your hand for a quick boost, she says.

Yoga your way to rest. Easing fatigue is as simple as lying on the floor, says Carrie Angus, M.D, medical director for the Center for Health and Healing at the Himalayan International Institute of Yoga Science and Philosophy in Honesdale, Pennsylvania. In yoga the flat-on-your-back position is appropriately called the corpse pose.

Simply lie flat with your feet separated about 24 inches apart and your hands relaxed alongside your body with your palms up.

"Just lie there for about five minutes and breathe slowly," suggests Dr. Angus. If you take a class in hatha yoga, the most popular form, it will probably start and end with that pose. "You're utterly at rest, letting your tensions go."

You can modify the corpse pose by putting a pillow under your knees for comfort. Or put cushions under the small of your back, suggests Dr. Angus. If you're not used to yoga, you may have a tough time lying flat on a hard floor for that long, she notes.

Chronic Fatigue Syndrome: Reclaim Your Life

There's tired and then there's bone-aching, want-to-hibernate-in-bed-all-day, mind-blurring fatigue. If you've had deep-down fatigue like that for four months or more, you might have Chronic Fatigue Immune Dysfunction Syndrome (commonly referred to as chronic fatigue syndrome).

This mysterious disorder, defined as persistent fatigue that's not a result of ongoing exertion and isn't helped by rest, grabs you by the collar and doesn't let go. No one knows just what triggers chronic fatigue syndrome, but doctors do know that eight out of nine of those who get it are women, says Jacob Teitelbaum, M.D., clinician and researcher on the treatment of chronic fatigue syndrome at Anne Arundel Medical Center in Annapolis, Maryland, and author of *From Fatigued to Fantastic!*

How do you know if you have chronic fatigue syndrome? Only a specialist can tell for sure, and even some M.D.'s will disagree. But you should look for a diagnosis if you've experienced at least four out of the following seven symptoms: short-term memory loss, sore throats, muscle pain, joint pain, headaches, unrefreshing sleep and tiredness after exertion that lasts for more than 24 hours.

Chronic fatigue can be a puzzling disorder, notes Dr. Teitelbaum, who himself once had chronic fatigue syndrome. "Usually, women who've been diagnosed with chronic fatigue look fine, so they don't get the same understanding as, say, someone diagnosed with cancer would. To have an illness that leaves you disabled and unable to do the basic things in life—and then having to fight for compassion because there's no blood test to diagnose the disease—is very sad," he adds.

If you do have CFS, it might seem like nothing can ease your crushing exhaustion. But Dr. Teitelbaum recommends some definite steps toward feeling better. Here's his how-to list.

Supplement your health. Taking certain vitamins and minerals gives your energy-zapped body a boost, says Dr. Teitelbaum. He recommends getting a weekly shot of 1,000 micrograms of B_{12} for ten weeks. That's because a shortage of B_{12} can cause fatigue, confusion, muscle aches, numbness of the arms and legs and poor memory. If you can't get the injection, Dr. Teitelbaum recommends taking a 1,000-microgram supplement of B_{12} once a day.

In addition, here's what he suggests for daily vitamin and mineral supplements.

- 300 milligrams of magnesium in the form of magnesium glycinate, magnesium chloride or magnesium lactate—supplements that help muscles relax. (People with heart or kidney problems should not take supplemental magnesium.)
- 18 milligrams of iron, which helps battle the shortage-of-red-blood-cells problem, anemia. (Anemia can cause a tiredness that further aggravates chronic fatigue.) Additional iron also helps improve mental clarity.
- 5 milligrams of manganese. According to Dr. Teitelbaum, it's not clear how manganese functions, but it does seem to work in conjunction with other vitamins and minerals to help combat CFS symptoms.
- 2 to 3 milligrams of copper. You need this mineral because lack of copper can cause joint inflammation as well as other kinds of inflammation, according to Dr. Teitelbaum.

Go with the (H$_2$O) flow. Because dehydration often accompanies chronic fatigue and even makes it worse, getting plenty of water every day is vital, according to Dr. Teitelbaum. People with CSF often have a malfunctioning hypothalamus, which is the part of the brain that controls thirst, body temperature and other vital functions such as blood pressure, he notes. To prevent dehydration, Dr. Teitelbaum recommends a slight increase in salt intake as well as an increase in your water consumption. You will need to carry a water bottle with you wherever you go to remind yourself to keep drinking. He recommends that you try to get at least 64 to 96 ounces of water each day. That's about 8 to 12 full glasses.

Beware of food allergies. For reasons unknown to doctors, many women's chronic fatigue is made worse by food allergies, says Dr. Teitelbaum. To see if that's the case with you, he suggests avoiding the most common problem foods: milk, wheat, eggs, citrus, sugar, alcohol, chocolate and coffee. Before you feel better, you'll probably go through a withdrawal period and feel worse for the first seven to ten days after cutting these foods out of your diet, he notes. But be patient. After ten days of deprivation, Dr. Teitelbaum says, you can start reintroducing one of the eliminated foods every few days to figure out which ones are contributing to the problem.

Go for the garlic. Garlic is an effective anti-infectious agent. That's important, says Dr. Teitelbaum, because chronic fatigue makes you exceptionally susceptible to bowel infections, including parasitic, yeast and bacterial infections.

Garlic has the active infection-fighting ingredient allicin, but you should eat it raw if you want to get the antiviral benefit, Dr. Teitelbaum notes. Here's one way that he recommends: "Crush one to two cloves of garlic, add it to a small amount of olive oil to taste and dip your bread into it instead of using butter."

Stroll toward relief. Getting out and walking every day, even for just a few minutes, is vital in helping someone with chronic fatigue feel energized, says Dr. Teitelbaum. Women with chronic fatigue are often out of condition because they feel too tired to exercise, which simply results in further deconditioning, he says.

"Start with three minutes of walking a day and increase that every three days by three to five minutes," advises Dr. Teitelbaum. "If you feel better the next day, good. But if it feels like you've been hit by a truck, cut back the amount and do as much as you can." Assuming that you can steadily increase your walking time, you might be striding along for a half-hour or so by the end of the month.

INSOMNIA: SAFE SOLUTIONS

Just as you have many reasons for not being able to sleep at night, there are many types of insomnia, says John Zimmerman, Ph.D., owner of Sleep Recording Services and laboratory director of the Sleep Disorder Center, both in Reno, Nevada, and a polysomnographer at the Mountain Medical Sleep Disorders Center in Carson City, Nevada.

For instance, some women have the kind of insomnia where it just takes a lot of time to fall asleep—often, more than 20 to 30 minutes. Others wake up from sleep repeatedly—usually twice or more every night. And then there are some women with insomnia who fall asleep soon enough but wake up between 2:00 and 5:00 A.M. and can't fall back to sleep.

What links these different kinds of insomnia? They're all symptoms of some other problem in your life, says Dr. Zimmerman. Insomnia could be a sign of anxiety, which results in delayed sleep, or a sign of depression, which usually results in the form of insomnia where you wake up very early and can't fall asleep again.

Insomnia could also be a sign of dropping estrogen levels, says Alex Clerk, M.D., director of the Stanford University Sleep Disorders Clinic. "We have found that after age 30, women begin to have more complaints of insomnia than men do. We don't know why, but we suspect that a slight decrease in the female hormone estrogen—starting at around that age— is one thing that can contribute to it."

Another condition linked with women's insomnia is menopause, says Irina Zhdanova, M.D., Ph.D., research scientist in the Department of Brain and Cognitive Sciences at the Massachusetts Institute of Technology in Cambridge. During menopause, some women are frequently awakened by night sweats, notes Dr. Zhdanova. For others, the psychological stress of going through that change of life is enough to cause insomnia, she adds.

Another reason that insomnia goes hand-in-hand with aging is that older people have decreased levels of melatonin, a hormone that helps regulate sleep. This hormone begins decreasing with age in both men and women, Dr. Zhdanova notes.

Whatever your age, if you have a problem with insomnia, you might be lured by claims of sleeping-pill producers that the solution to restless nights can be found in a bottle. But according to Dr. Zimmerman, you can easily build up a psychological dependence on sleeping pills if you believe that you can't fall asleep without them. "Every sleep researcher says don't use sleeping pills for more than a few weeks, and then only for sleep to help you through a traumatic event," he cautions.

Besides, doctors and researchers say that there are safe and natural ways to reclaim a sound slumber. Here's what they recommend.

Exhale deeply for deep sleep. Taking long, abdominal exhalations while sitting up in bed at night can help lull you to sleep, says Dr. Miller.

To do this, breathe out through your nose. When you inhale, let your head nod slightly upward, and when you exhale, drop your head slightly downward. This movement stimulates the reflex in the brain that controls sleep, says Dr. Miller.

Try a lullaby. If you listen to soothing music, maybe you won't obsess about the fact that you can't fall asleep, says Crowe. "Go for rather predictable music with simple, slow melodies," she advises. This way, your mind is centered on the music and not mulling over whatever happened during your day.

Lighten up. Getting a dose of early-morning sunlight adjusts your body's inner alarm clock so that you'll want to fall asleep earlier that night, says Michael Terman, Ph.D., director of the winter depression program and the light therapy unit at Columbia-Presbyterian Medical Center in New York City.

If you wake before dawn or if you can't get out into direct sunlight, spend a half-hour in front of a light box first thing in the morning, suggests Dr. Terman. That helps normalize your body's inner alarm clock. (For details on using a light box, see page 212.) "People often oversleep because it took them a long time to fall asleep the night before," he says. "But the light therapy moves your internal clock to an earlier hour. If you can get up earlier, you'll start feeling drowsy earlier in the night."

Keep yourself in the dark. A natural way of increasing your sleep-inducing natural melatonin is to keep your bedroom as dark as possible at night, says Suzanne Woodward, Ph.D., associate professor of psychiatry at Wayne State University School of Medicine in Detroit. It's darkness, not sleepiness, that spurs melatonin production in the brain, she notes. "Pull down the shades and wear an eye mask. When it's bright, you suppress the natural melatonin given off by your brain."

Ask about melatonin supplements. If all else fails, taking melatonin supplements can be a remedy for insomnia, but only if you have a melatonin deficiency and only if it's taken cautiously with a doctor's supervision, advises Dr. Zhdanova. "The main danger is that melatonin is not regulated by the FDA (Food and Drug Administration), so you can't be sure that you're getting pure melatonin." If you take melatonin, stop if you experience headaches, dizziness or nightmares.

Although people over age 50 do have a melatonin deficiency, it would be a good idea to have a doctor test you for a deficiency before you start taking melatonin, Dr. Zhdanova adds. The problem is, the test is not widely available.

LUPUS: BIG HELP FROM A LITTLE SEED

Nothing's more disheartening than having a good friend turn on you. And that's sort of what happens with lupus, an incurable disease that can inflame your small blood vessels, kidneys, skin, joints and other tissues.

Lupus is an autoimmune disease, like rheumatoid arthritis or multiple sclerosis, in which the body attacks its own tissues as if they were foreign substances, says Lawrence DuBuske, M.D., clinical instructor of allergy and immunology at Harvard Medical School Brigham and Women's Hospital in Boston.

Lupus strikes women five times as often as it does men. Most people who get it are in their twenties to forties. Among the first symptoms are tiredness, a butterfly-shaped rash on the face and a rash on the body due to sun exposure, says Dr. DuBuske.

A new, more sophisticated blood test is helping doctors detect this disease, says William Clark, M.D., chief of nephrology at Victoria Hospital in London, Ontario. Since lupus is sometimes confused with arthritis, this

---

How I Healed Myself **Naturally**

Acupuncture:
When the Point's Better Health

Gwenn Chriss, 53, a social worker in Plymouth, Minnesota, credits acupuncture with relieving the debilitating symptoms of lupus.

"Though I'd been showing symptoms of lupus for 25 years, I finally got to the point where I thought I couldn't work anymore," says Chriss. "Then I tried acupuncture. For the first six months, I had acupuncture treatments three times a week. Then, for a year, it was twice a week. Now I go once a week.

"I can't go for more than eight days without treatment because of increased joint pain and muscle pain and trouble sleeping," she notes.

"I used to swim a mile three times a week until the fatigue and pain became too bad. Then I could only swim one to two lengths of the pool. After four months of acupuncture, I was able to swim three-quarters of a mile. Now my rheumatologist believes that the treatments are what has made me not only able to work but has kept me off steroids, which are very damaging medications. My quality of life has significantly improved."

test is an important diagnostic tool. So be sure that your doctor gives you the blood test if she suspects lupus, advises Dr. Clark.

If you do have lupus, you should be in regular contact with a rheumatologist, no matter how mild your case is, cautions Dr. DuBuske. You can't say, "I'm cured" and never see a doctor again, he notes.

But even if you're getting medical treatment, here's one way to ease the course of lupus.

Give yourself flax. Putting 30 grams (about one ounce) of crushed flaxseed a day over food or in juice helps control blood vessel inflammation, a common side effect of lupus, says Dr. Clark. "Flax is a rich source of lignins, which is a form of fiber. Lignins prevent inflammation of blood vessels in people with lupus." And if blood vessels are inflamed, you increase your risk of severe kidney damage, he adds.

In a Canadian study, nine people with lupus who had kidney disease were given ground flaxseed with their cereal or juice for a course of 12 weeks in daily doses of 15, 30 or 45 grams. Although doctors saw improvement in symptoms at all three doses, they saw the most consistent benefits in people getting 30 grams of flaxseed. Dr. Clark recommends that you buy flaxseed in the form of crushed seeds (available at health food stores), and store it in little bags in the refrigerator.

WATER RETENTION: DEFLATE BLOATEDNESS

It's bad enough that your pants have felt a bit snug lately. Add a case of water retention just before your period and you're lucky if you can zip them up lying flat on the bed.

You can blame bloating on a drop in the female hormone progesterone in the seven to ten days before your menstrual cycle. This hormone depletion causes you to store salt and therefore retain water throughout your body, says Suzanne Trupin, M.D., head of the Department of Obstetrics and Gynecology at the University of Illinois College of Medicine at Urbana-Champaign. The result is abdominal bloating and distension. Also, your breasts may feel sore, your eyes get puffy and your hands, feet and face swell when you're retaining a lot of water.

A bit of premenstrual water retention is only normal, but even so, there are ways to prevent feeling waterlogged. Here's how.

Throw out the salt. Try not to add salt to any of your food, notes Dr. Trupin. She recommends taking in just 1,000 milligrams of salt a day, which is about 2,500 milligrams less than what the average adult uses. To reach this goal, leave the saltshaker alone and avoid high-sodium packaged foods. Eat fresh foods or choose low-salt and no-salt versions of prepared foods.

Too much salt in your diet adds extra sodium to your body fluids, which stalls the mechanism that pushes water out of your cells. So your cells end up plumping up with water, getting larger and making you feel bloated, explains Dr. Trupin.

Chug liquids. It may seem like the wrong way to go, but you can actually reduce water retention by drinking more. Have at least eight glasses of water a day to help dilute sodium in the body, suggests Dr. Trupin. Drinking a lot of water also helps the kidneys do their job more efficiently—that is, to get rid of waste products such as sodium that the body doesn't need, she notes.

Make some weedy tea. Drinking dandelion-leaf tea is a dandy way of ridding the body of excess water, says Dr. Fugh-Berman. In other words, it helps you urinate more frequently. "You could make the tea from the dried herb or mix some tincture into water or juice," she says. But just take it for a few days. And don't have any at all if you're on diuretic high blood pressure medication such as hydrochlorothiazide, she advises. Because blood pressure medication also flushes liquids from your body, you could have excess fluid loss if you combine it with dandelion-leaf tea.

You can make dandelion tea out of the root or the whole herb. Add one cup boiling water to one teaspoon dandelion. Let it steep for five minutes before straining. Drink a cup of the tea two or three times a day.

SOURCES
AND CREDITS

"A Typical Ornish Diet Menu" on page 135 is adapted from *Everyday Cooking with Dr. Dean Ornish* by Dean Ornish, M.D. Copyright © 1996 by Dean Ornish, M.D. Reprinted by permission of HarperCollins Publishers, Inc.

The list of yin, yang and neutral foods on page 144 was adapted with permission of Sterling Publishing Co., Inc., 387 Park Avenue South, New York, NY 10018 from *Chinese System of Food Cures* by Henry C. Lu, Ph.D. Copyright © 1986 by Henry C. Lu.

"A Typical Traditional Chinese Medicine Diet Meal" on page 147 was adapted from *The Tao of Nutrition* by Maoshing Ni, Ph.D., C.A., with Cathy McNease, B.S., M.H. Copyright © 1987 by Maoshing Ni and Cathy McNease. Reprinted by permission of Seven Star Communications.

The list of yin, yang and neutral foods on page 149 was adapted from *Holistic Health through Macrobiotics* by Michio Kushi with Edward Esko. Copyright © 1993 by Michio Kushi and Edward Esko. Reprinted by permission of Japan Publications, Inc.

The "Asian Diet Pyramid" on page 157 was adapted from the graph "The Traditional Healthy Asian Diet Pyramid" by Oldways Preservation & Exchange Trust. Copyright © 1995 by Oldways Preservation & Exchange Trust. Reprinted by permission.

The "Mediterranean Diet Pyramid" on page 162 was adapted from the graph "The Traditional Healthy Mediterranean Diet Pyramid" by Oldways Preservation & Exchange Trust. Copyright © 1994 by Oldways Preservation & Exchange Trust. Reprinted by permission.

INDEX

Underscored page references indicate boxed text. **Boldface** references indicate illustrations.

Margaret Muir emigrated from England to Australia to raise her family. After a career in diagnostic cytology she completed a writing degree and is now a full-time author. Like her previous novel *Sea Dust*, this book draws on her love of Yorkshire and in particular the moors and villages around Leeds where she grew up.

Visit the author's website at:
www.margaretmuirauthor.com

THE TWISTING VINE

In Yorkshire, Lucy Oldfield works as a maid at Heaton Hall. But when Lord Farnley's daughter dies, a shadow is cast over its future . . . Feeling insecure and unable to overcome temptation, Lucy steals an expensive French doll from her dead mistress. When the Hall is put up for sale and the staff dismissed, Lucy returns to Leeds. There, she falls victim to the deceit of an admirer, finding herself with a child to support. And then a chance meeting with a gentleman on a train leads to an offer that appears to be too good to be true . . . But will Lucy find herself subjected to even more heartache?

Books by Margaret Muir
Published by The House of Ulverscroft:

SEA DUST